# Health Informatics

*(formerly Computers in Health Care)*

Kathryn J. Hannah  Marion J. Ball
Series Editors

Springer
*New York*
*Berlin*
*Heidelberg*
*Barcelona*
*Hong Kong*
*London*
*Milan*
*Paris*
*Singapore*
*Tokyo*

# Health Informatics Series
## *(formerly Computers in Health Care)*

*Series Editors*
Kathryn J. Hannah   Marion J. Ball

*(continued after Index)*

Kathryn J. Hannah     Marion J. Ball
Margaret J.A. Edwards

# Introduction to Nursing Informatics

## Second Edition

With 47 Illustrations

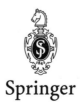

Springer

Kathryn J. Hannah, PhD, RN
Vice President, Health Informatics
Sierra Systems Consultants, Inc.
Calgary, Alberta T3B 2A6
*and*
Professor, Department of Community
  Health Science
Faculty of Medicine
University of Calgary
Calgary, Alberta T2N 4N1, Canada

Marion J. Ball, EdD
Professor, Department of Epidemiology
University of Maryland School of Medicine
*and*
Vice President
First Consulting Group
Baltimore, MD 21201, USA

Margaret J.A. Edwards, PhD, RN
Margaret J.A. Edwards and Associates, Inc.
52 Cordova Road SW
Calgary, Alberta T2W 2A6, Canada

*Series Editors:*

Kathryn J. Hannah, PhD, RN                Marion J. Ball, EdD

Library of Congress Cataloging-in-Publication Data
Hannah, Kathryn J.
    Introduction to nursing informatics/Kathryn J. Hannah, Marion J.
Ball, Margaret J.A. Edwards.—2nd ed.
        p.  cm.—(Health informatics series)
    Includes bibliographical references and index.
    ISBN 0-387-98451-8 (hardcover: alk. paper).
    1. Nursing informatics.  I. Ball, Marion J.  II. Edwards,
Margaret J.A.  III. Title.  IV. Series: Health informatics
(New York, N.Y.)
    [DNLM:  1. Information Systems nurses' instruction.  2. Nursing.
WY 26.5 H2431  1998]
RT50.5.H35  1998
610.73'0285—dc21                                        98-17983

Printed on acid-free paper.

Production coordinated by Chernow Editorial Services, Inc., and managed by Victoria Evarretta; manufacturing supervised by Thomas King.
Typeset by Best-set Typesetter Ltd., Hong Kong.
Printed and bound by R.R. Donnelley and Sons, Harrisonburg, VA.
Printed in the United States of America.

9 8 7 6 5 4 3 2

ISBN 0-387-98451-8                SPIN 108759-78

Springer-Verlag  New York Berlin Heidelberg
*A member of BertelsmannSpringer Science+Business Media GmbH*

*The three authors of this book share many experiences, interests, and values. The strongest of these shared values is a firm belief in marriage and family. We dedicate this book to our husbands, Richard Hannah, John Ball, and Craig Edwards, who are our respective life partners, our friends, and our greatest individual sources of support. We also dedicate this book to our families, especially the youngest generation, which represents the future: Richard Steven Hannah, Alexis Marion Concordia, Michael John Concordia, Erica Adelaide Concordia, Alexander John Ball, Ryan Jokl Ball, Maryn Joy Edwards, and John Kurt Edwards.*

# Series Preface

This series is directed to health care professionals who are leading the transformation of health care by using information and knowledge. Launched in 1988 as Computers in Health Care, the series offers a broad range of titles: some addressed to specific professions such as nursing, medicine, and health administration; others to special areas of practice such as trauma and radiology. Still other books in the series focus on interdisciplinary issues, such as the computer-based patient record, electronic health records, and networked health care systems.

Renamed Health Informatics in 1998 to reflect the rapid evolution in the discipline now known as health informatics, the series will continue to add titles that contribute to the evolution of the field. In the series, eminent experts, as editors or authors, offer their accounts of innovations in health informatics. Increasingly, these accounts go beyond hardware and software to address the role of information in influencing the transformation of health care delivery systems around the world. The series also will increasingly focus on "peopleware" and the organizational, behavioral, and societal changes that accompany the diffusion of information technology in health services environments.

These changes will shape health services in the next millennium. By making full and creative use of the technology to tame data and to transform information, health informatics will foster the development of the knowledge age in health care. As coeditors, we pledge to support our professional colleagues and the series readers as they share advances in the emerging and exciting field of Health Informatics.

Kathryn J. Hannah
Marion J. Ball

# Preface

The first book in the Computers in Health Care series, *Nursing Informatics: Where Caring and Technology Meet*, was published more than a decade ago. Both editions have provided experienced nurse informaticians with a detailed discussion of advanced concepts in nursing informatics. Since the publication of that book, we have been repeatedly asked by those who want to enter this exciting field, "How do we get started in Nursing Informatics?" This book in its first edition was the answer to that question. This new edition continues to address this same question.

This book is intended to be a primer for those just beginning to study nursing informatics, providing a thorough introduction to basic terms and concepts. We have listened to feedback about the first edition from readers. The book has been completely reorganized and restructured. New material has been added and new information incorporated. The book introduces terms and concepts foundational to nursing informatics as well as provides an introduction to the Internet. An overview of nursing use of Information Systems is provided. The book includes an exploration of the most common applications of nursing informatics in clinical nursing practice (both community- and facility-based settings), nursing education, nursing administration, and nursing research. It also provides insight into practical aspects of the infrastructure elements of the informatics environment. An overview of professional nursing informatics education and the future for nurses in health informatics concludes the book.

Although readers will no doubt find diverse uses for this book, we have written it with three principal uses in mind:

*University and College Baccalaureate Nursing Programs and Health Information Science Programs*: to acquaint undergraduate students in nursing and health information science with the field of nursing informatics. This book provides students with a fundamental understanding of the field of nursing informatics necessary for them to be able to use computers and information management strategies in their practices, to make informed choices related to software/hardware selection and implementation strategies, and to use the more advanced volumes in the Springer-Verlag series.

*Nursing Administrators*: to familiarize themselves with the field of nursing informatics in preparation for implementing computerized solutions for information management in their institutions. The practical guideline will assist the manager in making informed decisions regarding system selection/development, implementation, and use.

*Reference*: to involve nursing unit managers and staff in the implementation of computer applications and automated information management strategies in their workplaces. This book would be used to familiarize staff with the field of nursing informatics. In addition, the practical application information provided would help them to facilitate implementation and use of the computer application.

We believe that this book and the companion volume, *Nursing Informatics: Where Caring and Technology Meet*, provide comprehensive coverage of nursing informatics.

We hope that through this book we can introduce newcomers to the excitement of nursing informatics and share our enthusiasm for this rapidly evolving field.

Kathryn J. Hannah
Marion J. Ball
Margaret J.A. Edwards

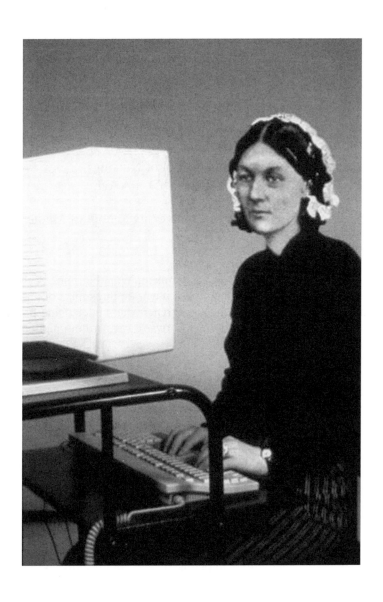

**Florence Nightingale at the Keyboard**

# Florence Nightingale at the Keyboard

Concept: MARYANN F. FRALIC, RN, DrPH, FAAN,
The Johns Hopkins University School of Nursing
Visualization: BARBARA FRINK, RN, PhD, FAAN,
The Johns Hopkins Hospital
Production: The Johns Hopkins University School of Medicine,
Department of Pathology

To win support for her work in the Crimean War, Florence Nightingale analyzed statistics and drew diagrams to illustrate the impact of nursing on soldiers' mortality. An early nurse researcher, she modeled and presented outcomes data in a simple and straightforward way, without modern information technology.

Think what she would have done with a high-powered PC and a fast modem! Think of what she could have accomplished!

Today we have incredible information technologies available to us. It is our responsibility as nurses to use these tools wisely, on behalf of our patients and our profession. We have the tools, and we have the template and the legacy that Florence Nightingale gave us. Our challenge now is to creatively blend the two for the next generation of nursing practice, shaping the future of nursing education, nursing research, nursing management, and—centrally—clinical nursing care.

Nursing informatics holds the capabilities and competencies we need—to track and measure outcomes, to support decisions, and to create evidence-based practice. And we must master nursing informatics in the era we are entering, the era of telehealth, where we will be "wired health care professionals," linked by computers to people, places, and resources—in a word, "telenurses."

Think of what we can do, what we can accomplish!

# Contents

# Contributors

*Steven C. Ball, BA, MSc*
Consultant, Edmonton, Alberta, Canada

*Ann Casebeer, PhD*
Assistant Professor, Department of Community Health Science, Faculty of Medicine, University of Calgary, Calgary, Alberta, Canada

*Judith V. Douglas, MHS*
First Consulting Group, Baltimore, MD, USA

*Richard S. Hannah, PhD*
Director, Canadian Medical Multimedia Development Centre, and Professor, Faculty of Medicine, University of Calgary, Calgary, Alberta, Canada

*Jo Ann Klein, RN, MS*
President, Mid-Atlantic Network Associates, Inc., Reisterstown, MD, USA

*Kathy Momtahan, RN, PhD*
Staff Scientist, Network Edge Technology Group, Nortel, Ottawa, Canada

*Cheryl Plummer, RN, MSc*
Consultant, Sierra Systems Consultants, Inc., Calgary, Vancouver, British Columbia, Canada

# Part I
# Foundations of Nursing Informatics

# 1
# Nurses and Informatics

## Introduction

We have entered the information age! Banks and stock markets move and track billions of dollars around the world every day through information systems. Factories and stores buy, build, sell, and account for the products in our lives through information systems. In schools, computers are being used as teaching tools and as instructional resources for students in such varied disciplines as astronomy, Chinese, and chemistry. The airline industry uses information systems to book seats, calculate loads, order meals, determine flight plans, determine fuel requirements, and even fly the planes and control air traffic. The information age has not left the health industry untouched. Moving beyond standard data processing for administrative functions common to all organizations such as human resource, payroll, and financial, information systems now play an important role in patient care by interpreting electrocardiograms, scheduling, entering orders, reporting results, and preventing drug interactions (by cross-referencing drug compatibility and warning appropriate staff). In addition, information systems are now being more widely used in support of population health and public health activities related to health protection (e.g., immunization), health promotion (e.g., well baby clinics), disease prevention (e.g., smoking cessation or needle exchange programs), and health monitoring or surveillance (e.g., restaurant inspection or air quality monitoring). Nurses have always had a major communication role at the interface between the patient/client and the health system. This role is now labeled information management, and nurses are increasingly using information systems to assist them to fulfill this role in clinical practice, administration, research, and education.

Before attempting to talk about the role of nursing in informatics, let us first establish definitions of nursing and "nursing informatics."

## What Is Nursing?

Nursing is emerging as a professional, practice discipline. Based on the work of theorists, nursing practitioners see its goals as the promotion of adaptation in health and illness and the facilitation of achievement of the highest possible individual state of health (Rogers, 1970; Roy, 1976). These early theoretical models have provided the impetus for the development of current approaches to the classification of phenomena of concern to nursing care (see Chapter 6 for a detailed discussion of nursing classification and nomenclature systems).

The practitioner of nursing has many roles and responsibilities. Among these roles are those of interface between the client and the health care system and that of client advocate in the health care system. Nursing functions can be considered under three major categories:

- Managerial, which includes establishing nursing care plans, keeping charts, transcribing orders and requisitions, and scheduling patient appointments for diagnostic procedures or therapy
- Delegated tasks, which include physical treatments and administration of medications under the direction of a physician
- Autonomous nursing functions, which include interpersonal communication skills, application of the psychological principles of client care, and providing physical care to patients.

It is the third category of nursing activities that is the core of nursing practice. In this category of autonomous activity nurses use their knowledge, skills, judgment, and experience to exercise independent decision making related to the phenomena for which nurses provide care and the nursing interventions that effect those phenomena and influence patient care outcomes.

## What Is "Medical/Health Care Informatics?"

Before we explore the nature of hospital and nursing information systems, we need to review the definitions of health, medical, and nursing informatics. Francois Gremy of France is widely credited with coining the term *informatique medical, which* was translated into English as *medical informatics.* Early on, the term *medical informatics* was used to describe "those collected informational technologies which concern themselves with the patient care, medical decision making process" (Greenburg, 1975). Another early definition, in the first issue of the *Journal of Medical Informatics*, proposed that medical informatics was "the complex processing of data by a computer to produce new kinds of information" (Anderson, 1976). As our understanding of this discipline developed, Greenes and Shortliffe (1990) redefined medical informatics as "the field that concerns itself with the cognitive, information processing and communication tasks of medical practice, education, and research, including the information science and the technology to support these tasks. . . . An intrinsically inter-disciplinary field . . . [With] an applied focus, . . . [addressing] a number of fundamental research problems as well as planning and policy issues."

One question consistently arose "does the word *medical* refer only to physicians or does it refer to all health care professions?" In the first edition of this book, the premise was that the word *medical* referred to all health care professions and that a parallel definition of medical informatics might be *those collected informational technologies which concern themselves with the patient care decision making process performed by health care practitioners*. Thus, because nurses are health care practitioners who are involved in the patient care, decision-making process that uses information captured by and extracted from the information technologies, there clearly was a place for nursing in medical informatics. Increasingly, as research was conducted and medical informatics evolved, nurses realized there was a discrete body of knowledge related to the nursing and the use of informatics. In the early 1990s, other health professions began to explore the use of informatics in their disciplines. Mandil (1989) coined the phrase "health informatics," which he defined as the use of information technology (including both hardware and software) in combination with information management concepts and methods to support the delivery of health care. Thus, health informatics has become the umbrella term encompassing medical, nursing, dental, and pharmacy informatics, among others. Health informatics fo-cuses attention on the recipient of care rather than on the discipline of the caregiver.

## Nursing's Early Role in Medical Informatics

The nurse's early role in medical informatics was that of a consumer. The literature clearly shows the contributions of medical informatics to the practice of nursing and patient care. Early developments in medical informatics and their advantages to nursing have been thoroughly docu-mented (Hannah, 1976; Chapter 3, this volume). These initial developments were fragmentary and generally restricted to automating existing functions or activities such as automated charting of nurses' notes, automated nursing care plans, automated patient monitoring, automated personnel time as-signment, and the gathering of epidemiological and administrative statis-tics. Subsequently, an integrated approach to medical informatics resulted in the development and marketing of sophisticated hospital information systems that included nursing applications or modules. More recently, as models of health services delivery have shifted toward integrated care delivery across the entire spectrum of health services, integrated informa-tion systems have been developed. These enterprise systems are intended to provide a comprehensive, lifelong, electronic health record that integrates the information generated by all of a person's contacts with the health services delivery system. Such systems support evidence based nursing practice, facilitate nurses' participation in the health care team, and document nurses' contribution to patient care outcomes.

## The Development of Nursing Informatics

Nursing informatics, as originally defined (Hannah, 1985, p. 181) referred to the use of information technologies in relation to those functions, within the purview of nursing, that are carried out by nurses when performing their duties. Therefore, any use of information technologies by nurses in relation to the care of patients, the administration of health care facilities, or the educational preparation of individuals to practice the discipline is considered nursing informatics. For example, nursing informatics would include, but not be limited to

- The use of artificial intelligence or decision making systems to support the use of the nursing process
- The use of a computer based scheduling package to allocate staff in a hospital or health care organizations
- The use of computers for patient education
- The use of computer assisted learning in nursing education
- Nursing use of a hospital information system
- Research related to what information nurses use in making patient care decisions and how those decisions are made.

As the field of nursing informatics has evolved, the definition of nursing informatics has been elaborated and refined. Graves and Corcoran (1989) suggested that nursing informatics is "a combination of computer science, information science, and nursing science designed to assist in the management and processing of nursing data, information and knowledge to support the practice of nursing and the delivery of nursing care."

## The Impact of Informatics on Nursing

As we mentioned earlier, nursing informatics has moved beyond merely the use of computers and is increasingly referring to the impact of information and information management on the discipline of nursing. Nurses form the largest group of health care professionals in any setting having a health information system. Therefore, when providing patient care, nurses make use of an information system more often than any other group of health care professionals. (The advantages to the practice of nursing that come from information systems are described in detail in Chapters 7 and 8.)

The nursing profession is recognizing the potential of informatics to improve nursing practice and the quality of patient care. New roles are evolving for nurses. Hospitals are now beginning to hire nurse consultants to help in the design and implementation of information systems. Nurse educators are using information systems to manage the educational environment. Computer based information systems are used to instruct, evaluate, identify problem areas of specific students, gather data on *how* each student learns, process data for research purposes, and carry out continued education! Nurse researchers, who have been using the computerized software for data manipulation for many years, are turning their attention to the problems of identifying variables for data sets essential to the diagnosing of nursing problems, choosing nursing actions, and evaluating patient care. As Figures 1.1 and 1.2 illustrate, there is no doubt that *we have reached the information age in nursing.* We must now prepare for the full impact of informatics on nursing.

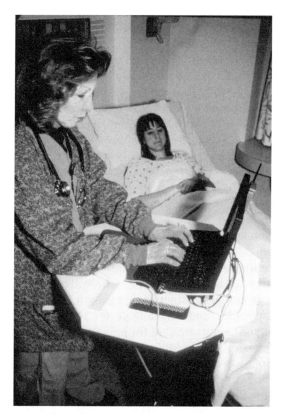

FIGURE 1.1. Nursing informatics at the bedside. (Photograph courtesy of Aironet Wireless Communications, Inc.)

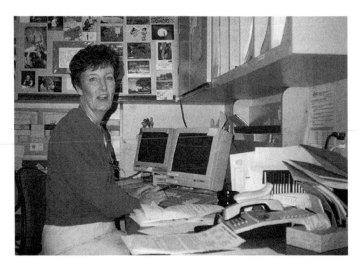

FIGURE 1.2. Nursing informatics at the nursing station. (Photograph courtesy of Clinicare Corporation.)

## Future Implications

Technology has historically relieved people of backbreaking drudgery and dreary monotony, providing them with more free time to pursue personal relations and creative activities. Nurses, too, when relieved of routine and time consuming clerical or managerial chores, can devote more time to the unique problems of individual patients. It is conceivable that the managerial and clerical category of nursing tasks will be done by information systems. In addition, robotics (e.g., lifting and turning patients, delivering medications or meals, and recording temperature, pulse, and other physiological measurements) might assist with the physical care category of nursing tasks. Similarly, decision support systems may actively assist with nursing judgments.

Relieved of routine and less complex chores, the professional nurse in an environment enhanced by information systems will be expected to carry out higher level, more complex activities that cannot be programmed. Nurses will be held responsible and accountable for the systematic planning of holistic and humanistic nursing care for patients and their families. Nurses will also be responsible for the continual review and examination of nursing practice (using innovative, continuous quality improvement approaches), as well as applying basic research to finding creative solutions for patient care problems and the development of new models for the delivery of nursing care. Increasingly, nurses will provide more primary care through community based programs providing health promotion and early recognition and prevention of illness. Nurse's role, as patient educator will also be extended by means of multimedia programs and the Internet. At the same time nurses will need to assume a greater responsibility for assisting the public to become discriminating users of information as they select, sort, interpret, evaluate, and use the vast volumes of facts available across the Internet.

Nurses will still be needed to assess, plan, carry out, and evaluate patient care, but advances in the use of information technology will create a more scientific, complex approach to the nursing care process. They will have to be better equipped by their education and preparation to have a more inquiring and investigative approach to patient care. Evidence based nursing practice will become the standard for nursing practice. As information systems assume more routine clerical functions, nurses will have more time for direct patient care. Accordingly, nursing needs to be part of future developments in nursing informatics with strong input regarding such decisions as

1. Which patient care related, nursing functions could be accomplished by nursing informatics?
2. What information do nurses need to make patient care decisions?
3. What information do caregivers from other health professions require from nursing?
4. To what extent can nursing informatics support improvements in the quality of nursing care received by patients?
5. How can the financial and emotional costs of care to patients be reduced using nursing informatics?

The implication is that nursing will continually need to reassess its status and reward systems. Presently, a nurse gains status and financial reward by moving away from the bedside into supervisory and managerial roles. If more of these functions are taken over by the computer, then nursing must reappraise its value system and reward quality of care at the bedside with prestige and money. Some movement in this direction is already beginning, for example, the movement toward employment of clinical nurse specialists prepared at the master's degree level to work at the bedside. However, this movement seems to be too little and too slow.

## Summary

The role of the nurse will intensify and diversify with the widespread integration of computer technology and information science into health care agencies and institutions. Redefinition, refinement, and modification of the practice of nursing will intensify the nurse's role in the delivery of patient care. At the same time, nurses will have greater diversity by virtue of employment opportunities in the nursing informatics field.

Nursing's contributions can, and will, influence the evolution of health  care informatics. Nursing will also be influenced by informatics, resulting in a better understanding of our knowledge and a closer link of that knowledge to nursing practice (Turley, 1997). As a profession, nursing must anticipate the expansion and development of nursing informatics. Leadership and direction must be provided to ensure that nursing informatics expands and improves the quality of health care received by patients within the collaborative interdisciplinary venue of health informatics.

## References Cited

Anderson, J. Editorial. *Journal of Medical Informatics* 1976;1:1.

Graves, J.R., and Corcoran, S. The study of nursing informatics. *Image* 1989;21:227–231.

Greenburg, A.B. Medical informatics: Science or science fiction. Unpublished (1975).

Greenes, R.A., and Shortliffe, E.H. Medical informatics: An emerging academic discipline and institutional priority. *Journal of American Medical Association* 1990;263(8):1114–1120.

Hannah, Kathryn J. The computer and nursing practice. *Nursing Outlook* 1976;24(9):555–558.

Mandil, S. Health informatics: New solutions to old challenges. *World Health* 1989;Aug–Sept;2:5.

Rogers, M.E. *An Introduction to the Theoretical Base of Nursing Practice.* Philadelphia: F.A. Davis, 1976.

Roy, Sister Callista. *Introduction to Nursing: An Adaptation Model.* Englewood Cliffs, N.J.: Prentice-Hall, 1976.

Turley, J.P. Developing informatics as a discipline. In: Gerdin, U., Tallbers, M., and Wainwright, P. (eds.) *Nursing Informatics: The Impact of Nursing Knowledge on Health Care Informatics.* Amsterdam: IOS Press, 1997:69–74.

# 2
# Anatomy and Physiology
# of Computers

J. Craig Edwards

## Basic Computer Ideas

For most people the inner workings of a television are a mystery, but that does not stop them from using and enjoying television. In the same way, it is not necessary to understand all the details of computer technology before it can be used to great advantage. This chapter is intended to give an adequate understanding of computers, thus enabling the reader to take confident advantage of whatever computer technology is available.

There are generally two main parts to any computer system:

1.  Hardwares: The term that describes the physical pieces of the computer, commonly grouped in five categories:
    *   Input: Data must be placed into the computer before the computer can be useful.
    *   Memory: All information processing takes place in memory.
    *   Central Processing Unit (CPU): The actual "brain" of the computer, which coordinates all the activities and does the actual information processing.
    *   Storage: The information and the programs can be saved for future use.
    *   Output: Processed information is of little value to people unless they can see it.

Hardware can be considered the anatomy of a computer, its physical, mechanical portion.

2.  Software: The term that describes the nonphysical pieces. It can be grouped into two categories:
    *   Operating Systems: These are standard activities that need to be done consistently and reliably. These processes are the building blocks for computer functions.

- Application Programs: These are packages of instructions that combine logic and mathematical processing and use the building blocks of the computer. Programs are what make computers valuable to people.

Software can be considered the physiology of a computer, the instructions that make its anatomy function properly. These pieces of a computer are described later in more detail, but it is important to have a mental picture of a "computer" in mind before we proceed. It is also helpful to understand some computer terminology (or jargon) that can overwhelm or confuse.

## Common Computer Terms

- Chip refers to a small piece of silicon that has electronic logic circuits etched into it. A chip can hold thousands of circuits in something that is about one-quarter of an inch on each side (see Figure 2.1). The chip is the fundamental physical piece used for computer memory and central processing units (CPU; see later in this chapter).
- RAM and ROM are the two types of memory that a computer uses. ROM stands for **R**ead-**O**nly **M**emory. This memory has information already stored in it by the computer manufacturer and nothing is allowed to change that information. RAM stands for **R**andom-**A**ccess **M**emory. This memory has no information in it but is available for any program to store information.
- Bit is the smallest part of computer memory. It can hold exactly one piece of information that has only two possible values, either a one (1) or a zero (0). This "two-value" system is called a binary system.
- Byte is the fundamental grouping of bits used to make up computer memory. By grouping bits together and setting these bits to either 0 or 1

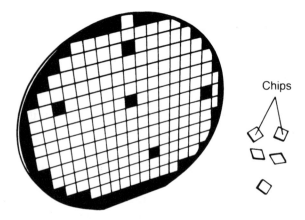

**FIGURE 2.1.** Silicon wafer.

in different combinations, a coding scheme can be built to represent information. The byte is the basic measuring unit for memory capacity or storage capacity. ✗

- Kilo, mega, and giga are prefixes that represent certain multipliers. Although "kilo," in scientific notation, means "1000" ($10^3$), its value is changed to "1024" ($2^{10}$) when talking about computer memory or storage. Numbers that are powers of 2 (e.g., 4 is a power of 2, being $2^2$) are chosen because the computer uses a binary system. Thus, one kilobyte of computer memory represents 1024 (1 × 1024) bytes, two kilobytes represent 2048 (2 × 1024) bytes, and so on. One megabyte represents 1,048,576 (1024 × 1024) bytes and one gigabyte represents 1,073,741,824 bytes (1024 × 1024 × 1024). Although it is not accurate, most people tend to still give kilo, mega, and giga their normal values of $10^3$, $10^6$, and $10^9$ when referring to computers.
- Megahertz (MHz) is the term describing the frequency that the central processing unit's internal clock uses for its timing control (CPU; see later in this chapter).

Computer technology has had an explosive growth during the past several decades. The computers that used to fill their own special-purpose rooms have been replaced today by computers small enough to fit on a desk ("desktop" model), on one's lap ("laptop" model), and in the palm of one's hand (palmtop computers). This trend is expected to continue. It is probable that what is described next will be considered obsolete in just a few years.

## Input (Hardware)

- *Keyboard* is the most common way that a person gives information and commands to a computer. It looks like a typewriter; its surface is filled with keys that are either numbers, letters, or control functions (such as "Home" and "Delete").
- *Touchscreen* is a technique that lets people do what comes very naturally—point with a finger. When a special sensing device is fitted around the perimeter of a monitor, the computer can calculate where someone's finger has pointed on the screen.
- *Light pen* is another pointing technique. By using special types of monitors, an attached pen (see Figure 2.2.) can be used (instead of a finger) to point to places on the screen.
- *Mouse* is yet another pointing device and perhaps the most common one. By moving a mouse around on a flat surface, a person also causes a marker (called the "cursor") on the computer screen to move. When that marker is resting on a certain desired place on the screen, a button on the mouse is pressed to signal the computer that something has been "pointed to."

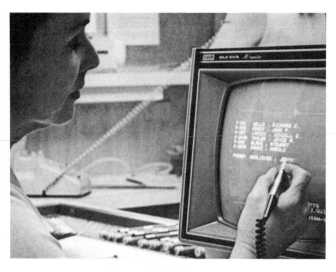

**FIGURE 2.2.** Light pen.

- *Voice* is a technology that is evolving rapidly. By using a microphone and some special application programs, a person can speak in a natural way and have that speech recognized by the computer. The words could be numbers (i.e., "One"), commands (i.e., "Print"), or just text (i.e., "The" "dog" "was" . . .).
- *Pen-based* technology translates the normal model of pen and paper for use with a computer system. With special computer screens and pens, a person can print or write on the screen with the pen and have the computer recognize what is written. Nothing is physically marked on the screen by the pen, but the computer senses and traces out the pen's movements. It then tries to recognize letters or numbers from those traces.

## Memory (Hardware)

The two basic types, ROM and RAM, were defined earlier. Generally, a computer has a sufficient amount of ROM built in by the manufacturer. ROM is preloaded with the low-level logic needed to run the computer. RAM is something that can be purchased separately and installed as needed. Most computers have a starting amount of RAM preinstalled. Application programs are loaded, when called for, into RAM. The program will execute there and store information in other parts of RAM as it needs. Today, application programs are growing in their RAM requirements as more logic and function is packed in them.

# Central Processing Unit (CPU) (Hardware)

There are several types of CPU chips. In the personal computer world, the Intel Corporation is probably the most recognized manufacturer with, first, its 80 × 86 series of CPU chips (i.e., 80,386, 80,486, ...) and then, its Pentium™ chip series. In the large computer world, IBM (International Business Machines) is probably the most recognized name. The Alpha chip, which DEC (Digital Equipment Corporation) began producing in 1992, is the one of the newest, most powerful processor chips yet.

All CPUs have three basic elements: a control unit, an arithmetic logic unit (ALU), and an internal memory unit. The ALU performs all the mathematical operations, the control unit determines where and when to send information being used by the ALU, and the internal memory is used to hold and store information for those operations. The CPU has an internal system clock that it uses to keep everything in synchronized order. The clock's speed is described in terms of frequency, using megahertz (MHz), so that a CPU might be described as having a clock speed of 200 MHz or 233 MHz. Generally, the faster the clock, the faster the CPU can process information.

# Storage (Hardware)

The memory of a computer is not the place to store information and programs for a long time. ROM is read-only (unwriteable) and therefore not of any use. RAM holds programs and information but only so long as the computer is turned on; once turned off, all information in RAM is gone. Computers use other means for long-term storage, the most common methods being magnetic and optical. Magnetic devices are standard in computers; optical devices require additional equipment.

- *Floppy Disk* (or "floppy") is the term that describes several sizes of material that can be magnetically encoded to store information and programs. This material is housed in a protective jacket. Floppy disks come in different sizes but the two most common are 3.5 inches ("three and a half") and 5.25 inches ("five and a quarter"). The computer has different-sized slots or openings where these floppy disks can be inserted as needed. The amount of information that these disks can hold varies. Most commonly now, the 5.25 inch floppy holds 1.2 megabytes of information and the 3.5 inch floppy holds 1.44 megabytes (although 2.88 megabyte floppies are available). Some manufacturers are offering floppy drives and disks that can store 120 megabytes of information. Floppies are reusable; old information on the floppy can be erased and new information stored in its place. Floppies are removable from the computer.

- *Hard Disk Drive* is the term that describes a device that magnetically encodes much more information than a floppy can, but is not removable from the computer. A typical size on personal computers, for example, is 1.2 gigabytes of capacity. Most often, a person will not see a hard drive; the drives are usually inside a computer and not removable. Hard disks are reusable.
- *Removable Disk Drive* is the same kind of device as a hard disk drive with similar storage capabilities. The difference is that the magnetic storage media can be removed and replaced, just as with a floppy drive.
- *Tape* describes a media that can magnetically encode a lot of information. In many ways, tape in a computer system is used like audio tape. Computer tape is typically used to store a copy of important information, to be recovered in the case of a major problem with the computer. Tape is packaged in different ways, from large reels to small cartridges. Tape is reusable.
- *Optical storage* is a term that covers several devices that store information optically, not magnetically. A common example is a CD-ROM (Compact Disc-Read Only Memory). Capacities of 500 megabytes or more are available. Reusable optical storage is becoming more common as manufacturers agree on storage standards.

## Output (Hardware)

- *Monitor* is the most common way that a person sees the information and instructions from a computer. It looks like a television screen and comes in different sizes. Most monitors today have color displays. On small computers called laptops ("small enough to fit in your lap"), the monitor is a flat screen that ordinarily uses liquid crystal display (LCD) technology. Some other names for the monitor are "VDT (video display terminal)," "CRT (cathode ray tube)," screen, and display. Illustrations of what a monitor and keyboard may look like are shown in Figure 2.3.
- *Printers and plotters* are two ways that the computer can put the processed information, such as a report or a chart, onto paper for people. The most common device in offices is the laser printer, capable of putting either text (like a report) or graphics (like a chart) onto standard sizes of paper.

## Operating Systems (Software)

Operating systems are the basic control programs for a computer. All the basic logic required for using a computer, such as the monitor, the printer, and the floppy drive, is contained in the operating system. Because the operating system handles those computer parts, it is unnecessary for application programs to do so. An example in the personal computer world is Microsoft Corporation's Windows™ operating system.

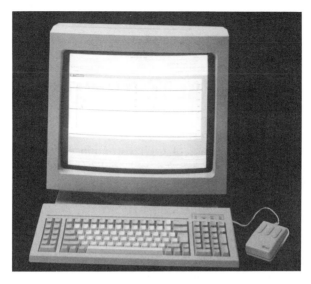

**FIGURE 2.3(A).** Monitor, keyboard, and mouse.

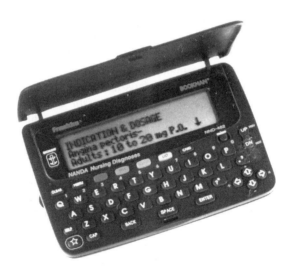

**FIGURE 2.3(B).** Another type of monitor and keyboard. (Photo courtesy of Franklin Electronic Publishing.)

## Application Programs (Software)

Application programs are packages of instructions and operations that take raw data and process them into information. Applications focus on working with people to produce information that is important to them. Some examples of applications are word processing, spreadsheets, and desktop publishing.

## Graphical User Interface (GUI) (Software)

This interface is a special type of software in common use today. It can be part of the operating system software or it can be a complete application program on its own; at times, a GUI (pronounced "gooey") seems to straddle the line between operating and application software. The basic design of any GUI is that it stands between the operator of the computer and the computer itself and acts as the go-between. Any GUI has two primary goals: to shield the operator from needing a great amount of technical knowledge to use the computer effectively and correctly, and to give a consistent "look-and-feel" to application programs (if they are designed for it).

Accomplishing the first goal means that an operator can perform all necessary technical tasks (e.g., copying data files between disks, backing up information) by pointing at icons (little pictures) on the screen. These icons represent the actual tasks that can be done. For example, by pointing to an icon that represents a desired data file and then dragging that icon over onto another icon that represents a printer, a person can print the file. Note that because of the GUI's capabilities, the person did not have to know the correct operating system commands to print the file.

Accomplishing the second goal means that any application program can be designed so that it is less difficult for a person to learn how to use it. Basically, the GUI defines a standard set of functions that it will provide (e.g., open a data file, save a data file, print a data file) and gives standard ways for application programs to use these functions. If application programs are designed and built to use these functions whenever possible, then a person only has to learn *once* how to open a data file. Any other program that uses the GUI functions will have the same "look-and-feel"; a person can open a data file in the same manner. Doing things in a consistent, predictable way not only reduces a person's learning time but increase a person's comfort level and productivity. Figure 2.4 is an example of what a main menu for a nursing software package looks like.

## Databases and Relational Database Management Systems (Software)

A database is a data file whose information is stored and organized so that it can be easily searched and retrieved. A simple analogy is a filing cabinet drawer. The difference between a file and a database is the same difference

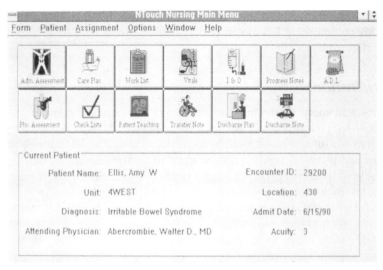

**FIGURE 2.4.** GUI-type menu.

between a file drawer that has reports dumped into it in any old way and a drawer that has neatly labeled file folders, arranged in meaningful order, with an index that shows where to store a report. In both cases, we know the information we need is in the file drawer. Only in the second case (i.e., the database) are we confident that we can find that information quickly and easily.

A database management system (DBMS) is a set of functions that application programs use to store and retrieve information in an organized way. Over the years, different ways to organize information have been used, e.g., hierarchical, network, indexed. The way that it is used most frequently now is called *relational*. A relational DBMS stores information using tables (i.e., rows and columns of information). This approach allows very powerful searches to be done quite easily.

## Terminals, Workstations, Standalone, Networks

### *Terminals*

In the early days of computer technology, an organization usually required only a single large-capacity computer to handle its information needs. These computers were called "mainframes." They required a trained staff to maintain and run them and were quite expensive to purchase and upgrade (i.e., add more memory, more disk storage, etc.). People gave information and commands to the mainframe through a "terminal," essentially just a keyboard and monitor; the terminal had no processing capability of its own. The number of terminals that a mainframe could handle was limited and this could create lineups of people, waiting their turn to submit computer requests.

## *Workstations*

Advances in computer technology, such as IBM's personal computer introduced in 1981, dramatically changed this situation. Now it was possible to have a powerful computer right in the office, and for far less money. What is more, all its resources and power were under the control of, and totally available to its user. As people began to move toward personal computing, computer manufacturers built more powerful workstations. Soon, these powerful workstations became small enough to be easily moved, promoting the idea of "mobile computing." Today, laptop computers easily allow computer technology to be available at the point of care (see Figure 2.5 Chapter 7 for more discussion).

## *Standalone*

By "standalone," we mean that all the pieces of a computer that are needed to gather, process, display, (possibly store), and output information are physically connected, and, if needed, could be moved as a complete unit to another location. This is the usual setup for most home and small business computer systems,. This setup is inexpensive and quite simple to manage. While it makes sense to use a "standalone" computer, it is often better for a computer to be part of a network.

## Local Area Networks (LANs)

A network is a way of connecting computers so that several benefits can be realized. Local Area Networks (LANs) are a way to connect computers that are physically close together, i.e., in the same local area. This does not just mean in the same room, but also in the same building, or in several buildings that are close together. LANs use three things to connect computers: a physical connection (like wire), a network operating system, and a communication scheme.

There are several ways to physically connect computers. Most common is coaxial cable, very similar to the kind used by cable television. Another way is to use wire similar to telephone cable ("twisted pair"), and the latest way uses fiberoptic cable (light is used in place of electricity). The very latest methods are wireless; they use either radio transmission or infrared light for the connection. Each method is suited for different situations and is part of the consideration when a network is built.

There are several network operating systems available today that provide the necessary processes to allow computers to talk with each other and to

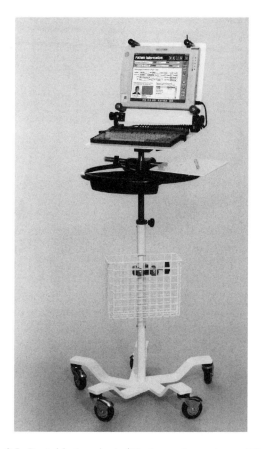

**FIGURE 2.5.** Portable terminal. (Photograph courtesy of Prologix.)

share information and programs. The communication schemes are properly called *protocols*. This is a standard way for the computers in a network to talk with each other and to pass information around. There are three main ways to connect computers in a network: star, ring, and bus configurations. These are called network topologies, which represent different physical arrangements of the computers (see Figure 2.6). Just as with the physical connecting medium (i.e., coaxial cable vs. twisted pair), each topology has its strengths and weaknesses. These must be considered when a network is built.

## *Benefits of a Network*

The important benefits of a network are shared information, shared programs, shared equipment, and easier administration. It is technically possible for any computer on a network to read and write information that another computer has in its storage, i.e., its hard disk. Whether that com-

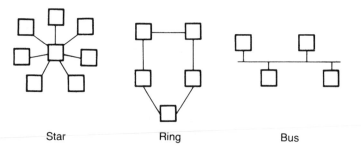

Star            Ring            Bus

**FIGURE 2.6.** Network typologies.

puter is *allowed* to do so is an administrative matter. This means, though, that information can be shared among the computers on the network. Programs can also be used by computers on the network no matter where those programs are physically stored. It is also possible (and usually desirable) for computers on a network to share equipment like printers. A diagram of how a system might be connected is shown in Figure 2.7. Technically, any computer on the network can print its information on a printer that is physically connected to another computer somewhere else. By sharing expensive office equipment, an organization reduces its expenses. Finally, administration of computers on a network is simplified because all the other computers can be examined, helped, and maintained from one computer.

## Wide Area Networks (WANs)

Wide area networks (WANs) are extensions of local area networks. There are two kinds of WANs. The first one attaches or connects a single computer to a preexisting LAN; this kind is called "remote LAN attachment."

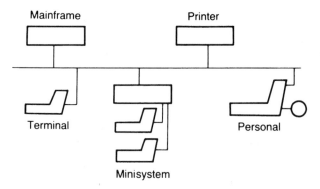

**FIGURE 2.7.** Example of resource sharing on a network.

The second one connects or "bridges" two or more preexisting LANs. Both WANs allow a computer to use information or equipment no matter where they are located in the organization. An interesting point about WANs is the options that can be used to connect LANs together. Instead of being limited by the length of cable that can be placed between computers, WANs can communicate via satellite and earth stations. This literally means that a person could be using a computer in Africa and working with information that is on a computer in Iceland and not really know or care about that fact. To that person, the information appears to be on their own computer.

## Open Systems

"Open systems" is the idea that it should be possible to do two things: run a particular program on any brand of computer and connect any collection of computers together in a network. However, because of the development of computer technology, this is difficult to accomplish.

Most computers were initially developed as "closed" systems; that is, a manufacturer built the computer, wrote the operating system, and wrote the application programs to run on the computer. Each computer manufacturer saw tremendous sales advantage from this strategy. The result was several computers that were similar in function but very different in how those functions were executed. It was not easy to buy an application program from a vendor and run it on two different brands of computers. It was a torturous exercise to get two different brands of computers to talk with each other.

For people who simply want to buy and use computer technology, "plug and play" is the ideal mode. This means that a computer could be purchased from vendor X, a second computer from vendor Y, a program bought from vendor Z, and a printer from vendor A, and all these parts could be connected and used with the same ease that people expect with stereo system components. The way to achieve this ideal is through standards. Just as stereo components are built to use a standard voltage, produce or use a standard type of signal, and connect with standard plugs and cables, computers and application programs need to use certain standards for communication protocols and file access. This "plug and play" mode is getting closer today because of vendors' and manufacturers' support and adoption of standards.

## Client/Server Computing

As we have seen, computers come in a variety of sizes and with various processing capacities. Some computers are better suited than others for different tasks. For example, personal computers, because of the physical size of their hard drives, have a limit to their storage capacity. On the other hand, the mainframe-type computer was designed to handle tremendous amounts of information and therefore has large storage capacity. Where does it make more sense to store a large data set?

This brings us to client/server computing. The essence of "client/server computing" is to assign to each computer the tasks for which it is best qualified, or, in other words, to use the right tool for the job. Capitalize on the strengths of one computer for task A, and use a different computer more suited for task B. A personal computer works well with people; it is fast, and has color and good graphical display capability. It could be the primary interface device for people and computer systems. Mainframe computers have huge storage capacity, great speed, and large processing power. This could be the place to store, process, and retrieve from the vast amount of information that a large organization might have. In a network, client/server computing really makes sense.

## *Remote Access Computing*

Computers can be connected together in a network but, increasingly, mobile computing requires that computers be able to access and connect to other computers from almost anywhere. This is possible through the use of the telephone system and special computer communication devices called "modems" (see Figure 2.8.) "Modem" is short for "modulate-demodulate." The computer that, at the moment, is sending information uses its modem to "modulate" its electronic signal into a form that can be carried over the telephone system; the computer that is receiving that information uses its

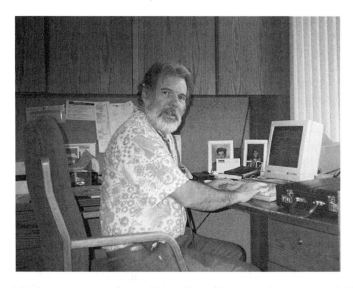

FIGURE 2.8. Remote access from clinic office. (Photograph courtesy of Clinicare Corporation and Health Plus Medical Clinic, Calgary, Alberta, Canada.)

modem to "demodulate" the telephone signal. Information can be exchanged at speeds that allow effective long-distance computing.

## Summary

As promised, we have not gone into great detail about computer technology. We have also not included a bibliography because technology is changing every day. We recommend that the interested reader visit any library or local bookstore to find up-to-date information on computer technology.

# 3
# History of Health Care Computing

## Introduction

Since the beginning of time, people have invented tools to help them. Tracing the evolution of computers gives us a clearer historical vantage point from which to view our fast changing world. This approach also identifies informatics as a tool that will advance the goal of high quality nursing care. From a historical perspective, however, it is difficult to identify the true origin of computers. For instance, we could go back in time to the devices introduced by Moslem scientists and to the mathematicians of the fifteenth century. An example is Al-Kashi, who designed his plate of conjunctions to calculate the exact hour at which two planets would have the same longitude (de S. Price, 1959; Goldstine, 1972). A more familiar example is the first rudimentary calculating tool, the Chinese abacus. This is still a rapid and efficient method of handling addition and subtraction.

## Historical Development of Computers

### Before 1950

The early nineteenth century had its share of men and women whose ideas were far ahead of the engineering, technological, and tooling abilities necessary to build calculating or computing machines. The groundwork for computerization was laid by Boole (1815–1864), who expanded the Leibnitz mathematical logic (binary numbers), and by Babbage (1791–1871), who invented the analytical machine in 1842.

It was not until the twentieth century that manufacturing made it possibile to carry out those ideas. Differential analyzers were developed in Germany and Russia during the 1930s. By 1940 there were about seven of these primitive analog computers in operation throughout the world. In 1939, Howard H. Aiken, of Harvard University, and Claire D. Lake of

IBM, developed an automatic-sequence-controlled calculator. In 1944 they developed the Harvard Mark I. The Mark I was an electromechanical digital machine that would do arithmetic computations (using punched cards) and store results. One hundred times faster than any manual operation, it could run 24 hours per day and accomplish 6 months' work in that time period.

George R. Stibitz, at the Bell Telephone Laboratories, set up yet another type of electromechanical computer using relay machines. It was possible, using this device, to calculate and produce firing and bombing tables and related gun control data. This prompted the Ordnance Department of the U.S. War Department to underwrite a development program at the Moore School of Electrical Engineering, University of Pennsylvania, which resulted in the production of the ENIAC in 1946. The ENIAC used vacuum tubes and electronic circuits and was the first electrical computer with no moving parts.

John von Neumann is credited with the concept of the stored computer program that revolutionized programming techniques. Augusta, Lady Lovelace, daughter of Lord Byron, is known as the "Mother of Programming" because of her pioneering work on the mathematical logic for Babbage's Difference Engine, his analytical machine (see Figure 3.1).

The invention of the general purpose, high speed electronic computer and the work by von Neumann marks the close of the early development of the computer. These first generation computers, although bulky, expensive, and less than totally reliable, provided useful results and excellent experience for both users and developers of the computer.

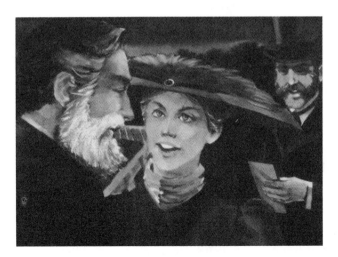

FIGURE 3.1. Augusta, Lady Lovelace, the Mother of Programming.

## The 1950s

The transistor, invented by Shockley in 1948, was used to develop a second generation of computers. These second generation computers were smaller, produced less heat, were more reliable, and were much easier to operate and maintain. Second-generation computers moved into the business and industrial world where they were used for dataprocessing functions such as payroll and accounting. The rapidly expanding health care industry began using computers to track patient charges, calculate payrolls, control inventory, and analyze medical statistics.

During the decade of the 1950s, Blumberg (1958) foresaw the possibilities of automating selected nursing activities and records. Little action was taken then because the existing computer programs were inflexible, computer manufacturers had a general lack of interest in the health care market, and hospital administrators and nursing management had a general lack of interest and knowledge about such equipment.

## The 1960s

In the 1960s, universities were bursting at the seams as members of the post World War II baby boom entered college. The philosophy of "education for all" left educators searching for a way to provide more individualized and self-paced instruction. The computer seemed to hold great promise. At the University of Illinois, Dr. Donald Bitzer was working on a display screen that would increase the graphics resolution available on the PLATO (Programmed Logic for Automated Teaching Operations) computer system that he developed.

During 1965 and 1966, the "third generation" of computers was introduced. These third generation computers were identifiable by their modular components, increased speed, ability to service multiple users simultaneously, inexpensive bulk storage devices that allowed a greater amount of data to be immediately accessible, and rapid development of systems.

## The 1970s

The development of the silicon chip paved the way for the development of minicomputers and personal computers. The silicon chip allowed very large amounts of data to be stored in a very small space. This development allowed the total size of computers to be significantly reduced.

## The 1980s

Personal computer technology augmented and replaced the large and cumbersome hardware of the 1970s. Research and development in computer technology was aimed at "open systems." This additional technological advance served the nursing profession because it systematized and simplified the process of data entry, storage, and retrieval.

## The 1990s

In the 1990s, information technologies, including personal computers and workstations, combined with telecommunications technologies such as local and wide area networks to create client/server architectures. Client/ server architecture integrated and capitalized on the strengths of hardware, software, and telecommunications capacities, allowing users to navigate through data across many systems. These linkages were vital to breaking the barriers between different systems. The open flow of information among systems (see details in Chapter 2 of this book): contributed to many developments in nursing informatics.

## Introduction of Computers into Health Care

Health care trailed government and industry in the initial exploration of the feasibility of computer usage and in actual installation of computers. One reason for the delay was that first and second generation computers were not well suited for the data processing needs of hospitals. A second reason was that only about 250 of the largest hospitals had in-hospital punched card installations. These hospitals were usually the first targets of computer salesmen. The potential of the hospital market was simply not understood by the computer manufacturers.

When focusing on the use of computers in health care, computers traditionally grew up in the accounting area where most hospital computer systems still have their roots. Patient care requires continuous and instantaneous response as opposed to the fiscal methodology where timing is less critical. To achieve successful utilization of computers in health care, both needs must be addressed.

## The 1950s

In the very late 1950s a few pioneering hospitals installed computers and began the development of their application software. Some hospitals had help from computer manufacturers, especially IBM. Then, in 1958–1959, John Diebold and Associates undertook an in depth feasibility study of hospital computing. The study was conducted at Baylor University Medical Center. The final report identified two major hospitalwide needs for computerization: (1) a set of business and financial applications, and (2) a set of hospital–medical applications that would require on line terminals at nursing stations and departments throughout the hospital. Such a system could be used:

- As a communications and message-switching device to route physicians' orders and test results to their proper destinations
- As a data-gathering device to capture charges and patient medical information
- As a scheduler to prepare such items as nursing station medication schedules
- As a database manager with report preparation and inquiry capabilities.

These functions are often collectively called hospital information systems (HISs), medical information systems (MISs), and sometimes hospital–medical information systems (HMISs). The first term (or its acronym, HIS), is used in this book.

## *The 1960s*

Although a few hardware manufacturers offered some business and financial application packages for in hospital processing in the early 1960s, it was not until the mid-1960s that other vendors began to see the potential of the hospital data processing market. The hardware vendors in the 1960s (e.g., IBM, Burroughs, Honeywell, UNIVAC, NCR, CDC) were committed primarily to selling large general-purpose computers to support clinical, administrative, communications, and financial systems of the hospitals.

The 200- to 400-bed hospitals that installed computers in the late 1960s for accounting applications found their environments growing more complex, which resulted in a constant battle just to maintain and update existing systems to keep pace with regulating agencies. Many hospitals of this size turned to shared computer services.

In 1966, Honeywell announced the availability of a business and financial package for a shared hospital data-processing center. IBM followed quickly the next year with SHAS (Shared Hospital Accounting System). The availability of this software was an important factor in establishing not-for-profit and for-profit shared centers during the next five years. There are still many shared-service companies (e.g., SMS, McAuto) specializing in hospital data processing. These companies continue to provide useful services, particularly to smaller hospitals. These companies prospered not only because of their computer and systems products and services but because smaller, single hospitals were unable to justify, employ, and retain the varied technical and management skills required for this complex and constantly changing environment.

The first hospital computer systems for other than accounting services were developed in the late 1960s. The technology that attempted to address clinical applications was unsuccessful. Terminal devices such as keyboard overlays, early cathode-ray tubes, and a variety of keyboard and card systems were expensive, unreliable, and unwieldy. Also, hardware and software were scarce, expensive, and inflexible. Database management systems, which are at the heart of good information software today, had not yet appeared. During this period, some hospitals installed computers in offices to do specific jobs (Ball and Jacobs, 1980). The most successful of these early clinical systems were installed in the clinical pathology laboratory (Ball, 1973). Most of the hospitals that embarked on these dedicated clinical programs were large teaching institutions with access to federal funding or foundation research money. Limited attempts were made to integrate the accounting computer with these standalone systems.

In the mid-1960s, Lockheed Missile and Space Company and National Data Communications (then known as Reach) began the development of HISs that would require little or no modification by individual hospitals. This was the forerunner to the product that is now marketed by Elipsys.

About 1965, the American Hospital Association (AHA) began to conduct four or five conferences per year to acquaint hospital executives with the potential that the computer holds for improving hospital administration. The AHA also devoted two issues of its journal solely to data processing. These AHA activities served to crystallize a market (i.e., hospitals ready for data processing) and to encourage existing and new firms to enter the marketplace.

## The 1970s

In the early 1970s, with inflation problems and with cost reimbursement becoming more strict, some large hospitals that had installed their own computers with marginal success changed to the shared service. By this time the shared companies had improved upon earlier accounting software and could carry out tighter audit controls. Most importantly, however, the companies developed personnel who understood hospital operations and could communicate and translate the use of computer systems into results in their client hospitals. This added a dimension of service that is seldom offered or understood by the major hardware vendors. As a result, the business opportunities for the service companies increased. Over time, these companies have expanded their scope of services from fiscal applications and administrative services to clinical and communication applications.

Major hardware changes took place as the minicomputer entered the scene. This was quickly followed by the introduction of the personal computer in the late 1970s. Technological developments have resulted in a steady trend toward microminiaturization of computers. Personal computers are now more powerful than the original ENIAC. These personal computers have invaded homes, schools, offices, nursing stations, and administrative offices to a degree never dreamed possible. The linking of these personal computers, using local area networking technology, provided a better alternative to many of the processes formerly carried out by one large general purpose computer.

Many major mainframe hardware companies moved rapidly into the personal computer as well. Simultaneously, the service companies began to develop on site networking systems to handle data communications and specialized nonfinancial applications. They began to expand their scope of data retention to support clinical applications that required a historical patient database.

## The 1980s

In the 1980s, very specific personal computer based systems were developed. These systems did not replace but instead complemented a variety of alternatives in various health care environments. Thus, awareness of computer concepts by health care professionals became even more essential.

## The 1990s

In the 1990s, the advent of powerful, affordable, portable personal computers made information management tools accessible to support highly mobile, remote activities, especially in community health. At the same time, the power of networks and database technology has made possible linkages of health data in widely separated locations. There also was a growing emphasis on information management across health enterprises. Accompany this was a recognition of the importance of patient/client centred, integrated data as apposed to departmental focused data. Such linkages and shift in focus created the possiblity of a longitudinal, lifelong health record, encompassing health care encounters by individuals with all sectors of the health care system.

# History of Nursing Use of Computers

## Nursing Education

The seminal work in the use of computers in nursing education was conducted by Maryann Drost Bitzer. In the early 1960s, Maryann Bitzer (Mrs. Donald Bitzer) wrote a program that was used to teach obstetrical nursing. Her program was a simulation exercise. It was the first simulation in nursing and one of the first in the health care field. Bitzer's (1963) master's thesis showed that students learned and retained the same amount of material using the computer simulation in one-third the time it would take using the classic lecture method. This thesis (1963) has become a classic model for subsequent work by herself and many others, including two of the authors (K.J.H. and M.J.E.) of this volume. Bitzer's early findings have been consistently confirmed. She was later project director on two Department of

Health Education and Welfare (HEW)-funded research projects. These projects undertook evaluative studies that documented the efficacy of teaching nursing content using a computer. Until 1976 Bitzer was associated with the Computer-Based Education Research Laboratory at the University of Illinois in Urbana, Illinois, where she continued to develop computer-assisted instruction lessons to teach nursing.

In the 1970s many individual nursing faculties, schools, and units developed and evaluated computer-assisted instruction (CAI) lessons to meet specific institutional student needs. Most of the software created was used solely by the developing institution.

The use of computers to teach nursing content has been a focal point of informatics activity in nursing education. However, the need to prepare nurses to use informatics in nursing practice is just as important. This aspect was pioneered in 1975 by Judith Ronald of the School of Nursing, State University of New York at Buffalo. Ronald developed the course that served as a model and inspiration for courses developed later. Ronald's enthusiasm and her willingness to share her course materials and experiences have greatly facilitated the implementation of other such courses throughout North America. In Scotland, Christine Henney of the University of Dundee undertook similar activities aimed at promoting computer literacy among nurses.

## *Nursing Administration*

The use of computers to provide management information to nurse managers in hospitals has been promoted on both sides of the Atlantic. Marilyn Plomann of the Hospital Research and Educational Trust (an affiliate of the American Hospital Association) in Chicago was actively involved for many years in the design, development, and demonstration of a planning, budgeting, and control system (PBCS) for use by hospital managers. In Glasgow, Scotland, Catherine Cunningham was actively involved in the development of nurse-manpower planning projects on microcomputers. Similarly, Elly Pluyter-Wenting (from 1976 to 1983 in Leiden, Holland), Christine Henney (from 1974 to 1983 in Dundee, Scotland), Phyllis Giovanetti (from 1978 to the time of writing in Edmonton, Canada), and Elizabeth Butler (from 1973 to 1983 in London, England) have been instrumental in developing and implementing nurse scheduling and staffing systems for hospitals in their areas.

In the public health area of nursing practice, Virginia Saba (a nurse consultant to the Division of Nursing, Bureau of Health Manpower, Health Resources Administration, Public Health Service, Department of Health and Human Services) was instrumental in promoting the use of management information systems for public health nursing services. The objective of all these projects has been to use computers to provide management information to help in decision making by nurse administrators.

## *Nursing Care*

Much research on the development of computer applications for use in patient care was conducted during the 1960s. Projects were designed to provide justification for the initial costs of automation and to show improved patient care. Hospital administrators became aware of the possibilities of automating actual health care activities besides business office procedures. Equipment became more refined and sophisticated. Health care professionals began to develop patient care applications, and the manufacturers recognized the sales potential in the health care market.

Nurse pioneers who have contributed to the use of computers in patient care activities have been active on both sides of the Atlantic. In the United Kingdom, Maureen Scholes, chief nursing officer at The London Hospital (Whitechapel), began her involvement with computers and nursing in 1967 as the nurse member of the Steering Team that directed and monitored The London Hospital Real-Time Computer Project. This project resulted in a hospital communication system providing patient administration services, laboratory services, and x-ray services using 105 visual display units in all hospital wards and departments.

Elizabeth Butler was associated with the Kings College Hospital from 1970 to 1973. As the nursing officer on a medical unit, Butler was involved in developing and implementing the computerized nursing care plan system for the Professional Medical Unit, and of the nursing care plan system for all wards and specialties in the 500-bed general area of the hospital. In Dundee, Scotland, Christine Henney worked with James Crooks (from 1974) on the design and implementation of a real-time nursing system at Ninewells Hospital.

In the United States, Carol Ostrowski and Donna Gane McNeill were both associated with the development of the Problem Oriented Medical Information System (PROMIS) at Medical Center Hospital of Vermont under the direction of Lawrence Weed. From 1969 to 1979, Donna Gane McNeill was a nurse clinician on the PROMIS project. As such, McNeill managed the first computerized nursing unit, developed content for PROMIS, as well as developed function and tasks for the computer. She also conducted a comparison between computerized and noncomputerized units. From June 1976 to December 1977, Carol Ostrowski served as director of audit for the PROMIS system. She was responsible for implementing the components that supported concurrent audit of medical and nursing care and the environment that guided and evaluated patient care.

In the United States, Margo Cook also began her association with computers in nursing in 1970 when she was employed at El Camino Hospital, Mountain View, California. Cook participated as the nursing representative on the team that developed and implemented the Medical Information System (still marketed by Elipsys). As nursing implementation coordinator, Cook was responsible for identifying and addressing the needs of all nursing units at El Camino. Often she functioned as interpreter between the computer analysts and nurses. Eventually she assumed senior level responsibility for the MIS maintenance and development. In 1983 Cook left El Camino to become senior consultant of Hospital Productivity Management Services. In 1976 Dickey Johnson became computer coordinator at Latter Day Saints Hospital in Salt Lake City, Utah. Johnson's reponsibilities involved coordination between the computer department and other hospital users in planning, development, implementation, and maintenance of all programs either used by, or affecting, nursing personnel. In 1983, Johnson was the nursing representative on the hospital's Computer Committee that was actively involved in planning, designing, and implementing a hospitalwide computer system. Projects which Johnson was responsible for included order entry, nursing care plans, nurse acuity, and nurse staffing.

In Canada, from 1978 to 1983, Joy Brown and Marjorie Wright, systems coordinators at York Central Hospital in Richmond Hill, Ontario, were actively involved in designing, coding, and implementing the computerized patient care system at their hospital. They were also responsible for the training of many nurse users on the system. Beginning in 1982 at Calgary General Hospital in Calgary, Alberta, Wendy Harper, assistant director, Nursing Systems, was responsible for all aspects of the nursing applications on the hospital information system being installed in that hospital.

Nurses have recognized the potential for improving nursing practice and the quality of patient care through nursing informatics. These applications facilitate charting, care planning, patient monitoring, interdepartmental scheduling, and communication with the hospital's other computers. New roles for nurses have emerged. Nurses have formed computer and nursing informatics interest groups (see Appendix B) to provide a forum through which information about computers and information systems is communicated worldwide.

## *Nursing Research*

In the 1960s, nursing researchers began using computers to store data and maintain complex data sets without error.

## Communicating Nursing Developments

Kathryn Hannah, of the University of Calgary, was the first nurse elected to the Board of Directors of the Canadian Organization for the Advancement of Computers in Health (COACH). In that capacity, with the assistance of David Shires of Dalhousie University (and at that time program chairman for the International Medical Informatics Association), Hannah was instrumental in establishing the first separate nursing section at an International Medical Informatics Association (IMIA) meeting (Medinfo '80, Tokyo).

Previously, nursing presentations at this international conference had been integrated into other sections. In 1982, based on the success of this Tokyo workshop, which Hannah also chaired, a contingent of British nurses led by Maureen Scholes mounted an International Open Forum and Working Conference on "The Impact of Computers on Nursing." The international symposium on the impact of computers on nursing was convened in London, England in the fall of 1982, followed immediately by an IMIA-sponsored working conference. One outcome of the working conference was a book that documented the developments related to nursing uses of computers from their beginning until 1982. The second outcome was the consensus that nurses needed a structure within an international organization to promote future regular international exhanges of ideas related to the use of computers in nursing and health care. Consequently, in the spring of 1983, a proposal to establish a permanent nursing working group (Group 8) was approved by the General Assembly of IMIA. In August 1983, the inaugural meeting of the IMIA Working Group on Nursing Informatics (Group 8) was held in Amsterdam, The Netherlands.

In 1992, the working group recommended a change of bylaws and began its transformation to a nursing informatics society within IMIA. This society continues the organization of symposia every three years for the exchange of ideas about nursing informatics, the dissemination of new ideas about nursing informatics through its publications, the provision of leadership in the development of nursing informatics internationally, and the promotion of awareness and education of nurses about nursing informatics.

In the United States, in 1981, Virginia Saba was instrumental in establishing a nursing presence at the Symposium on Computer Applications in Medical Care (SCAMC). This annual symposium, while not a professional organization, provided opportunities for nurses in the United States to share their experiences. In 1982 the American Association for Medical Systems and Informatics (AAMSI) established a Nursing Professional Specialty Group. This group, which was chaired by Carol Ostrowski, provided the benefits of a national professional organization as a focal point for discussion, exchange of ideas, and leadership for nurses involved in the use of computers. Subsequently, AAMSI merged with SCAMC to become the American Medical Informatics Association (AMIA). This organization continues to have a very active nursing professional specialty group.

## Summary

In spite of their wide usage, computers are historically very young and did not come into prominence until 1944 when the IBM-Harvard project called Mark I was completed. This was followed closely by the development, in 1946, at the University of Pennsylvania of the ENIAC I, the first electronic computer with no moving parts. Subsequent refinement and expansion, accompanied by development of the silicon chip in 1976, has raised the possibility that, by the end of the decade, microcomputers could be as common in our homes as television sets. During the 1950s, computers entered the health care professions. They were primarily used for the purposes of tabulating patient charges, calculating payrolls, controlling inventory, and analyzing medical statistics. A few farsighted individuals saw the possibilities of automating selected nursing activities and records. However, little action was taken because of the inflexibility and slowness of the equipment, the general disinterest of the manufacturers in the health care market, and the lack of knowledge concerning such equipment among hospital management, hospital administrators, and nursing management.

By the 1960s, hospital administrators had been exposed to the possibility of automating actual health care activities; besides the existing business office automation, equipment had become more refined and sophisticated, and the manufacturers had recognized the sales potential in the health care market. The major focus in the 1960s was on the research aspect of computer applications for patient care; the business applications for auditing functions in the health care industry were becoming well established. Projects were designed to provide justification for the initial costs of automation and to display the variety of areas in which computers could be used to facilitate and improve patient care. Nurses began to recognize the potential of computers for improving nursing practice and the quality of patient care, especially in the areas of charting, care plans, patient monitoring, interdepartmental scheduling, and communication and personnel time assignment. These individual computer applications or modules, which were developed to support selected nursing activities, were later integrated in modular fashion into various hospital information systems. Today these hospital information systems are widely promoted and marketed by computer vendors.

Simultaneously, advances in the uses of computers in educational environments were initiated during the 1960s. The major focus in this decade was on showing the efficacy of computers as teaching methods. During the 1970s, many projects were designed to compare student learning via computer with learning via traditional teaching methods. The mid-1970s also saw the development of the personal microcomputer, and, during the latter years of that decade, their widespread dissemination throughout society. During the 1980s nursing educators were scrambling to develop software for use with this technology. In fact, the hardware technology has advanced beyond nursing educators' capacity to use it all.

Major contributions by nurses to developments leading to the use of computers in nursing were also discussed. Our apologies to those nurses whose activities were unknown to us. If readers know of other nurses whose contributions merit inclusion in future editions, the authors would be pleased to receive such information.

The future demands that computer technology be integrated into the clinical practice environment, education, and research domains of the nursing profession. The ultimate goal is always the best possible care for the patient.

## *References*

Ball, M.J. *How to Select a Computerized Hospital Information System.* New York: S. Karger, 1973.

Ball, M.J., and Jacobs, S.E. Information systems: The status of level 1. *Information Systems* 1980:179–186.

Bitzer, M.D. *Self-Directed Inquiry in Clinical Nursing Instruction by Means of PLATO Simutated Laboratory.* Report R-184, Co-ordinated Science Laboratory. Urbana: University of Illinois, 1963.

Blumberg, M.S. Automation offers savings opportunities. *Modern Hospital* 1958;91:59.

de S. Price, D.J. An ancient Greek computer. *Scientific American* 1959;200(6):60–67.

Goldstine, H.H. *The Computer from Pascal to von Neumann.* Princeton: Princeton University Press, 1972:5, 69.

# 4
# Telecommunications and Informatics

The convergence of telecommunications and informatics has opened up a new world of communication service delivery and health information for consumers and health professionals. This chapter is designed to provide a basic understanding of the Internet, intranets, and extranets.

## What Is the Internet?

At the most basic level, the Internet is the name for a group of worldwide computer based information resources connected together. It is often defined as a network of networks of computers. According to the Internet Society, there are more than 6 million sites (computers) connected throughout the world. Every day, it is estimated that more than 5000 sites join the Internet.

One of the major challenges in using the Internet is that there is no clear map of how all those networks are connected. There is also no master list of what information or resource is available where! Because there is no overall structured grand plan, the shape and face of the Internet is constantly changing to meet the needs of the people who use it. The Internet can be likened to a cloud in this way; it's amorphous, without boundaries and constantly changing shape and space.

Although the thought of all those computers joined together is mind boggling, the real power of the Internet is in the people and information that all those computers connect. The Internet is really a people oriented community that allows millions of people around the world to communicate with one another. The computers move the information around and execute the programs that allow us to access the information. However, it is the information itself and the people connected to the information that make the Internet useful.

# Connecting to the Internet

Access to a telephone line, a modem, and a computer is required to connect to the Internet. There are four basic ways to connect to the Internet: make a direct connection over dedicated communications lines; use a personal computer to connect to a university or hospital computer system that has Internet access; buy time and connections from a commercial Internet service provider; or use an indirect service provider.

## *Direct Connection to the Internet*

A direct or dedicated connection wires a personal computer directly to the Internet through a dedicated machine called a router or gateway. The connection is made over a special kind of telephone line. The gateway identifies the personal computer as an "official" Internet computer that must remain on-line all the time. This type of direct connection is very expensive to install and maintain. For this reason, it is usually used only by large companies or institutions rather than by individuals or small businesses.

## *Connecting Through Another's Gateway*

Another way to connect to the Internet is to use a gateway that another company or institution has established. In this case, a company or university or hospital that has an Internet gateway allows individuals to connect to the Internet using their system. The connection is usually made through a modem or remote terminal. This type of access is often available to students through the computing services department of their university. Many hospitals and health services organizations also allow staff access to the Internet through the institution's facilities. To use an institution's access, each user will need a login id and password. For the individual, this is the best type of access to have if full Internet access is available. An organization maintains the computer system and the Internet connection and, most importantly, pays for the connection.

## *Connecting Through a Commercial Service Provider*

Connecting to the Internet through a service provider is much the same process as using another's gateway. The service provider builds and maintains the gateway and sells Internet connection access to individuals and small companies. Service providers usually charge a flat fee for membership, usually so many dollars per month for so many hours of Internet access per month. Some providers also charge based on the amount of extra time spent connected to the Net or on the amount and size of e-mail messages sent.

Although this section has focused on commercial service providers, many cities and towns also have free community computing services called "FreeNets." These services function much like using another's gateway. The major advantage is they are free. The main disadvantage is that FreeNets do not provide full Internet access. FreeNets generally supply e-mail and newsgroup access but not the ability to search databases or connect to remote host computers.

## Connecting Through an Indirect Service Provider

On-line services such as America Online, Compuserve, Sympatico Delphi, and Prodigy have supplied, for some time now, a place for experimentation with new software, discussion groups, and file transfers. They all offer Internet access in varying degrees. The advantage, again, is that the internetworkings of connecting to the Internet are hidden to the user, so connecting is a simple process. Some of the disadvantages are that full Internet access is not available through all on-line providers, and on-line service fees generally include not only a membership fee but also connect time charges. Some on-line service providers not only charge for connect time, but also for numbers of characters transferred as files.

## What to Look for When Choosing an Internet Provider

There are several basic elements to consider when getting access to the Internet through a provider. First, what kind of personal computer is to be used for the connection? Generally, providers are most comfortable supporting PC-compatible computers. The processing power and storage capacity of the computer are also important. Some of the Internet facilities (i.e., World Wide Web) make strong demands on the computer's resources.

Second, what is the individual's level of technical knowledge and comfort when working with the computer? There may be levels of technical details not understood by computing nonprofessionals. Some Internet providers, for a fee, will help you install the connection software on your computer and get it working.

Third, look for a provider with a local telephone number that is used to connect. Some providers advertise 1–800 numbers. The point here is to avoid additional telephone charges. Without a local number, additional charges to a telephone company will result.

Fourth, what set of Internet services or tools does the provider offer? Be sure to check the details of what is offered and what, if any, additional charges there might be for things such as number of e-mail messages sent, etc.

Fifth, what is the cost of this connection? Be sure that all the restrictions and assumptions are fully identified. Last, what kind of technical support does the provider offer? Make sure of the support policy of the provider (i.e., 24 hours a day, business hours only, etc.).

## Internet Addresses

To look for information or people on the Internet, it is vital to understand Internet Addressing. Every person and every computer that is on the Internet is given a unique address. All Internet addresses follow the same format: the person's userid (user-eye-dee) followed by the @ symbol, followed by the unique name of the computer. For example, one of the author's university-based Internet address is

**marge@cs.athabascau.ca**

In this example, the userid portion is **marge** and the unique computer name is **cs.athabascau.ca**. That unique computer name is also called the *domain*. The same author also has an Internet account with a service provider. That address is

**edwardsc@cal.cybersurf.net**

In general, an Internet address has two parts, the userid and the domain, put together like this:

**userid@domain**

This combination needs to be unique on the entire Internet so that the right person receives the right message!

## Internet Applications

### *Electronic Mail*

Electronic mail (or e-mail) was the first Internet application and is still the most popular one. E-mail is a way of sending messages between people or computers through networks of computer connections. E-mail is not limited to just the Internet. E-mail messages can be moved through gateways to other networks and systems, such as Compuserve or America Online. Many hospitals and health care agencies already have an internal e-mail system and, with a little work by the employer, employees can send and receive messages from other organizations and individuals via the Internet.

E-mail on the Internet is analogous to the regular postal system but faster in delivery of mail. E-mail combines a word processor function and a post office function in one program. Here's a typical scenario. When an e-mail program is started, a command is used to begin a new message. The message is typed into the computer along with the recipient's e-mail address and the return address. Then, the message is "sent"; this is something like dropping a letter in the regular postbox. The electronic post office in the personal system takes over and passes the message on. Electronic packets of data carry the message toward its ultimate destination mailbox. The message will often have to pass through a series of intermediate networks to reach the recipient's address. Because networks can and do use different e-mail formats, a gateway at each network will translate the format of the e-mail message into one that the next network understands. Each gateway also reads the destination address of the message and sends the message on in the direction of the destination mailbox. The routing choice takes into consideration the size of the message and also the amount of traffic on various networks. Because of this routing, it will take varying amounts of times to send messages to the same person. On one occasion, it might be only a few minutes; on others, it might be a few hours.

**Anatomy of an E-Mail Message**

E-mail messages will always have several features in common regardless of the program used to create the e-mail. A typical e-mail message includes a "From:" line with the sender's electronic address, a date and time line, a "To:" line with the recipient's electronic address, a "Subject:" line, and the body of the message. If there are any spelling or punctuation mistakes in the recipient's address, the message will be sent back from the electronic postoffice. The "Subject:" line is the place to give a clear, one-line description of the message. This description is usually displayed when someone checks their e-mail. Then they can decide how quickly they want to read the message!

If the message has been copied to others, their addresses will appear after the "Copies to:". Copying or forwarding messages to others is easy to do with most mail programs. For this reason, be very prudent in what is said in a message. There is no way to know where it will end up because there is no control over the message once it is sent.

**Legal Issues**

Privacy, libel, and copyright are legal issues that can affect e-mail users. Understand that privacy is not assured with electronic mail. There are no legal requirements that prevent an institution or company from reading incoming and outgoing e-mail messages. For individuals using an employer's equipment, this is especially applicable. In addition, once a message has been sent, there is no control over the what the recipient may do. The recipient may send a copy to someone else without the knowledge of the message's originator. Also, do not assume that messages received are private. The sender may have sent that same message to others without using the "Copies to:" function. A final note about privacy: even though a mail message has been deleted from a mailbox, don't assume that it has been completely erased. Many institutional and company policies require regular backups of their computer system disks, which generally hold incoming and outgoing mail messages. It is possible that copies of individual users' messages were taken during a regular system backup. Be aware that e-mail records can be subpoenaed.

A second legal issue for e-mail users is libel. Libel is applicable within e-mail messages and newsgroups. Take care with all comments. What you say can be held against you. Finally, copyright law applies to transferring files and information. It is illegal to distribute copyrighted information by any means, including electronic transfer. It is not uncommon to find material that has been scanned by a user for personal use and then distributed through e-mail. Unless the copyright owner has granted specific permission for the transfer of such material, it is illegal to do so.

## *Mailing Lists*

Mailing lists are an extension of e-mail. When an e-mail message is sent to someone, their address is indicated. When an individual or organization consistently want to mail to the same group of people, a special recipient name called an *alias* can be set up. For example, a hospital could create an alias called "nursing" that lists the e-mail addresses of all the directors of nursing. To send a message to all the directors of nursing, simply specify "nursing" in the "To:" line and the same message will be sent to everyone on that list (alias). The directors of nursing can use this method to have an electronic discussion group. One director sends a message about a certain topic that is distributed to all those users identified by the alias "nursing" (all the other directors of nursing). When another director wants to respond to the topic, a message is sent again to "nursing" and all the directors of nursing receive it.

A mailing list is like an alias that contains hundreds or thousands of users from all over the Internet. Any message sent to the mailing list "alias" will automatically be sent to everyone on the mailing list. Everything that anyone says through the mailing list goes to everyone on the mailing list. Mailing lists facilitate electronic discussion groups. Each mailing list resides at a specific computer and is looked after by a human administrator. The host computer is responsible for distributing incoming messages to all mailing list members. The administrator is responsible for maintaining the mailing list. Some mailing lists are also moderated. In these lists, there is a moderator who reviews each incoming message for appropriateness and either passes it through for distribution or rejects it. Some moderators will also prepare *digests*, something like an issue of a magazine. The digest will be a whole set of messages and articles in one package, making it much easier to keep up with the messages.

These mailing lists are maintained in two ways, either manually by a person or by a program. In the manual approach, the list administrator takes care of adding or deleting addresses from the master distribution list. In the program approach, you send messages to the address of a computer that provides this service. The most common mailing list administration program is called *Listserv* (standing for **List server**).

## *Newsgroups*

Discussions take place on the Internet using both mailing lists and newsgroups, but there is a significant difference between the two methods. A mailing list discussion comes directly to an individual's electronic mailbox, just like a letter is delivered by a postal service. However, the messages that form discussions in newsgroups are only sent to the newsgroup administrator, who then sends them to Internet newsgroup system sites (not individual subscribers). Individuals then read the messages in the newsgroup at a particular system site in the same way as walking down the hall to read the messages posted on a bulletin board. In fact, the origin of newsgroups was as a bulletin board service where messages could be posted for all to see.

### What Is Usenet?

Usenet (User's Network) is made up of all the machines that receive network newsgroups. A machine that receives these newsgroups is called a Usenet Server. Any computer system that wants to carry newsgroups of interest to that site can be a Usenet server.

Instead of forwarding all messages to all users on a mailing list, Usenet forwards all messages (called *articles* to keep up the newspaper analogy) not to individual subscribers, but to other Usenet servers who forward them on until all machines that are part of Usenet have a copy of the article (message). Individuals then use programs called "newsreaders" to access the newsgroup through their own computers. A typical Usenet server receives more than 20,000 articles per day. To organize all these articles, they are assigned to specific newsgroups. Newsgroups are further collected into hierarchies, similar to the domains described in relation to e-mail addresses.

Every Usenet server subscribes to specific newsgroups. Not all newsgroups are available on all Usenet servers. Some newsgroups are moderated. This means that articles cannot be posted directly to the newsgroup. Instead, all messages sent to this newsgroup will be automatically routed to the volunteer moderator. The moderator then decides what articles to send on to the newsgroup. Articles may be edited by the moderator or grouped with other articles before they are forwarded to the newsgroup. In some cases, the moderator may decide not to forward an article at all. Moderators exist to limit the number of low-quality articles in a newsgroup, especially all those "me too" or "I agree" type of articles.

**Reading Articles**

To read the articles posted to a newsgroup, a program called a newsreader is used. A newsreader is the interface to Usenet that allows individuals to choose the newsgroups to which they wish to belong, or select and display articles. When using a newsreader, articles can be saved to a file, mailed to someone else, or printed. Responding to the article's author or the newsgroup is also done through the newsreader program. There are a number of common newsreader programs: **rn, trn, nn,** and **tin.**

Newsgroups and mailing lists exemplify the power of the Net. An individual has the ability to call on the resources and creativity of people around the world to help. As well, individuals can contribute their experience and share their knowledge with others. This borderless Global Village is the true spirit of the Internet.

## *Telnet and FTP*

The Internet can make it as easy to use a computer on the other side of the world as it is to use a personal computer. A special program called *telnet* is used to connect to a remote computer (called a *host*). That computer can then be used as easily as using a terminal in the room next to it. An account or a password may be needed to connect to the remote computer. Telnet acts as a go-between for the originating computer and the other remote computer. Whatever is typed on the originating computer keyboard is passed on by telnet to the other computer. Whatever is displayed on the other computer screen is passed back to the originating computer and appears its screen. The originating screen and keyboard appear to be connected directly to the other remote computer.

To access a remote computer, its telnet address, sometimes but not always the same as its e-mail addrdess, is needed. Generally, if a remote computer allows telnet connection, the address is not freely distributed for security reasons. Some remote hosts offer a public service. If one of these types of hosts is accessed, often the program starts by itself, without the need to enter a userid or password. Once a userid and password have been validated, an individual can take advantage of all the resources provided by the host computer. For example, CINAHLdirect, a telnet application, allows the user to search its electronic databases from a remote location, such as a home. Searches are done in the same manner as they would be in a library using the CD-ROM version of CINAHL. Search results can be printed from the remote computer, in the home, hospital, or university.

*FTP* (File Transfer Protocol) is technically the set of specifications that support Internet file transfer. Practically, however, FTP is used to refer to a service that allows a file to be copied from any Internet host to another Internet host (usually a personal computer). Therefore, FTP is another Internet application that allows access to a remote host computer. Telnet allows direct login to the remote computer, making an individual's computer a terminal of the host. FTP, however, only allows access to the file names on a remote computer and the ability to then copy (download) them to a remote computer. FTP is one of the most widely used Internet services. All types of information and computer software are available on the Internet, and FTP provides the means to copy these onto your own computer. The possibilities are endless: statistics programs, computer games, text files, sound, and even video clips.

The only problem is that you must have a valid userid and password to access the remote host and copy files, just as you needed for telnet. To facilitate the distribution of information on the Internet, many computers have been set up to be an *Anonymous FTP host*. The systems administrator of an Anonymous FTP host designates specific directories as open to the public and creates a user login called *anonymous* (or sometimes *guest*). Anyone who wants to can log in to that computer with the userid *anonymous* and their e-mail address as the password. Any of the files found in the public directories can then be copied onto another computer. Those directories, however, are the only ones that the user *anonymous* can see. All other files and directories on the computer are invisible and not accessible. For example, personnel files, research data files, and licensed software are kept out of the public directories.

## World Wide Web

The latest service to be developed in the evolution of attempts to make sense of all the Internet resources is the *World Wide Web* (variously called WWW, W3, or the Web). The goal of WWW development was to offer a simple, consistent, and intuitive interface to the vast resources of the Internet. WWW tries to provide the intuitive links that humans make between information, rather than forcing people to think like a computer and speculate at possible file names and hidden submenus as do the previous services. A short history of the development of the WWW will help to understand its services.

### History of the Web

In 1989, researchers at CERN (the European Laboratory for Particle Physics) wanted to develop a simpler way of sharing information with a widely dispersed research group. The problems they faced are the same as those you face in using the previous information retrieval systems. Because the researchers were at distant sites, any activity such as reading a shared document or viewing an image required finding the location of the desired information, making a remote connection to the machine containing the information, and then downloading the information to a local machine. Each of these activities required running a variety of applications such as

FTP, Telnet, Archie, or an image viewer. The researchers decided to develop a system that would allow them to access all types of information from a common interface without the need for all the steps required previously. Between 1990 and 1993, the CERN researchers developed this type of interface, WWW, and the necessary tools to use it. Since 1993, WWW has become one of the most popular ways to access Internet resources.

## Hypertext

To navigate around the World Wide Web, a beginning understanding of *hypertext* is essential. Hypertext is text that contains links to other data. For example, when doing a literature search using the hard copy of CINAHL, the first search term is selected and looked up. After reading through the listings, another idea for a search term becomes apparent. Traditionally, the user marks the first page (to facilitate returning at a later time) and turns to the new term. At the bottom of the listings of the second term is a note that says "see also" and gives several other words to follow. In a hypertext document, it is unnecessary to wait until the end to find the links; they may be anywhere in the document. Links in hypertext documents are marked either with color bars, underlining, or use of square brackets with numbers, so that they stand out. Whenever a word is marked as hypertext, it can be selected and immediately the link will be made to another document related to the word or phrase. When finished looking at the linked document, simply go back to the previous text with the click of a mouse button, where the program has kept its finger in the page.

This is what makes the Web so powerful. A link may go to any type of Internet resource. For example, the link can go to a text file, a Gopher site, a Telnet session, or a UseNet newsgroup. Another powerful feature of the Web is that hypertext allows the same piece of information to be linked to hundreds of other documents at the same time. The links can also span traditional boundaries. A hypertext document related to a specific professional group may contain links to information in many different disciplines. For example, in Figure 4.1, the text "Student Health Services" is underlined. If that text is selected, the next screen to appear would be the Web page that describes Student Health Information. If "Headaches" was selected, the link would be made to an on-line document about headaches and headache management.

## Web Browsers

To access the Web, a Web browser program is needed on the computer. A Web browser program knows how to interpret and display the hypertext documents that it finds on the Web. There are many browsers on the market. Graphical user interface (GUI) or windows-based browsers include *Netscape*™, Microsoft Corporation's *Internet Explorer*™, and *Mosaic*™. To

## University of Montana HEALTHLINE Server

 This server under MAJOR construction! Please excuse our mess!

Welcome to The University of Montana **Student Health Services** HEALTHLINE

Is the high-fiber theory just another dietary fad? Do you have trouble sleeping? Suffer from migraine headaches? Interested in learning more about the proposed Clinton Health Care Plan? Are you concerned about proper labeling and advertising of food/health products? What steps should you take before, during, and after a natural disaster? Interested in Electronic Books for the Blind and other similar projects? The answer to these questions and much more are available through HEALTHLINE.

**FIGURE 4.1.** The Web Home Page of Healthline. (Reprinted with permission from Edwards, M.J.A., The Internet for Nurses and Health Professionals, Second Edition, New York: Springer-Verlag, 1997, p. 44.)

use these browsers, the hypertext links are highlighted and the user simply "points and clicks" with a mouse. There are also text-based browsers such as *Lynx*. With a text-based browser, each link is given a number enclosed in a square bracket [3]. To select a link, simply enter the number of the desired link.

All Web sites have a welcome page, called a home page, that appears when the site is first accessed. The home page may just give the name of the site but usually contains a list of resources and links available at the site.

The World Wide Web project also developed a standard way of referencing an item whether it was a graphics file, a document, or a link to another site. This standardized reference is called a *Uniform Resource Locator* (URL). The URL is a complete description of the item including its location. A typical URL:

**http://healthline.umt.edu:700**

The first part of the URL, which ends with the colon, is the protocol that is being used to retrieve the item. In this example, the protocol is HTTP (hypertext transfer protocol), used for the Web. Other protocols are self-evident: gopher for Gopher sites, FTP for FTP sites, and so on. The next part is the domain name of the computer that you need to connect to (healthline.umt.edu). This tells you that the information is on a computer in the education top-level domain (edu). The computer is located at the University of Montana (umt) and the server name is healthline.

**Search Engines**

Search engines, such as Lycos or Alta Vista, send out software agents called spiders that crawl the nooks and crannies of the Web, building indexes that can be scanned in seconds. Various search engines come up with different results and different presentations, so several may be used when searching any one topic. A major problem in searching the Internet is the sheer volume of information. Alta Vista, the fastest search engine, takes 6 days to sweep the Net once. Complementing these databases are searchable directories such as Yahoo! and Magellan. In these directories, broad subject areas such as sports or food or health are winnowed into subcategories. The next-generation search engines, Meta-search engines such as Metacrawler, simultaneously load queries into many search engines at the same time.

## Intranets and Extranets

As was stated earlier, the real power of the Internet is in the people and information that all those computers connect. Many organizations have taken the concepts and tools of the Internet and have applied them within their own structures. The organizations, in effect, create private internets that are called *intranets*. Information and people can then be connected in the same easy fashion as on the larger public Internet. Organizations thus have all the advantages for information sharing and communication for their people without the security concerns of using the public Internet. If organizations then selectively allow outside agencies to connect to their intranet, they have now created an *extranet*. This extranet can allow several organizations with common purpose to easily share information on an "extended intranet."

## Summary

The integration of telecommunications and health informatics has made a powerful impact on health care delivery. We have only begun to see what is possible when telecommunications meets health informatics. Specific applications of the Internet to health care (i.e., telehealth) are described in Chapter 8.

## Additional Resources

Edwards, M. *The Internet for Nurses and Allied Health Professionals.* New York: Springer-Verlag, 1997.

# Part II
# Nursing Use of
# Information Systems

# 5
# Enterprise Health Information Systems[1]

## Introduction

Health care institutions generate massive volumes of information that must be collected, transmitted, recorded, retrieved, and summarized. The problem of managing all these activities for clinical information has become monumental. As a result, computer based hospital information systems (HISs) were designed, tested, and installed in hospitals of all sizes. The original purpose of HISs was to provide a computer-based framework to facilitate the communication of information within a hospital setting. Essentially, an HIS is a communication network linking terminals and output devices in key patient care or service areas to a central processing unit that coordinates all essential patient care activities. Thus, the HIS provides a communication system between departments (e.g., dietary, nursing units, pharmacy, laboratory, etc.); a central information system for receipt, sorting, transmission, storage, and retrieval of information; and a high speed, data processing system for fast and economic processing of data to provide information in its most useful form.

The management of information in the hospital setting and its environs is a critical component in the process of health care delivery. The problem of information management has been complicated by an exponential increase in the amount of data to be managed, in the number of stakeholders in the process, and in the requirements for real time access and response. In the United States, 12%–15% of the cost of health care is attributed to the costs associated with information handling (Office of Technology Assessment, 1995). The cost of information handling in the hospital setting has lead to the use of computers in an attempt to provide more data at lower costs. Estimates of the costs of information handling vary between 25% and 39%

---

[1] This chapter is based in part on material previously published by Hannah, Kathryn J., and Hammond, W.E. The Evolution of Clinical Information Systems. In: Ball, Marion J., and Douglas, J. (eds.) *Clinical Information Systems That Support Evolving Delivery Systems.* Redmond: Spacelabs, 1997.

of the total cost of health care (Jackson, 1969). Most health informatics professionals agree that a reasonable cost for the electronic information handling is at least 3%–5% of the operational budget for an institution.

Information systems currently being used in health care environments can be broadly categorized into three types. The first type is composed of those systems that are limited in objective and scope. They most often exist as a standalone module and address a single application area. Examples of such a system are the nursing workload measurement systems currently being used in many hospitals. The Medicus and GRASP systems serve a specific function and therefore would fall into this category of system. In the hospital environment, systems that are commonly included in this category are dedicated clinical laboratory systems, dedicated financial systems, and dedicated radiology, EKG, pulmonary functions, pharmacy, and dietary systems. In a public health setting a standalone immunization system is a good example of this category of system.

The second type of information system is composed of hospital information systems, which usually consist of a communications network, a clinical component, and a financial/administrative component. The overall communications component integrates these three major parts into a cohesive information system. A typical hospital information system in this category may have computer terminals at each nursing station as well as terminals that are in, or accessible to, each ancillary area in the hospital. The terminals are tied together through one or more large central computers, which may be on- or off-site.

The third type of information system for use in health environments, Enterprise Health Information Systems (EHISs), are just beginning to emerge. Such systems capture and store comprehensive, lifelong, patient information across the entire continuum of health services. These records are captured and stored in multiple media including audio, image, animation, or print. The records may be stored centrally, either in total or in and abstracted format, using a data warehouse approach. Alternatively, these records may be physically stored at the point of capture and logically linked into a virtual record that is only physically assembled as required to meet care requirements.

## Hospital Information Systems (HISs)

Early computer applications for hospitals dealt with administration and financial matters. Later applications included task oriented functions such as admission/discharge/transfer (ADT), order entry, and result reporting. With the availability of minicomputers, various departmental service-related systems such as laboratory, radiology, and pharmacy were developed. Few, if any, of these systems were electronically connected. The subsequent development of Hospital Information Systems (HISs) was a factor of technology (hardware and software), people (developer and user), and economics.

An implicit assumption in the development of Hospital Information Systems is that the ability of complete, accurate, and timely data delivered at the point of care to the person providing that care will result in a higher quality of care at a more efficient cost. Support for this assumption is provided by simple observation; e.g., such systems should eliminate redundant tests, eliminate the need to reestablish diagnoses, increase awareness of drug allergies and adverse events, increase awareness of the medications the patient is taking, and enhance communication among those involved with the patient's care. There are four main functions typical of such hospital information systems:

- Recognize both sending and receiving stations, format all messages, and manage all the message routing (this is called message switching)
- Validate, check, and edit each message to assure its quality
- Control all the hardware and software needed to perform the first two functions
- Assemble transaction data and communicate with the accounting system

The first hospital computer systems that were developed in the late 1960s were geared to batch accounting to meet the complexity of third-party billing, cost statistics, and fiscal needs. The technology of that era was unsuccessfully applied to clinical systems. Terminal devices, such as cathode-ray tubes, were expensive and unreliable. Also, hardware and software were limited, expensive, and highly structured. Database systems had not appeared. During this period, some hospitals installed standalone computers in clinical departments and in business offices to do specific jobs. The most common clinical example is laboratory reporting. Most of the hospitals that embarked on these clinical programs for standalone systems were large teaching institutions with access to federal funding or other research grants. Usually there was no attempt made to integrate the accounting computer with the standalone departmental computer—this came much later.

The 200- and 400-bed hospital that installed computers in the late 1960s for accounting had varied success. During that period accounting needs became more complex, and this trend continues. The result is a constant battle just to maintain and change existing systems to keep pace with regulating agencies. Many hospitals of this size turned to a shared computer service such as Shared Medical Systems. The reason these companies prospered was not only because of their products and services but also because a small hospital simply cannot justify employing and retaining the technical staff and management skills necessary for this complex, conflicting, changing environment.

In the early 1970s, with rampant inflation and restricted cost reimbursement, some large hospitals that had installed their own computers with marginal success changed to the shared service. By this time, the shared companies had better accounting software and audit controls. Most importantly, these companies developed field personnel who understood hospital operations and were able to communicate and translate the use of computer systems into results in their client hospitals. This added dimension of service that is not offered or understood by the hardware vendors increased business opportunities for the service companies. Many of these companies, in turn, increased their scope of services beyond fiscal to clinical and communication applications.

The hardware vendors of the 1960s (e.g., IBM, Burroughs, Honeywell, NCR) committed themselves to large general purpose computers that attempted to support clinical, communications, and financial systems. In the 1970s, technology such as the minicomputer and personal computer was generally accepted as providing a better alternative to the approach than the large general-purpose computer. And, in fact, the major hardware companies are moving in this direction. In this same time frame, the service companies began to develop on site minicomputers to handle data communications and specialized nonfinancial applications. They began to expand their scope of data retention to support clinical applications that required a historical patient database. In other words, hospital information systems vendors and service providers migrated toward a similar concept.

Current hospital information systems grew out of developmental work that took place during the 1970s. Functional specifications, system design, and technology selection were driven by the immediate problem at hand. Hospital information systems were designed to deal primarily with the problem of moving transaction oriented data throughout an institution. The business functions for which software applications were developed included admission/discharge/transfer (ADT), order entry/result reporting, and charge or cost capture. In most cases, administrative and financial personnel who had responsibility for the accounting systems controlled the systems. Mainframe technology was utilized as the best hardware platform for providing an extensive network.

Gradually, HISs evolved into communication networks linking terminals and output devices in key patient care or service areas to a central processing unit that coordinates all essential patient care activities. The difference among systems that fall into this category is not in their communications, but in the complexity of the integration of their application functions. Some systems have more sophisticated provisions for validating, checking, editing, formatting, and documentation than others. Some respond faster and offer a better variety of displays. These variations are differences in the communication and presentation aspects of the system. Other systems provide more complex integration of the application structure and data retention. One example of this is the total integration of information from the lab, radiology, pharmacy, and medical records, which then interacts with the nursing stations, thereby providing communication from order entry to result reports. Another difference in hospital information systems is the orientation toward the data content: some systems are oriented around the financial and administrative data, and others are organized around patient care data. In the latter case, administrative and financial data and functions are derived from patient care information. More patient information, such as history, physical, and progress data, is contained in these systems because they emphasize integration of direct clinical information.

## Components of HIS

### Administrative and Financial Modules

Accounts receivable, accounts payable, general ledger, materiel management, payroll, and human resources applications are the minimum management functions required of the administrative and financial modules of a hospital information system. Accounts receivable at a minimum consists of charge capture for transmission to another system. Other accounts receivable functions include utilization review; professional and technical component billing; proration of revenue; corrections and late charges; adjustments and payments; account aging by method of payment, by category of patient and category of physician, by date of encounter, by inpatient/outpatient and by date of payment; and collections, including delinquent accounts report, collection comments, dunning letters, turnover letters, and collection agency reports. Miscellaneous software applications are required to support other management functions such as environment and energy control, marketing, fund raising, and public relations.

Departmental management functions include inventory control of supplies, drugs, and perishables; item tracking of such things as specimens, charts, and films; revenue and utilization statistics; word processing; electronic mail; budget and actual monthly financial statements for use in variance analysis; workload analysis and personnel scheduling; and human resources and payroll.

### Admission/Discharge/Transfer Modules

Admission/Discharge/Transfer is the core of any hospital information system. At a minimum, this module must establish a patient record, provide a unique encounter identification number, and document the place of encounter. Other functions include bed availability; call lists; scheduling; collection of demographic data, referral data and reason for admission;

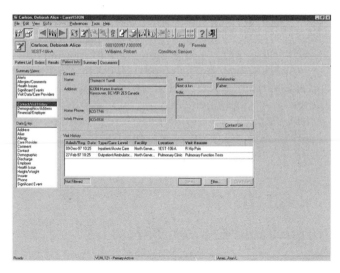

**Figure 5.1.** Admission profile. (Photograph courtesy of Health Vision.)

precertification; verification of benefit plan and ability to pay; and preadmission orders and presurgery preparation procedures (see Figure 5.1).

The admission process includes: update pre-admission/appointment data; create the hospital account number; collect admitting diagnosis; initiate concurrent review; notify dietary, housekeeping, and human services; collect/initiate orders; notification of orders/requisitions; bed assignment; notification of arrival to all interested parties; census with locators by patient name, identification number, account number, nursing station, physician group (includes primary, admitting, referring, and consultants); organize work flow by data to be reviewed, reports to be completed, and reports to be verified/signed; bed control; room charging including variable services/ room and multiple patients/day; concurrent review including utilization, quality assurance, and risk management; transfer of patient including bed control and discontinue orders; pending discharge, including notify next admission, prepare discharge medications and contact home health provider; discharge, including verify diagnoses and procedures, discharge summary, patient instruction, and return appointments; and case abstracting, including diagnosis/procedure coding, diagnosis related group statistics, and retrospective review.

## Order Entry Module

Order Entry Module is a module in a hospital information system (HIS) by which doctors or nurses enter clinical orders or prescriptions using terminals located in patient care areas. Orders are transmitted through the computer system to the recipient for immediate implementation. Using this module, errors at the time of input of the orders are theoretically minimized, and the efficiency of data transmission in hospitals increases. Order entry can occur at either the point of care or at a centrally located terminal. Increasingly, caregivers are seeking systems that allow for order entry at the point of care.

Order entry is a function common to almost all service departments in the hospital. At a minimum, orders may be entered in a batch mode as a method of charge capture. The full functionality includes: initial order capture of procedure, urgency, frequency, scheduling (beginning date, time and duration), performer, ordering physician and comments; order verification; order sets; activation of preorders; check for inappropriate orders including frequency by patient, match to diagnosis, negated by medications and credential verification; order followup including look up patient by requisition number, list overdue pending orders and list continuing orders due to expire; initiate work, including insertion on work to be done list by service department and nursing station, print requisition, queue for scheduling, and print labels; and enter charge if billing on order entry (see Figure 5.2).

An important capacity of order entry system is the ability to provide feedback to caregivers at the time they enter orders. For instance, at the University of Tokyo Hospital, when a physician prescribes an inappropriate

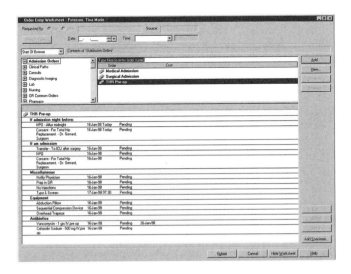

**Figure 5.2.** Order entry. (Photograph courtesy of Health Vision.)

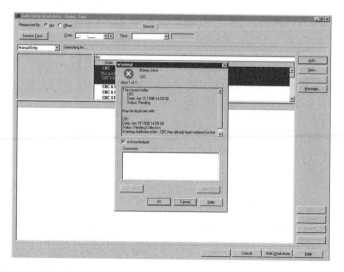

**FIGURE 5.3.** Order Alert. (Photograph courtesy of Health Vision.)

dosage, the system provides a warning. The system also has the ability to alert physicians when they order too many clinical tests without sufficient justification. Because the hospital is a teaching hospital, there are many young physicians in training programs. The education and training of physicians is a very important function of the hospital. These interns and resident physicians often lack professional self-confidence, are insecure in their clinical judgment, or are excessively curious. Consequently, they tend to order more clinical tests than are required by more experienced physicians. This has been a problem from financial perspective of the hospital because the insurance body will not provide compensation for these excessive tests. The warning alert on the order entry system had remarkable effects, and the number of clinical tests ordered decreased approximately 30% following system implementation. The warning system was evaluated by interviewing the users and all agreed that the system gave them a chance to reconsider the necessity of the clinical tests, which had some educational value (see Figure 5.3).

## Result Reporting Module

Result reporting requirements vary markedly among departments. Minimum result reporting consists of notification that a procedure is complete. Other functionality includes: cancel procedure; entry of result including flag process complete and bill; enter normal/abnormal range (numeric, coded or text); check data for accuracy through edit tables and internal consistency such as delta checks; and report result including immediate result reporting,

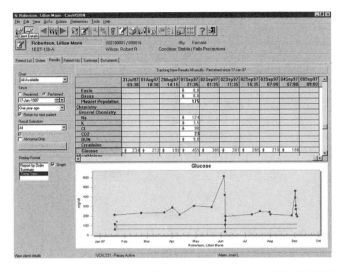

**FIGURE 5.4.** Results reporting. (Photograph courtesy of Health Vision.)

flow sheets or graph, related calculated results, and physician prompts (see Figure 5.4).

## Scheduling

Scheduling of admissions, surgery, outpatient encounters, and diagnostics is critical for the smooth, integrated working of the health care facility. The outpatient scheduling permits the preadmission ordering of tests and preoperative diagnostic assessments and of coordinating the performance of those tests and assessments with the admission. Effective management of the mix of patients and length of time for encounters is facilitated by a good scheduling system. Patient notification of pending appointments reduces no-show rates.

## Specialized Support for Clinical Functions

Software application programs are required to provide specialized support for departmental services. Some examples are as follows:

- Clinical laboratory tasks include accession numbering, collection list, specimen tracking, specimen logging, automatic capture of results from instruments, and quality control: processing controls, calculation of means and standard deviation for a test, analysis of patient trend, technologist verification, check for drug/test interactions, and protocols (see Figure 5.5).

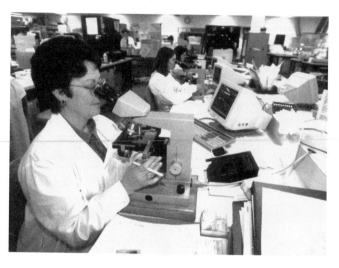

**FIGURE 5.5.** Laboratory applications. (Photograph courtesy of Sunquest.)

- Radiology tasks include result reporting (preliminary, final, amended results), electronic signature, reference file, and images of various types.
- Pharmacy tasks include verification of order by pharmacist, dual result reporting by pharmacy (number dispense) and by nurse (number administered), unit dose tracking (fills and returns), IV admixture, and chemotherapy protocols.
- Nursing systems must provide nursing assessment, nursing diagnoses, nursing interventions, and care plans including medication administration records, nursing workload, and nursing note of client outcomes.
- Medical records requires that the system provide a list of all diagnoses, an encounter-oriented summary abstract, time-oriented summaries (flow sheets), utilization review, and longitudinal studies (see Figure 5.6).
- Dietary tasks include meal planning, menu selection, food distribution, inventory, ordering, nutrition management, and drug–food interactions.
- Consultation programs, which should be available, include bibliographic retrieval, calculations, modeling, decision support systems, protocols, and health knowledge bases such as the PDR, Emergency procedures, and Poison Index.
- Critical Care areas have special needs for electronic data capture for patient monitoring and charting.
- Patient support should include security, privacy, confidentiality for patient data, information sheets for patient education and awareness, concern for general patient welfare, reminders of appointments, admissions, tests, and health maintenance reminders.

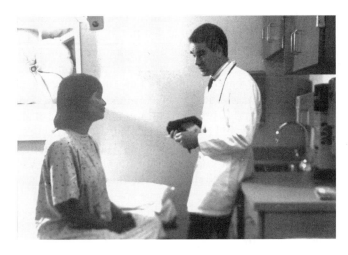

**FIGURE 5.6.** Medical documentation. (Photograph courtesy of Cerner Corporation and Ron Berg Photography, Kansas City, Missouri.)

## Issues Related to HISs

There were many problems encountered in early implementation efforts. The organizational discipline required to implement hospital information systems was complicated by departmental priority differences and, sometimes, departmental autonomy. Systems functions that support patient care requirements, when given top priority, most often conflicted with existing administrative systems or at least could not communicate with these legacy systems. Computers traditionally started in accounting, and most hospital applications still have their roots in this area. The operations cycle of patient care is continuous and instantaneous. Fiscal methodology and timing are intermittent and historical. To achieve successful utilization of information systems in health care, both these disparate needs must be recognized and served.

As indicated previously, currently available, commercial hospital information systems are built primarily around the framework of technologies, design philosophies, and health care delivery models of the 1970s. As new concepts and new technology have become available, these classic systems have been modified, most usually on a superficial level, to accommodate these changes. Most of these systems were designed with no thought of an electronic patient record and certainly no concept of a longitudinal cross sectoral, multidisciplinary, patient specific record.

In fact, most of these systems, even today, retain only the data for a single hospitalization and then for only a few months after discharge. The primary orientation of these systems remains financially driven, problem focused, and task oriented. These systems use a mainframe computer, a central database, and character-based terminals. Few of these systems support a unified patient problem list and complete, integrated studies and therapy data sets. Current systems are primarily an automation of the manual system for documentation of hospital care. The design philosophy reflects the flow of documents as the primary communication. The traditional paper chart still exists in even the most computerized hospitals of today. No major systems exist today in which all data and the management of those data is fully computerized.

During the 1980s, major issues in health care delivery systems surfaced. Most vendors moved into integrated distributed networking and shared configurations. The initial expectations associated with general purpose computers for developing hospital information systems were not met in the time frame anticipated by early studies. Some of the reasons for this failure to meet expectations are these:

- The complex information and communication structure, which is required to deliver patient care in hospitals, was grossly underestimated.
- The hardware and software of the 1960s, 1970s, and 1980s were grossly inadequate, rigid, unreliable, and very expensive.
- The staffing requirements in terms of systems and data processing professionals who could manage, define, communicate, and implement systems in hospitals were grossly underestimated.

However, one more technological advance was necessary. The development of relational database management systems for use in patient care was imperative for nursing to fully exploit technology. As McHugh and Shultz (1982) suggested:

Hospital nursing departments have followed the frozen asset path for their data resources. Information contained in existing modular and turnkey systems cannot be easily merged with other computer-stored information.

Experienced users of computers in business abandoned the traditional modular approach to computer file handling that is still being marketed by some vendors to the health care industry. Database management systems have long been available that can

1. Reduce data redundancy
2. Provide quality data
3. Maintain data integrity
4. Protect data security
5. Interface relatively easily with technological advances
6. Facilitate access to a single integrated collection of data for many applications by multiple user groups.

# Enterprise Health Information Systems (EHISs)

## *Evolution of Health Enterprises*

Most recently, health care organizations and health services delivery systems internationally are under enormous pressure from all sides (see Figure 5.7).

There is a decrease in the revenue available to fund health services delivery; the explosion of new treatments, new programs, and new technologies is accompanied by citizens' increasing demands and expectations of their health system and reflected in such changing health services delivery modalities as managed care; drug costs are rising; population demographics are characterized by the rising average age; there is a shifting health services delivery paradigm from acute care to community based care; and employee expectations for remuneration and compensation are resulting in rising labor costs. Simultaneously, there are also expectations that the efficiency and effectiveness of health services delivery will improve while the quality of care is maintained or even improved.

For all these reasons, health services delivery systems around the world are under enormous pressure to change. However, decisions about health care organizations and health care delivery systems must not be

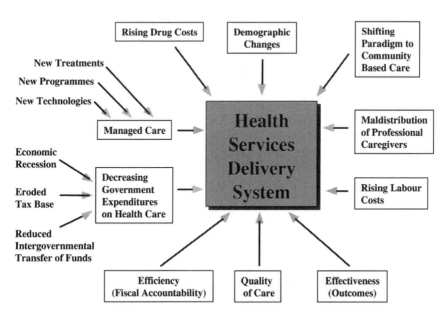

**FIGURE 5.7.** Pressures on National Health Care Systems. (Adapted from Hannah, Kathryn J. Transforming information: data management support of health care reorganization. *Journal of American Medical Informatics Association,* 1995;2(3):145–155.)

based on opinion, emotion, historical precedent, or political expediency. Data and information are essential to rational decision making and good management of the health services delivery system in any country. The restructuring of health systems worldwide must be based on data and information.

Health services, health care delivery systems, and health organizations around the world are undergoing reorganization and reengineering. Rational decision making about such activities must be based on information. Historically, the field of Medical Informatics has focused on individual patient care in acute care. Much less attention has been directed toward population based health care. Increasingly, the field is beginning to emphasize Health Informatics, which has a broader multidisciplinary focus on health services delivery including community needs assessment, population health status indicators, health promotion, and disease prevention in addition to the treatment of illness. Health Informatics can and should play a major role in the reengineering and restructuring that is occurring in many health care organizations and health services delivery systems. Many of the data presently available are inadequate for these tasks; therefore, current data must be transformed and future information requirements anticipated to support the reengineering of health care enterprises and organizations. Essential concepts are:

- The reconceptualization of health services delivery within a jurisdiction as one enterprise.
- Use of information engineering techniques.
- Development of a comprehensive information management strategy.
- The need to apply information management principles.
- The organizational implications of information management.
- A conceptual model for achieving added value as a by-product from health service delivery data.

Enterprise health information systems (EHISs) can be conceived of as tools intended for use by legislators, policy makers, managers, and caregivers within the health system to fulfill their responsibilities with regard to the delivery of health services to the population. New models for health care delivery, e.g., regionalized health care delivery enterprises such as those found in the United Kingdom, South Africa, and some Canadian provinces, and managed care such as is developing in the United States, have expanded the walls of the hospital and are requiring the development of integrated health services delivery enterprises that involve the hospital, extended care facilities, the community, public health, and a multidisciplinary team of caregivers (e.g., traditional healers, physicians, nurses, physiotherapists, nutritionists, dentists, social workers, educators, music therapists, psychologists, speech therapists). This new vision encompasses the concept of the electronic health record or computer based patient record that is patient centered and includes all data relating to a person's health or well being as well as a documentation of illness care. There is an evolution occurring from health care systems that only treat people when they are ill to health enterprises which support people's activities to protect, promote, and maintain their own health in addition to treating people's illnesses. All these changes require an altered approach to information management.

Future jurisdictional health information systems need to take into the account the fundamental principle that the reason a health care delivery system exists in any jurisdiction is to provide health services to its citizens. Thus, administrative and managerial information for use in operating the health care delivery enterprise should be a by-product of the care delivery process. One can envision a future environment in which current information about health facilities and health care delivery systems for use in enterprise planning and policies as well as resource allocation and utilization will need to be much more widely available to the professional care providers than in the past.

The responsibilities related to operating a health services delivery system, that is, a comprehensive health services enterprise, within a jurisdiction (community, state/provincial, or national), can be summarized into the following functional categories:

- Assess the health status of the population
- Set health goals and objectives
- Set strategic directions
- Provide programs and services
- Communicate with stakeholders
- Manage resources
- Evaluate the health services delivery system.

Such a comprehensive health services delivery enterprise requires a health information system that is defined in the broadest and most inclusive fashion possible. It should include the data and the most rudimentary media for gathering the data (e.g., pencil and paper) as well as all possible means of storing, processing, aggregating, and presenting the information. A jurisdictional health information system also should include the people who interface with the system, specifically those who

- Generate the data (i.e. the recipients of care and the caregivers)
- Use the data in its various forms (i.e., caregivers, health systems managers, policy makers, and legislators)
- Maintain the data and the means by which it is captured, stored, processed, aggregated, and presented (e.g., data gatherers, filing clerks, forms analysts, data entry clerks, computer operators, network managers).

The kinds of decisions that are facing health services enterprise managers are more complex than decisions required in the past. For example:

- Decisions are patient focused rather than discipline focused. The concept of multidisciplinary teams is increasingly being used within health care delivery, resulting in data that focus on the recipient of care rather than the provider of care.
- Previously, decisions within the health care delivery system have been focused within specific service sectors (acute care, public health mental health, long term care, insured services) but now are becoming focused within jurisdictions (community, state/provincial, or national), geographical areas that require a cross-sectoral perspective.
- Decisions affecting the entire health services enterprise require information about the entire health services enterprise.
- Decisions affecting even a part of the health services enterprise still require information about other parts of the health services enterprise because of the impact of interdependencies among the sectors; for example, early discharge programs in the acute care sector have a major impact on the home care delivery sector.
- Decisions to reduce expenditures on health services while maintaining the quality and maximizing the benefits to the health of citizens will require information about the outcomes of health services. There is a need to know whether or not what is done for, with, or to a client makes any difference in the health status of that client.

The role of the professional care provider (e.g., physicians, nurses, dentists, physiotherapists) in managing information in health care facilities is of necessity related to the role of the caregiver within the organization. In most health care delivery facilities, it is necessary to manage both the patient care and the patient care environment within the organization. Usually, caregivers manage patient care and managers administer the organization. Therefore, for some time, the caregiver's role in the management of information generally has been considered to include the capture and use of the information necessary to manage patient care, and caregivers have also been expected to provide the information necessary for managing the organization, e.g., resource allocation and utilization, personnel management, planning and policy making, and decision support. This dual responsibility has generated an increasing burden on caregivers to provide information because of the redundancy and duplication of information that they are expected to provide.

Health care delivery is information intensive. Caregivers handle enormous volumes of patient care information. In fact, caregivers constantly process information mentally, manually, and electronically. In every aspect of patient care, caregivers are continually engaged in problem solving using clinical judgment and decision making: assessing; identifying patient problems and diagnoses; determining appropriate action or interventions; evaluating; and reassessing and communicating. Care providers integrate information from many diverse sources throughout the organization to provide patient care and to coordinate the patient's contact with the health system. They manage patient care information for purposes of providing care to patients.

An implicit assumption in the development of Enterprise Health Information Systems is that the ability to deliver complete, accurate, and timely data at the point of care to the person providing that care will result in a higher quality of care at a more efficient cost. Support for this assumption is provided by simple observation, e.g., such systems should eliminate redundant tests, eliminate the need to reestablish diagnoses, increase awareness of drug allergies and adverse events, increase awareness of the medications the patient is taking, and enhance communication among those involved with the patient's care.

Modern health care delivery generates massive volumes of information that must be collected, transmitted, recorded, retrieved, and summarized. The problem of managing all these activities for clinical information has become monumental. As a result, computer based hospital information systems (HISs) were designed, tested, and installed in hospitals of all sizes. The original purpose of HISs was to provide a computer-based framework to facilitate the communication of information within a health care setting.

## Enterprise Wide Information Systems

In most countries, the model for health care is moving toward integrated delivery systems see Figure 5.8. This process could be enhanced by develop-

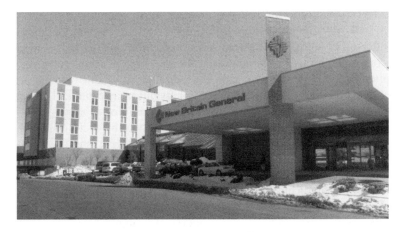

FIGURE 5.8. Enterprise wide integrated delivery systems service entire hospitals. (Photograph courtesy of Sunquest.)

ing an electronic health record that supports the patient, the primary care provider, physician, nurse, other caregivers, and hospital or other critical care setting, along with pharmacies, nursing homes, nursing, home health, payers, federal, state or province, and local authorities, accreditation and quality assurance agencies, and others. All these stakeholders must be integrated into a single, distributed system for maximum return on investment in information management systems. Requirements include the physical network to support such integration; an infrastructure to manage and regulate such a structure; standards for data interchange; a common data model defining the objects to be transmitted; and a common, clinically rich vocabulary.

Future systems must reflect the major paradigm shift in health services delivery models. The underlying philosophy must be patient centered: what are the requirements of a system whose primary purpose is to provide the mechanism for the most efficient and economical care possible for people receiving health services. Rather than using the computer to improve the current paper oriented systems, new systems must answer the question: Given the power of modern computation devices with massive storage and ubiquitous network linkages, graphical interfaces, image display capabilities, capacity for vast and instant data analyses, and personalization of function, what can and should the health care information system of tomorrow provide? Much of the functionality of current systems will still be required. The transmission of orders, processing of orders, and reporting of results still remain. Functional requirements of ADT, scheduling, department service management, supply replacement, inventory, materials management, and documentation still remain. Quality assurance should occur in real time, rather than recognizing days later that something was overlooked or that a mistake was made.

At an International Medical Informatics Association (IMIA) Working Group 10 workshop on Hospital Information Systems in 1988, Collen stated that the goal of a hospital information system should be to "use computers and communications equipment to collect, store, process, retrieve, and communicate relative patient care and administrative information for all activities and functions within the hospital, its outpatient medical offices, its clinical support services (clinical laboratories, radiology, pharmacy, intensive care unit, etc.), and with its affiliated [health] facilities. Such an integrated, multi-facility, [health] information system should have the capability for communication and integration of all patient data during the patient's service life time, from all of the information subsystems and all facilities in the medical system complex; and to provide administrative and clinical decision support." This statement is important because it recognizes that clinical information is not the property of a single facility but rather is part of a global resource that focuses on the patient centered record.

Hospital Information Systems (HIS) and the concepts underlying them are limited because they focus primarily on operational information and not on a comprehensive patient record. An Electronic Health Record (EHR) or Computer-based Patient Record (CPR) is one component of a larger Enterprise Health Information System that includes not only hospital functionality but also features of a comprehensive integrated delivery system. Using information from an HER, an Enterprise Health Information System can incorporate the use of aggregated health data for use in the management of the health services delivery system, i.e., assessing population health status, setting health goals and objectives, defining strategic directions, program planning and delivery, and resource allocation.

Health Service Enterprises also are able to exploit technological advances because of the networks that have become available. Now, the system is the network and the network is the system. Networks are enablers that allow health service enterprises to be virtual organizations. Until recently, the various communication barriers imposed by distance and time made concrete physical organizations essential and dictated management structures partitioned to allow each individual geographic facility to be managed independently. Today, management of virtual health enterprises is possible because the technology ties the various component health facilities together with communication networks. Distance, time, and location all become almost irrelevant.

A patient-centered record requires that all data relating to the patient and the patient's well being must be available at all times and accessible at appropriate locations. Data from all relevant sources must be integrated into a single record including but not limited to demographic data, data related to health determinants, and risk factors, along with diagnostic and treatment data from all contacts with the health enterprise (e.g., primary care providers; all members of the multidisciplinary health care team; home care; public or private acute care, long term care, or mental health facilities). This record will likely take the form of a virtual record and may well be stored in a variety of locations. Initial efforts at exploring such a concept are underway in a few environments, although experiences with Enterprise Health Information Systems (EHISs) over large geographic areas and numerous locations across multiple jurisdictions are limited. Initial prototypes or pilot projects are beginning to be reported in Germany, Taiwan, Europe, the United States, and Canada. In addition, the Canadian Network for the Advancement of Research, Industry and Education (CANARIE) is also examining ways to implement health projects using advanced telecommunication projects.

A common problem list, a complete drug profile, and patient allergies should be centrally stored, maintained, and accessible. Data must be readily shared among all the providers of care. The patient record must be a lifetime record, extending before birth to after death. The new HIS will contain character based data, image data, waveforms, drawings, digital pictures, motion videos, and voice and sound recordings. The networks tying these systems together must have a wide bandwidth to accommodate the volume of data, which must be exchanged in real time among facilities. Electronic mail could provide easy linkage among the providers requesting consults and discussing a patient's care. A clinically rich common medical and health vocabulary whose major purpose is communication needs to be created and used by all stakeholders. Confidentiality and privacy issues must be adequately supported with patient consent for the sharing of data.

The new systems must support source data capture, most specifically by primary care providers (e.g., midwives, nurses, physicians, dentists, acupuncturists, traditional caregivers, psychologists, social workers). Ideally, decision support systems would also be available at or near the point of care (see Chapter 6 for more discussion). Most computer support algorithms are useful only if they are interactive with the person making the clinical decision at the time of decision making. Workstations customized for physicians, nurses, and other clinical caregivers as well as administrators and researchers will be mandatory for tomorrow's systems. The move toward managed care increases the necessity for informed, algorithmic driven order sets. Decision support systems, operating in the background, will save much money as well as improving patient care. As an example, a typical physician session involving ordering tests and prescribing treatment may typically invoke several thousand decision rules. These decision rules need to be standardized and shared by the international community.

## Prerequisites for EHISs

A prototype for a EHS incorporating a multimedia, lifelong, multisite Computerized Patient Record was designed and implemented at the University Hospital in Grosshadern, Germany. The essential design elements identified included are described next.

## *Data Model*

The data model describes the medical concepts (e.g., blood pressure) that can be recorded in the electronic patient file and handled by the patient record system. The concepts are based on technical objects (e.g., figures, test, and video) whose properties and relations are explicitly defined in at data object dictionary.

## *Presentation Types*

Medical items must be modified, displayed, and communicated. A set of basic methods exists that allows the manipulation, presentation, and communication of medical items that are controlled by a large number of parameters. Presentations must be adapted to the specialized needs of individual patient care environments and corresponding patient care requirements. Examples of presentation types include, but must not be limited to, forms, graphs, images, text, and audio.

## Communication

The computerized medical record in an EHIS environment requires standardized protocols (e.g., HL7, EDI, EDIFACT, DICOM) for exchange of data among different systems.

## Interpreter

An interpreter provides analysis, presentation, and communication of patient data in the computerized patient record system. While global communication techniques make the creation of telemedicine (EHIS) records possible, there are still major barriers, notably the absence of data and communication standards and the lack of public acceptance (see Chapter 8 for more discussion).

Experience in Calgary, Canada, with a virtual health clinic has been developed through a collaboration of the Alberta Research Council, the University of Calgary, the Calgary Regional Health Authority, Clinicare Corporation, and the Lupus Society of Alberta. The overall strategy has been to focus on health care delivery to people with chronic relapsing-remitting conditions. Not only are these the most vulnerable citizens in society, but information is critical to their well being. In addition, the health care system may expend up to 30 times more resources on these individuals than on people without chronic conditions. Estimates indicate that up to 30% of the expenditure could be saved with appropriate use of information systems to ensure that hospitalizations are used effectively, medications are not overprescribed, and diagnostic testing is not redundant. The project was based on the premise that providing patients with information and self-management tools through the Internet is key to success in providing effective care more efficiently.

The goal of this project was to provide a secure, confidential environment for patients and their providers on the Internet. This environment provided a unique opportunity for the delivery and exchange of health care information. During the initial phase (January 1996 to 1998) modules were developed and tested for standard presentation of patient symptoms, laboratory evaluation, patient education, and communication with diverse care providers. Standard modules are under development for care providers, including family practitioners, specialists, nurses, and physiotherapists. The virtual health clinic can support software tools such as clinical practice guidelines that pertain to a given case, geographical information regarding resources which are useful for self-management, communication with key providers, and a secure site for the storage of medical information such as symptoms, signs, medications, and laboratory results. Patients and physicians are using the Virtual Health Clinic using an Internet/Intranet approach. The patient–caregiver dyad is the focus, and they have been included in planning and testing.

Thus, as illustrated by the preceding example, EHISs must have a broad multidisciplinary focus on health services delivery including community needs assessment, population health status indicators, health promotion, and disease prevention in addition to the treatment of illness. EHISs can and should support the reengineering and restructuring that is occurring in many health care organizations and health services delivery systems. Many of the data presently available are inadequate for these tasks; therefore, current data must be transformed and future information requirements anticipated to support the reengineering of health care enterprises and organizations using EHIS.

## Producing Value Added Information

Future EHISs need to take into the account the fundamental principle that the reason a health care delivery system exists in any jurisdiction is to provide health services to its citizens. Thus, administrative and managerial information for use in operating the health care delivery enterprise should be a by-product of the care delivery process. One can envision a future environment in which current information about health facilities and health care delivery systems for use in enterprise planning and policies as well as resource allocation and utilization will need to be much more widely available to the professional care providers than in the past.

As reengineering or restructuring proceeds, Information Products of interest to health system decision makers include:

- Residents: information about the health needs and health status of the population, their families, and communities
- Recipients: information about residents receiving services from the health services enterprise
- Providers: information about available persons and organizations with health service skills (health workforce)
- Services: information about the range of health-affecting interventions and activities available in the health system
- Programs: information about the objectives, target recipients/populations, resource allocation, and bundling of particular sets of services
- Resources: distribution of fiscal (financial), physical (facilities and equipment), human (people working within the health services enterprise), and information resources
- Utilization: use of resources by service provider (by whom are services provided), by service recipient (to whom are services provided), by program and by type of service.

# Impact of EHISs

The impact of EHISs, which provide health care information over wide areas in a secure manner, is profound. Such availability could potentially allow for data mining of information that would enable:

- Using the information to discover and analyze associations between disease entities and previously unknown risk factors (recorded in the patient history).
- Testing hypotheses regarding putative risk factors, or to study disease distribution using demographic data.
- Enabling a physician to do a comparative analysis of a particular patient's symptoms with the symptoms of other patients with similar or different diseases.
- More intelligent video consultations. During these consultation, along with the video, specialists in multiple locations could simultaneously see and annotation a patient's record.
- Improved outcome analysis.
- Decision support information.
- Better education of patients to manage their own health.

As we move into a new century, the major problems that hospitals have experienced with hospital information systems can be resolved, if the emerging health enterprises learn from the past experiences of others. They must realistically address the following issues:

- The complex information and communication structure related to patient care can be improved by redesigning and reengineering the functions and process of institutions to capitalize on the efficiencies permitted by modern information management techniques and equipment.
- Involve caregivers (including nursing) in the design and implementation stage.
- Every health enterprise should develop a strategic business plan that provides the foundation for its information management strategic plan. The information management strategic plan is implemented using tactical and operation plans.
- The development of client/server architectures and graphical user interfaces, working with powerful database software and proven application software that is flexible, can now be reasonably implemented.
- Staffing continues to be a major problem. Our academic institutions must address the need for health informatics preparation at all levels of education: undergraduate, graduate, and continuing education.
- With the arrival of reliable software and more graphical user interfaces, the use of information management technology can be expected to benefit the patient.

As we look toward enterprise information systems from the perspective of where health informatics has been, where it is now, what we have learned, and where we will be heading in the next century, there is no doubt that the following observations are true:

- Nursing will play a major role in EHIS development.
- Information management, as applied to a wide variety of health care disciplines, is a proven reality and will continue to expand for the foreseeable future.
- Financial data processing has been the mainstay in hospital computing, but is rapidly being superseded by clinical, administrative, management, and educational applications. In the future the core of enterprise health information systems will be the patient care data, with all other uses being value added reprocessing of these data.
- The introduction of client/server architectures and networks into the health arena is revolutionizing the older concepts of centralized data processing.
- Real-time distributed use, in conjunction with central data storage, data warehousing, or info-mart technology, will continue as a rapidly growing trend.
- Cost of hardware has decreased, making new options for the user increasingly feasible. Indeed, major technological changes will influence the entire medical and health science professions.
- Advances in technology will enable the use of multiple media to capture store and retrieve data and information
- Government policy statements will lead to further growth and support of health informatics. This has further implications for information management regarding rural medicine.
- A final prediction is that in the next century, caregivers, including nurses, will have personal workstations with capacity to access and navigate through databases in remote geographic locations.

Advantages for nurses accruing from the use of an EHIS include the following:

- Timesaving through reducing clerical activities, telephone calls between departments, and hand-written information transfer.
- Greater accuracy and speed of information transfer.
- Continuity of care through the current and status documentation available on the system for the nurse.
- Elimination of duplicate effort and more effective use of personnel provide financial savings for the patient and time savings for the nurse.
- More complete patient records and data for patient care, quality assurance, and research.

These advantages relate to nursing practice in the same way as the previously identified advantages of automation. Time saved from manual information processing tasks provides more time for the nursing process. More complete patient records, greater accuracy, and the increased speed of transferring information facilitate the nursing assessment. A more effective use of personnel and continuity of care can only result in better quality care for patients.

## Conclusion

Countries around the globe are searching for ways to simultaneously improve the delivery of health care and reduce the costs connected with providing this care. The ultimate goal of sustaining and improving the health status of the population of a local state, national, or even international community purportedly guides all such efforts. An interesting phenomenon surrounding the changes being undertaken in a number of health care systems emerges when even cursory comparisons of various attempts are drawn. Various countries demonstrate remarkable differences in approach, sometimes even the adoption of strategies that seem to move their health care systems in opposite directions (e.g., health reform initiatives within the British National Health Services, Canadian provincial health care systems, and the United States provide striking examples). Yet, these initiatives and many others all claim to support the improvement of health care and health status among their respective populations. The common goal is "Health for All." However, if health systems are changing in different ways for the same reasons, can all the strategies for change be effective ones? How will these be evaluated? How will the outcomes of the health systems and of health services be evaluated? Previous concepts of the scope of a Hospital Information System must change along with changes in the health care process and the restructuring of national and regional health systems. The functionality presently provided by such systems merely provides a base for beginning the development of the Health Information Systems of the future. Information is key and information systems are essential to enabling and informing the delivery of health services and the effectiveness of national health systems.

## *References*

Jackson, G.G. Information handling costs in hospitals. *Datamation* 1969;15:56.

McHugh, M., and Schultz, S. Computer technology in hospital nursing departments: Future applications and implications. In: Blum, B.I. (ed.) *Proceedings, Sixth Annual Symposium on Computer Applications in Medical Care.* Los Angeles: IEEE, 1982:557–561.

Office of Technology Assessment, Congress of the United States. Health Care Online: The Role of Information Technologies. Washington DC: US Government Printing Office OTA-ITC-624, Sept. 1995.

## *Additional Resources*

Adelhard, K., Eckel, R., Holzel, D., and Tretter, W. Design elements of a telemedical medical record. In: Cimino, J.J. (ed.) *Proceedings, AMIA Fall Symposium*, 1996:473–477.

Alvarez, R.C., Curry, J., Hodge, T., Chatwin, B.J., and Hannah, K.J. A provincial health information processing strategy: A case study. In: Lunn, K.C., Degoulet, P., Piemme, T.E., and Reinhoff, O. (eds.) *Medinfo '92 Proceedings*. Amsterdam: North-Holland, 1992.

Ballardini, L., Mazzoleni, M.C., Tramarin R., Caprotti, M. Remote management of a cardiac magnetic resonance imaging session by a low cost teleconsulting system. In: Cimino, J.J. (ed.) *Proceedings, AMIA Fall Symposium*, 1996:825.

CANARIE Inc. Towards a Canadian Health Iway: Vision, Opportunities and Future Steps. Ottawa, 1996.

Chang, I.F., Suarez, H.H., Ho, L.C., Cheung, P.S., and Ke, J.S. Nationwide implementation of telemedicine and CPR systems in Taiwan. In: Cimino, J.J. (ed.) *Proceedings, AMIA Fall Symposium*, 1996:878.

Donsez, Didier, Tiers, Gonzague, Modjeddi, Bijan, Beuscart, Regis. Improving the continuity of care: the ISAR—Telematics European Project. In: Cimino, J.J. (ed.) *Proceedings, AMIA Fall Symposium*, 1996:890.

Forslund, D.W., Phillips, R.L., Kilman, D.G., Cook, J.L. Experiences with a distributed virtual patient record system. In: Cimino, J.J. (ed.) *Proceedings, AMIA Fall Symposium*, 1996:483–487.

Hannah, K.J. Transforming information: Data management support of health care reorganization. *Journal of the American Medical Informatics Association*, 1995; 2(3):147–155.

# 6
# Nursing Aspects of Health Information Systems

## Nursing Information Systems

Motivation for the development and implementation of computerized hospital information systems has been financial and administrative, i.e., driven by the need to capture charges and document patient care for legal reasons The majority of systems marketed today have been motivated by those two factors. Historically, such systems have required a major investment in hardware (typically a mainframe), and, even though they have demonstrated significant improvement in hospital communications (with a corresponding reduction in paper flow), they have been characteristically weak in supporting professional nursing practice. These factors have prevented the level of acceptance by nurses that was originally foreseen. Only recently have developers and vendors begun to consider the nature of modern nursing practice and its information processing requirements (see Figure 6.1).

If one considers the original principles that Campbell (1978) identified when looking at the activities nurses perform when caring for patients, nursing roles fall into three global categories. The first is managerial roles or coordinating activities, for example, order entry, results reporting, requisition generation, and telephone booking of appointments. Current hospital information systems can help nurses with those activities. The second category is physician-delegated tasks. Current systems can capture these from the physicians" order entry set and then incorporate them into the patient care plan. The third category is the autonomous nursing function, characteristic of professional nursing practice, when knowledge unique to nursing is applied to patient care. Current systems are beginning to support nurses in fulfilling their responsibilities in this category. All three categories—managerial/coordinating, physician-delegated, and autonomous nursing function—must fit together to create a fully operational system. Current systems, while they release nurses to focus on professional nursing practice, fail to provide the appropriate support essential to professional nursing practice. The future will require decision-making support for professional nursing practice and the capture of information from the patient care plan

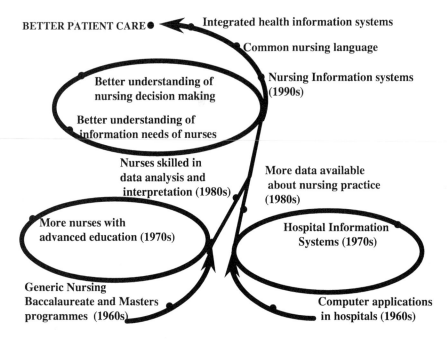

**FIGURE 6.1.** Evolution of Nursing Information Systems.

for nursing administration decision making related to nursing resource allocation.

From an economic point of view, the combination of the shrinking health care dollar and escalating health care costs makes it imperative that the productivity issues associated with nursing dollars spent be considered. To that end, a comprehensive nursing management information system is necessary. The major objective of such systems would be the provision of information upon which decisions can be made that will effectively and efficiently allocate nursing resources for the highest quality of patient care. Nursing management information systems need to integrate the clinical data about patients that ultimately impact on the cost of providing patient care. Historically, nursing costs have never been reliably projected because they did not incorporate fluctuating patient acuity levels and the associated needs for nursing care. Based on its integration of patient clinical data, the system will ultimately ascertain costs of nursing care for individual patients. This costing must incorporate multiple components such as quality and workload measurements, financials (payroll and general ledger), and staff utilization, as well as contractual obligations and costs. Such a nursing management system enables the development of productivity standards by which one can compare patient care outcomes as well as variance analysis, which enables the manager to rationalize deviations from the budget. Furthermore, when the nursing costs associated with patient type are accurately and reliably quantified, such a system has great potential in forecasting and long-range planning. This ability has potential for health care planning that incorporates costs associated with patient care groupings. On an operational level, the nursing management information system will include human resource capabilities such as staff profiles, educational levels, and scheduling, all of which facilitate effective development and deployment of nursing resources.

The overall goal must be developing a comprehensive, integrated nursing information system. Such a system will have the capacity to integrate with, and build upon, a variety of hospital information systems. It needs to be independent, but also compatible and capable of interfacing with existing installed hospital information systems. It will capitalize on the distributed processing concept, communication capacity of networks, and the power of client server architectures to provide clinical workstations for decision support. The achievement of such a goal will require the application and use of existing technology in an innovative manner.

Developments in nursing informatics must assist the nurse in the gathering and aggregating of nursing data to make decisions related to the nursing care of patients. Modern nursing practice no longer focuses on the assessment and care planning phase of the nursing process. Instead, it emphasizes decision making, and exercising clinical nursing judgment in patient care. Because of the growing complexity of patient care and the rising acuity level of patients in hospitals today, nurses have acquired an expanded repertoire of intervention skills. These nursing intervention skills reflect the autonomous aspects of nursing practice that are based on the body of nursing knowledge and the nurse's professional judgment. Autonomous nursing interventions are complementary to, not competitive with, physician-prescribed treatments.

How can technology help nurses care for patients? The ideal nursing system requires the technology for source data capture and considerable work by nurses on the development of the nursing knowledge base. Until recently, it was not possible to even consider such a system because the technology did not exist. Now that it does, the onus is on nursing to develop effective means of using the technology. From the nursing perspective, there are three major areas related to health information systems that need to be addressed in the immediate future. To provide information management assistance to nurses, the three areas of (1) source data capture, (2) nursing data standards, and (3) decision support systems must be addressed. These three areas are crucial to providing computer support for nurses in the delivery of patient care.

## Source Data Capture

In this context, source data capture means gathering data and information about patients where it originates, that is, with the patient. The concept of "terminals by the bedside" was introduced in the mid-1980s. Most experts agree that bringing the computer access closer to the patient, i.e., locating it at the "point of care," is a valid premise, and clinicians appear to favor the bedside terminal as a means to reduce much of the clerical workload and improve access to clinical data.

Point of care systems are still not in widespread use. Their potential has yet to be fully realized. As more facilities and organizations implement source data capture systems, including bedside terminals, the concept will gain acceptance in the industry and, in fact, become the standard for nursing systems. This conclusion is based also on the fact that significant funds are presently being channeled toward research and development of bedside and other "point of care" devices in Canada, the United States, and around the world.

## Criteria for Source Data Capture

Such technology must meet specific criteria. Specifically, it must permit nurses at the patient's bedside to interact with the main patient database and the main care planning system or hospital information system. It must have the capacity to interact with existing hospital information systems so that effort already expended in developing hospital information systems is not wasted. Such technology must be small and compact so as to occupy the minimum amount of space at the patient's bedside and, therefore, not interfere with the use of other important equipment necessary to the care of the patient. This technology must be rugged and durable. In addition, it must be constructed so that it can be disinfected between patients. Also, it must be easy and uncomplicated to use, and have high-resolution screens with graphics capability that can be read in the dark. Provision must be made for a variety of means of data entry, (e.g. bar code reader, physiological probe, digital camera, natural language, or keyboard). A volume control is necessary to mute any keyboard sounds. Moreover, because patients do not always stay in their beds, this type of technology must allow nurses the maximum degree of mobility to enter data wherever the patient may be. Two-way radio transmission of data should provide an acceptable level of security and confidentiality for patient information, perhaps by such means as encrypted data or irregular short burst transmissions. Much work remains to be done before a satisfactory system for source data capture is fully developed.

## Types of "Point of Care" Devices

Three types of "point of care" devices are presently available. The first is the standard stationary terminal. The most expedient approach to the concept of source data capture was to simply place a standard keyboard and monitor (i.e., a CRT) at the bedside; the Ulticare Systems uses this approach. The second type of terminal is specially designed for the purpose of source data capture. One variety of special-purpose terminal is a small footprint terminal, fixed at the bedside, and having special function keys for data input. The Criticom terminal is an example of this type of system. A second variety of specially designed "point of care" device is a hybrid solution that attaches to the wall in the patient's room when not in use but is portable and interactive within the patient's room. CliniCom's CliniCare is a good example of this type, as is the Ubitrex Terminal. The third type of device is a handheld portable terminal, not restricted to a particular space such as the patient's room. There is still far too little experience, in the health care field, with "point of care" or source data capture devices to allow consensus as to whether a fixed bedside terminal or a portable handheld terminal is best suited for both patient care and optimum system utilization. Portable devices are favored for a number of reasons, including better access by professionals, better control over access by patients, lower cost, and ease of service and maintenance.

## Uses of Source Data Capture in Health Care

The capacity for source data capture could be more greatly exploited by nurses if assessment guidelines and interview instruments were developed to be downloaded to the point of care device. Data input of responses in an interactive fashion at the patient's bedside would permit source data capture. More accurate documentation of patient care would be the first outcome. Ultimately, it should be possible to develop and deliver decision support systems for use at the patient's bedside. Clearly, the initial uses of such technology will be within acute care facilities. Eventually, extended-care facilities, long-term care facilities, occupational health, outpatient clinics, community health, and home care are prime areas for development of software for use with this technology. These areas have been sorely underserved by the health care computing industry primarily because until now the technology was unable to serve the highly mobile and geographically dispersed nature of practice in these fields of health care. With this technology, there is almost unlimited opportunity. It is also conceivable that this technology could be used in physicians' offices for hospital bookings and preadmission data gathering.

## Nursing Data Standards

Nurses continually use mental processes, often unconsciously, to organize information systematically by grouping data according to common features. We do this to make sense of the massive amounts of information with which we are daily bombarded. The problem arises because nurses do not have a common system or language to communicate precisely, even with each other. Lang has well described the situation: "If we cannot name it, we cannot control it, finance it, teach it, search it or put it into public policy" (Clark and Lang, 1992, p. 109). Because nursing has not had universally accepted methods for defining and collecting nursing data, nursing data has not been collected. For example, the patient discharge abstracts prepared by medical records departments in hospitals contain no nursing care delivery information. The abstracts, therefore, fail to acknowledge the contribution of nursing during the patient's stay in the hospital. The abstracts are used by many agencies for a variety of statistical and funding purposes. Patient discharge summaries need to include nursing workload data that recognize the personnel providing the care in addition to the substance of that care, i.e., the nursing components of patient care, the type of nursing care provided, and the impact of that care on patient outcome. Presently, much valuable information is being lost. This information is essential for nurses to be able to develop evidence-based practice. Data to support evidence-based practice is required not only for clinical practice, but also to inform evidence-based decision making by nurse managers. Therefore, as the development of nationwide health databases increases, it is vital that a minimum number of essential nursing elements be included in the databases.

There are a variety of concepts that interlink when considering the capture of nursing practice data. Figure 6.2 illustrates the derivation, from nursing practice, of nomenclature, language, classification systems, minimum data set, and the resulting feedback loop.

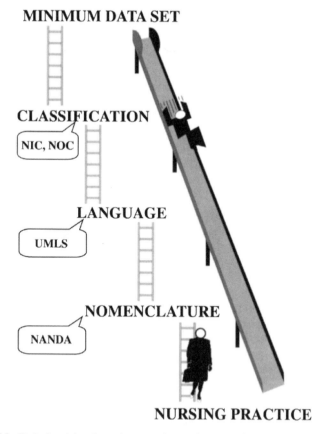

FIGURE 6.2. Relationship of nursing practice and nomenclature, language, classification, and minimum data set.

"The practicing nurse finds word (labels) for the elements of her/his practice. When these words are standardized among nurses, they can be called a nursing nomenclature. These word-labels can then be combined within a defined structure and systematic management to form a language system for nursing. From this point onward, the data that are labeled according to a nursing nomenclature, structured into a nursing language, and classified by means of common features, can be collated for inclusion in a nursing minimum data set which in turn can be fed back into nursing practice at the center of the spiral; and the continuos process of development, refinement and modification in response to external change begins again." (Clark and Lang, 1992, p. 11).

The following section describes the interaction of these concepts in the ways that different countries have addressed the need for nursing data standards.

# Historical Development

## *United States*

In the United States, a working conference was held in 1969 to develop that minimum basic set of data elements to be collected from all hospital records at the point of patient discharge from hospitals. Conference participants identified a need to organize information on the present operation of health care systems in a way that would help decision making about the control of rising health care costs, equitable distribution of services, and accountable resource use. At the same time, developments in the computer science field had made it possible to design programs to manage data (Murnaghan and White, 1970).

The idea of a Uniform Hospital Discharge Data Set (UHDDS) emerged from a discussion by key health care providers and health data users after a set of commissioned working papers were presented at that conference. In gaining consensus on the minimum data elements required by multiple users, the conferees focused on the justification of data elements in terms of availability, utility, reliability, and cost associated with collection of these data (Murnaghan and White, 1970). The UHDDS underwent testing, evaluation, and revisions in the early 1970s.

In 1974 the UHDDS was adopted and mandated by the Secretary of the Department of Health and Human Services for collection by the U.S. National Committee on Vital and Health Statistics (Abdellah, 1988; Pearce, 1988). Specific criteria, guidelines, and processes for development of minimum data sets have evolved, resulting in reviews of the UHDDS over the years (Abdellah, 1988; Pearce, 1988). These reviews resulted in the endorsement of the data elements, with significant changes to the definitions of procedures and diagnoses to promote uniform accurate data collection (National Center for Health Statistics, 1972, 1980).

The care items included in the UHDDS focus on physician-derived clinical data through the inclusion of medical diagnosis and procedures based on medical treatments. Absolutely *no* nursing clinical data were included in this data set. Patient care is not exclusively physician directed; therefore, a data set of this nature falls short of providing a complete, accurate representation of information related to the operation of hospitals. In response to the recognition of the information gap created by the exclusion of nursing data elements from the Uniform Hospital Discharge Data Set, Werley and colleagues developed the Nursing Minimum Data Set (NMDS) in 1985, building on initial work by Werley and colleagues in 1977. A Nursing Minimum Data Set (NMDS) was defined by Werley (1988) as "a minimum set of items of information with uniform definitions and categories concerning the specific dimension of professional nursing, which meets the information needs of multiple data users in the health care system" (p. 7). There were five purposes of the NMDS: establish comparability of nursing data across practice settings and geographic boundaries, capture descriptors reflecting the nursing care of clients and their families in a variety of settings, project trends in nursing care needs and resource use according to health problems, provide a database for nursing research, and provide data about nursing care for consideration by individuals involved in health policy decision making.

The NMDS, achieved through a consensus conference at the University of Wisconsin-Milwaukee School of Nursing, consisted of nursing care elements, patient demographic elements, and service elements. The nursing care elements of nursing diagnosis, nursing intervention, nursing outcome, and intensity of nursing care drew on the nursing process used by the nurse in the planning and provision of patient care in any setting. The patient demographic and service elements, except health record number and the unique number of the nurse provider, are data elements contained in the Uniform Hospital Discharge Data Set and would be accessed through linkage with this data set.

The North American Nursing Diagnosis Association (NANDA) has provided a formal structure for the development and testing of nursing diagnosis. NANDA has defined nursing diagnosis as ". . . *a clinical judgment about individual, family, or community responses to actual and potential health problems and life processes. Nursing diagnoses provide the basis for selection of nursing interventions to achieve outcomes of which the nurse is accountable*" (Carpenito, 1989).

NANDA has at least five levels of abstraction, moving from Level 1 (most abstract) to Level 5 (most concrete and deemed most clinically useful). The human response patterns constitute the most abstract level (Level 1) and provide the organizing framework for the system. There are nine Human Response Patterns, which are choosing, communicating, exchanging, feeling, knowing, moving, perceiving, relating, and valuing (Saba, 1993). In the second level of abstraction there are 29 categories. NANDA has a total of 104 diagnostic labels.

The Omaha Classification System is a client-focused management information system based on the nursing process. It illustrates the mutuality of the nurse–client relationship and provides a framework for integrating clinical data with other essential personnel and financial data in an automated information system. The client status segment of the system is called the Problem Classification Scheme (PCS). It consists of 44 patient problems considered to be community health client problems and nursing problems used for documenting community health nursing services. A problem is defined as *a clinical judgment about environmental, psychosocial, physiologic and health related behavior data that is of interest or concern to the client* (Martin and Scheet, 1992).

The Omaha System was developed during a series of four research contracts between the Visiting Nurses Association (VNA) of Omaha and the Division of Nursing, Public Health Service, U.S. Department of Health and Human Services from 1975 to 1993. The result was the development of the Problem Classification Scheme, Intervention Scheme, and Problem Rating Scale for Outcomes.

The Home Health Care Classification (HHCC) was developed at the Georgetown University School of Nursing from 1988 to 1991 to assess and classify home health Medicare clients to predict their need for nursing and other home care services, as well as measure outcomes and data on actual measures of resources employed (Saba, 1992, p. 50) NANDA's definition of nursing diagnosis was adopted for this method. Twenty Home Health Care Components provide the framework for the classification and coding of nursing diagnoses and nursing interventions. The components were empirically developed to categorize, process, and statistically analyze the data. The client status classification system of the HHCC is called Nursing Diagnosis. The HHCC coding structure links and maps the six steps of the care process. The HHCC of Nursing Diagnosis is structured and coded according to the tenth revision of the International Classification of Diseases (ICD-10), which was developed by the World Health Organization. ICD is the Classification used to develop Diagnostic Related Groups (DRGs) used by hospitals for reimbursement of in-hospital patient services by third-party payers.

Nursing interventions were defined in the HHCC: Nursing Interventions (HHCC:NI) as a nursing service, significant treatment, intervention, or activity identified to carry out the medical or nursing order (Saba, 1992). Nursing interventions were considered to be critical measures of the actual resources used. Nursing Interventions Classification (NIC) was developed by a large research team (the Iowa Intervention Project), led by McCloskey and Bulechek at the University of Iowa. This team defined nursing interventions as "any treatment, based upon clinical judgment and knowledge, that a nurse performs to enhance patient/client outcomes. Nursing interventions include both direct and indirect care; both nurse-initiated, physician-initiated and other-provider-initiated treatments" (McClosky and Bulechek 1996, p. xvii). Through literature review, expert opinion, and focus groups, 6 domains, 26 classes and 336 interventions were identified (Bulechek et al., 1994). Each intervention consists of a label, a definition, a list of activities for implementing the intervention, and a set of readings related to it.

NIC was coded to be consistent with the Current Procedural Terminology, the American Medical Association, and the Health Care Financing Administration's Common Procedure Coding System and was included in the Library of Medicine's *Metathesaurus for a Unified Medical Language.* Additionally, it has been endorsed by the ANA for inclusion in the proposed Unified Nursing Language System (McCloskey and Bulechek, 1996; McCormick et al., 1994). NIC provides a standardized language that can be used across settings and across health care disciplines (McCloskey and Bulechek, 1996). Both independent and collaborative interventions as well as basic and complex interventions were included.

A Nursing Outcomes Classification System (NOC) has also been developed in conjunction with the NIC through the Iowa Intervention Project (Johnson et al., 1997). The NOC should be watched for future development as its links to NIC and thus NANDA I and Omaha hold promise for a consolidated system. NANDA, The Omaha System, the Home Health Care Classification, and the NIC have been included in Unified Medical Language System (UMLS). The UMLS is a long-term research project developed by the U.S. National Library of Medicine to integrate clinical vocabularies from various sources so that data from each can be cross-referenced when needed.

## *Canada*

In Canada, the Management Information System (MIS) Group evolved through a merger of the Management Information System Project and the National Hospital Productivity Improvement Program in 1989. The MIS Group developed data collection guidelines that focus primarily on financial and statistical data with limited capture of patient clinical data. Besides demographic data, the clinical data are limited to resource consumption data and data required for record abstracts. These data are, again, limited to physician-derived data. Thus, there are *no* clinical nursing data elements captured and stored based on the MIS Guidelines.

The Hospital Medical Records Institute (HMRI) was founded in 1963 by the Ontario Hospital Association and Government of Ontario to develop a health care database. In 1977 the HMRI became an independent, federally chartered organization for the purpose of health care data management. The HMRI gathers data abstracted from patient hospital records and processes these data to provide information to health care providers, managers, and planners to aid in the delivery of health services (Youngblut, 1991). Because submission of abstracted medical record data to the HMRI is not mandated by all provincial health ministries, the HMRI database falls short of being a national database. The care items included in this data set are limited to physician-derived data including most responsible diagnosis, primary diagnosis, secondary diagnosis, and procedures. Noteworthy, again, is the *total absence* of clinical nursing data.

In the Canadian province of Alberta, the Alberta Association of Registered Nurses (AARN) has shown that it recognizes the importance of the development of an NMDS through initiatives that include (1) establishing the definition of an NMDS as a priority in the 1991–1992 year and (2) submission of a resolution to the Canadian Nurses Association (CNA) in June 1990 calling for a national consensus conference "to develop in Canada a standardized format (Nursing Minimum Data Set) for purposes of ensuring entry, accessibility, and retrievability of nursing data." This resolution was adopted for action by the CNA. Initiatives directed at the development of an NMDS in other provinces have not been reported in the literature.

At the Canadian national level, the CNA responded to the AARN's NMDS resolution by organizing an invitational conference, with national representation, held in Alberta in the fall of 1992. The focus of the conference was the discussion of the content for and issues related to the development of an NMDS. This was the first conference in Canada to be devoted solely to the discussion of this important topic.

In 1996, CIHI (Canadian Institute for Health Information) formed the Partnership for Health Informatics/Telematics, to give leadership to shaping the national agenda for information and technology standards in health care. The goals of the Partnership are to define and adopt emerging standards for health informatics and telematics to ensure the evolution of a nonredundant, nonconflicting set of standards for Canada; collaborate with other standards-setting organizations in Canada and internationally; and utilize the standards to enable the development of a national, longitudinal electronic health records, accessible to health providers, researchers, and policy makers as well as health monitoring and surveillance agencies (CIHI, 1997). One of the activities of a working group of the Partnership has been the development of the Canadian Classification of Health Interventions (CCI). The CCI differs from the classifications systems developed in the United States in that it is service provider and service setting neutral. This means that the same codes are intended to be applicable regardless of whether a physician, nurse, or respiratory technologist performed the intervention and whether the intervention was performed in an operating room, an emergency department, a clinic, or a practitioner's office. Service provider and service setting information are captured as separate data elements in the client record.

## United Kingdom

In the United Kingdom, in response to widespread discontent with the National Health Service (NHS) information system, and with the recognition of the need for information to enable clinicians to manage resources, a full-scale investigation of the NHS information system was undertaken in 1979. This investigation revealed problems with the collection, processing, timeliness, accuracy, and comparability of data. These findings gave rise to the Steering Group on Health Services Information. The major aim of this group was the production of relevant, timely, accurate information to assist health service managers. Further, the group attended to the need for consistency in definitions, and to aggregation and linkage of data sources to provide information (National Health Service/Department of Health and Social Security Steering Group on Health Service Information [NHS], 1982).

Through the formation of working groups consisting of members from the National Health Service, the Department of Health and Social Security, and the Office for Population, Censuses and Surveys, the Steering Group on Health Service Information completed its work. Guided by the aims previously outlined, the steering group identified, defined, and tested those data elements to be included in a national health services data set and developed strategies for the collection of these data. The activities of the Steering Group on Health Services Information culminated in the production of a seven-volume report referred to as "The Körner Report," outlining the collection of data and use of information about hospital clinical activity (NHS, 1982); ambulance services (NHS, 1984a); manpower (NHS, 1984b); activity in hospitals and the community (NHS, 1984c); services for and in the community (NHS, 1984d); and finance (NHS, 1984e).

The Körner data set, again, focuses on physician-derived clinical data, through the inclusion of codes for tracking the general practitioner, medical diagnosis, and operations, and this data set is devoid of nursing clinical data. However, Wheeler (1991) indicates that the Körner data set has evolved to include nursing elements, a step that reflects the changing role of nurses in the U.K. The specific nursing elements include "nursing episode," which reflects episodes for which nurses are totally responsible for care; "right of admission," which defines who admits the patient since nurses now have admitting privileges; and "nursing home operational plan," which reflects the planning intent and focuses on facilities offered by nurses in units run by nurses (Wheeler, 1991). Despite these developments these nursing data elements focus only on facilities and not on nursing activities.

The U.K. has been integrally involved in the International Council of Nurses (ICN) International Classification of Nursing Practice (ICNP) project. The ICNP project, begun in 1990, aims to develop a standardized vocabulary and classification of nursing phenomena (nursing diagnosis), nursing interventions, and nursing outcomes that can be used in both electronic and paper records to describe and compare nursing practice across clinical settings. An Alpha Version of the Classification of Nursing Phenomena and Nursing Interventions was released for further development and testing in 1996 and an outline for a Classification of Nursing Outcomes, in 1997 (Clark, 1997). It is anticipated that the Beta Version will be available in 1999. The Alpha Version has been circulated to all National Nurses Associations for feedback. In Europe, the TELENURSE Project, begun in 1996 to initiate the definition and implementation of a strategy to promote the use of common structures and processes across Europe, has translated the Alpha Version into several languages and is testing aspects of the use of the ICNP in electronic patient records (Clark, 1997; Yensen, 1996).

## Issues in the Development of a Nursing Minimum Data Set

As nurses embark on the development of nursing data standards, several issues emerge. Attention must be directed to the coordination and linkage of data. Three aspects of data linkage demand attention. First, the computer hardware must support database linkage. Second, the content of the nursing data standard must be developed in a way that lends itself to integration with other information. Finally, the ethics of data linkage with respect to patient information, including security confidentiality and privacy of data, must be addressed. Integration will be a key consideration as the developments in various countries converge. Once nursing data standards are developed, three more issues emerge: (1) promoting the idea to ensure widespread use, (2) educating the users to ensure the quality of the data that are collected, and (3) establishing mechanisms for review and revision of the data elements.

## Decision Support Systems

Nursing literature regarding decision support systems exhibits confusion and lack of clarity because of the various definitions and conceptualizations. It is characterized by authors who use the same term to refer to different concepts or who use different terms for the same concept. A broad definition, that has some professional consensus, is that computerized decision support systems (CDS or DSS) include "any computer software employing a knowledge base (facts and/or rules) designed for use by a clinician involved in patient care, as a direct aid to clinical decision making" (Langton et al., 1992, p. 626). There is a consensus among authors that decision support systems be used to extend the nurse's decision making capacity rather than to replace it. The majority of care planning systems now in use are not decision support systems. Standardized care plans, whether manual or computer based, only provide care for standardized patients! Standardized care plans neither enhance nor support nursing decision-making; on the contrary, their "cookbook" approach discourages active decision-making by nurses. Therefore, they are not congruent with a professional practice model of nursing.

A decision support system for nursing practice is intended to support nurses by providing them with information to facilitate rational decision-making about patients" care. In other words, decision support systems help nurses to maintain and maximize their decision-making responsibilities and focus on the highest priority aspects of patient care. The major caveat that must be considered in a professional practice model of nursing is that clinical judgment that considers contextual factors as well as the recommendations of decision support systems must be exercised. In addition, because the current status of computer technology and understanding human cognition restricts the performance of such systems, nurses must be discriminating users of these systems and ensure that the systems are providing appropriate recommendations before acting on the output of such systems.

Eddy (1990) believes that the complexity of modern health care has now exceeded the limitations of the unaided human mind. Decision support systems offer great potential to assist nurses to handle the volumes of data and information required. Pryor (1994) has identified six major uses of decision support:

1. Alerting: Alerting systems are those which notify the clinician of an immediate problem that calls for a prompt action or decision. These alerts are commonly clinician alerts that appear on the screen at time of entry of orders, assessments, or laboratory values. These systems may also provide management alerts based on problems with an individual patient (DRG cost overrun), or an individual clinician (use of expensive resources not generally warranted).

2. Interpretation: This type of CDS system is one that works to interpret particular data such as electrocardiogram or blood gases. A system such as this works by assimilating the data and transforming it into a conceptual understanding or interpretation. The interpretation is then presented to the clinician for use in decision making.

3. Assisting: A system that is used to speed or simplify clinician interactions with the computer is classified as an assisting system. These systems usually assist in the ordering or charting process by offering the clinician such things as standing order lists, patient-specific drug dosing, or appropriate parameters for charting based on earlier identified patient problems.

4. Critiquing: Systems that do this are primarily in the research stage and not yet available for implementation. This type of system is designed to critique a set of orders for particular problems. For example, a clinician might enter orders for a change in respirator settings which the system would then critique in light of the most recently entered blood gases. The clinician would be presented with an alternate set of orders and the rationale for changes made. The clinician would have the option of accepting or rejecting the changes suggested by the computer.

5. Diagnosing: This type of decision support system uses general assessment data to generate suggested diagnoses. These systems may then ask for additional data so as to rule out, rule in, or otherwise refine the list of diagnostic possibilities. Other systems that can be considered in this category are those that provide predictive scoring of mortality, estimation of treatment benefits based on effects of competing risks, or prediction of specific risks (pressure ulcers, falls).

6. Managing: The computer automatically generates the treatment or plan of care from assessment data and/or diagnostic categories and the nurse or physician then critiques the computer and its logic. While those systems with fixed protocols are easy to program and to implement, the lack of individualization leaves the clinician with the job of extensive critiquing. This type of system can be used in a developmental manner, however, so that clinicians give a rationale for changing the plan or the protocol and this is used to determine further data needs and decision rules so that the protocols are further refined. The variation in intervention and the rationale offered can be combined with data of outcomes of care, to determine which interventions are most effective in producing the desired outcome, so the refined protocols result in a progressively higher quality of care (p. 300).

## Knowledge Based Systems

All the six types of decision support systems outlined have are combined in a knowledge based or expert system. For the sake of simplicity, the term expert system is used here to encompass advisory systems and knowledge based systems. The purpose of expert systems is to recommend solutions to nursing problems that reflect the judgment of nurse experts regarding the most expedient response to nursing situations. Expert systems capture or encapsulate, in a computer system, the knowledge of a human expert within a particular domain of practice. Their function is to mimic the clinical reasoning and judgment of one specific human expert in the aggregation and interpretation of data in a precisely defined area of practice. Expert systems are characterized by use of artificial intelligence principles, specifically, symbolic representation of specialist knowledge to make decisions within a specified domain; the capacity to interrogate the user sensibly;

explanation of reasoning (rationale) underlying a decision on request by the user; and incorporation into the knowledge base of systematic feedback about the effects of decisions.

General approaches used as the basis for expert systems are knowledge engineering elicitation of a knowledge base and decision rules from an expert; actuarial data that are based on multiple observations of patient encounters; and objective probability that is based on the subjective judgment of multiple experts using heuristics, to determine what a reasonable professional nurse would decide in a particular situation. The components of an expert system include a knowledge base, an inference engine, a patient database, and a user interface. The knowledge base may incorporate that which constitutes empirically validated research; clinical experience based heuristics; and authority, tradition, and textbooks. An inference engine deals with the interpretation of knowledge using such techniques as logical deduction (decision rules), semantic networks, and logical relationships (Bayesian, probabilistic, or "fuzzy" logic). The patient database is composed of the data gathered from the patient who is the subject of the decisions. The user interface provides the capacity for natural language communication with the system to enable the user to pose questions and to enter and receive information. The most widely reported examples of nursing expert systems for use in clinical practice are the Creighton On-line Multiple Modular Expert System (COMMES), Cyber Nurse, and Computer-Aided Nursing Diagnosis and Intervention (CANDI).

There is still much work to be done, both in considering the implications of expert systems in a care giving environment and in actually developing and implementing expert systems. Issues that remain outstanding relate to legal liability, ethical concerns such as privacy, confidentiality and data integrity when using electronic patient records, and professional practice. Expert systems, integrated into nursing information systems and hospital information systems, informed by source data capture and made possible through nursing data standards, offer the potential to significantly impact the evidence-based practice of nurses to the end of enhancing patient care.

## Conclusion

As hospital information systems moved beyond the developmental stage and were marketed and installed on a wide scale, they provided nurses with access to a great deal of information about their practice and increased the time needed to analyze and consider this information. Simultaneously, the level of educational preparation of nurses began to rise with the proliferation of master's and doctoral programs that produced a cadre of nurses with much greater appreciation for, as well as sophistication and skill at, data analysis and research. We believe that the consequence of this concurrent evolution of both technology and the nursing profession will be advances of astronomical proportions in nursing practice. We are just beginning to initiate the cycle whereby information availability promotes greater under-standing of nursing decision making and diagnosis. This, in turn, not only facilitates a higher level functioning of nurses, but also generates additional information and further stimulates the cycle.

# *References*

Abdellah, F.G. Future directions: Refining, implementing, testing, and evaluating the Nursing Minimum Data Set. In: Werley, H.H., and Lang, N.M. (eds.) *Identification of the Nursing Minimum Data Set*. New York: Springer, 1988:416–426.

Bulechek, G.M., McCloskey, J., Titler, M., and Demehey, J. Nursing interventions used in practice. *American Journal of Nursing* 1994;94(10):59–63.

Canadian Institute for Health Information (CIHI). *Controlled Clinical Vocabularies: Background Document*. Ottawa, Canada: Canadian Institute for Health Information, 1997.

Campbell, C. *Nursing Diagnosis and Nursing Intervention*. New York: John Wiley and Sons, 1978.

Carpenito, L.J. Nursing Diagnosis. In: Arherican Nurses' Association, *Classification systems for describing nursing practice*. Working Papers (pp. 13–19). Kansas City, Mo.: American Nurses' Association, 1989.

Clark, J. The international classification for nursing practice: a progress report. Nursing Informatics. In: Gerdin, U., Tallberg, M., and Wainwright, P. (eds.) *The Impact of Nursing Knowledge on Health Care Informatics*. Amsterdam: IOS Press, 1997:62–68.

Clark, J., and Lang, N. Nursing's next advance: An international classification for nursing practice. *International Journal of Nursing* 1992;39(4):102–112, 128.

Eddy, D.M. Practice policies: Where do they come from. In: Clinical decision making: From theory to practice (series). *JAMA (Journal of the American Medical Association)* 1990;263:1265–1275.

Johnson, M., Maas, M., and Moorhead, S. *Nursing Outcomes Classification (NOC)*. St. Louis: Mosby, 1997.

Langton, K.B., Johnston, M.E., Haynes, R.B., and Mathieu, A. A critical appraisal of the literature on the effects of computer-based clinical decision support systems on clinician performance and patient outcomes. *Proceedings of the Annual Symposium on Computer Applications in Medical Care (SCAMC)* 1992:626–630.

Martin K.S., and Scheet, N.J. *The Omaha System: Applications for Community Health Nursing*. Philadelphia: W.B. Saunders, 1992.

McCloskey, J.C., and Bulechek, G.M. *Nursing Interventions Classification (NIC), 2nd Ed*. St. Louis: Mosby Year Book, 1996.

McCormick, K.A., Lang, N., Zielstorff, R., Milholland, D.K., Saba, V., and Jacox, A. Toward standard classification schemes for nursing language: Recommendations of the American Nurses Association Steering Committee on databases to support clinical nursing practice. *Journal of the American Medical Informatics Association*. 1994;1(6):421–427.

Murnaghan, J.H., and White, K.L. Hospital Discharge Data: Report of the conference on hospital discharge abstracts systems. *Medical Care (Suppl.)* 1970;8:1–215.

National Center for Health Statistics, *Uniform hospital discharge data: Minimum data set*. DHEW Publication No. PHS 80-1157. Hyattsville, 1980.

National Health Service/Department of Health and Social Security Steering Group on Health Services Information. *Steering group on health services information: First report to the secretary of state*. London, 1982.

National Health Service/Department of Health and Social Security Steering Group on Health Services Information, *Steering group on health services information: Second report to the secretary of state*. London, 1984a.

National Health Service/Department of Health and Social Security Steering Group on Health Services Information. *Steering group on health services information: Third report to the secretary of state*. London, 1984b.

National Health Service/Department of Health and Social Security Steering Group on Health Services Information. *Steering group on health services information: Fourth report to the secretary of state*. London, 1984c.

National Health Service/Department of Health and Social Security Steering Group on Health Services Information. *Steering group on health services information: Fifth report to the secretary of state*. London, 1984d.

National Health Service/Department of Health and Social Security Steering Group on Health Services Information. *Steering group on health services information: Sixth report to the secretary of state*. London, 1984e.

Pearce, N.D. Uniform minimum health data sets: Concept, development, testing, recognition for federal health use, and current status. In: Werley, H.H., and Lang, N.M. (eds.) *Identification of the Nursing Minimum Data Set*. New York: Springer, 1988:122–132.

Pryor, T.A. Development of decision support systems. In: Shabot, M.M., and Gardner, R.M. (eds.) *Decision Support Systems in Critical Care*. New York: Springer-Verlag, pp. 61–72. Cited in Braden, B.J., Corritore, C., and McNees, P. Computerized decision support systems: Implications for practice. In: Gerdin, U., Tallberg, M., and Wainwright, P. (eds.) *The Impact of Nursing Knowledge on Health Care Informatics*. Amsterdam: IOS Press, 1994:300–304.

Saba, V.K. Diagnosis and interventions. *Caring* 1992;11(3):50–57.

Saba, V.K. Nursing diagnosis schemes. In: Canadian Nurses Association. *Papers from the nursing minimum data set conference*. Ottawa, 1993:54–63.

Werley, H.H. Introduction to the Nursing Minimum Data Set and its development. In: Werley, H.H., and Lang, N.M. (eds.) *Identification of the Nursing Minimum Data Set*. New York: Springer, 1988:1–15.

Wheeler, M. Nurses do count. *Nursing Times* 1991;87(16):64–65.

Yensen, J. Telenursing, virtual nursing and beyond. *Computers in Nursing* 1996; 14(4):213–214.

## *Additional Resources*

Clark, J., and Lang, N. The International Classification for Nursing Practice (ICNP): Nursing Outcomes. *International Nursing Review* 1997;44(4):121–124.

Urden, L.D. Development of a nurse executive decision support database: A model for outcomes evaluation. *Journal of Nursing Administration* 1996;26(10):15–21.

Youngblut, R. Hospital Medical Records Institute (HMRI). *National Health Information Council* 1991;2(1):10.

Zielstorff, R.D., Estey, G., Vickery, A., Hamilton, G., Fitzmaurice, J.B., and Barnett, G.O. Evaluation of a decision support system for pressure ulcer prevention and management: Preliminary findings. *Journal of the American Medical Informatics Association, Symposium Supplement.* Nashville: Hanley & Belfus, 1997:248–252.
An overview of Healthcare Information Standards:
  http://www.cpri.org/docs/overview
NANDA home page:
  http://www.mcis.duke.edu:80/standards/HL7/termcode/nanda.html
UMLS home page:
  http://www.nim.nih.gov/research/umls

# Part III
# Applications of
# Nursing Informatics

# 7
# Clinical Practice Applications: Facility Based

## Introduction

New applications for facility based clinical practice continue to be the fastest growing area of interest in nursing informatics (see Figure 7.1). Although there are many technological advances discussed here, the areas of greatest interest are conceptual. Source data capture, the development and use of decision support and expert systems, and the development of a nursing minimum data set as they relate to facility based care are the most important issues. (See Chapter 6 for a full discussion). Although none of these concepts is easily categorized, the nursing process provides the structure for this chapter. Clinical applications of nursing informatics are related to assessment, planning, implementation, and evaluation.

## Assessment

Computerization helps in gathering and storing data about each patient. For example, assessment data can be physiological measures automatically charted through a patient monitoring system (Erb and Coble, 1995; Lyness et al., 1997). Other assessment data are added to the electronic patient record by departments such as the laboratory and radiology. The largest source of assessment data is from ongoing nursing assessment. The following section briefly describes these sources of assessment data.

## *Patient Monitoring*

The major area of development for automated patient monitoring originally was coronary care. In coronary care units and pacemaker clinics, computers were initially used to monitor electrocardiograms, analyze the information, and reduce former volumes of data to manageable proportions (generally some type of graph). The computers were also programmed to

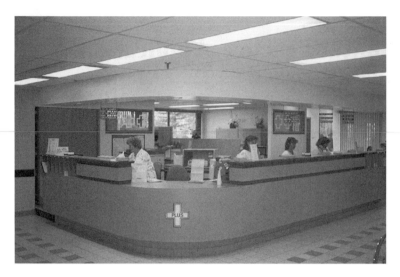

**FIGURE 7.1.** Facility based nursing informatics. (Photograph courtesy of Clinicare Corporation.)

recognize deviations from accepted norms and to alert attending personnel to the deviation by some indication, for example, an alarm or light.

In addition to arrhythmia monitoring, computers in acute care areas, such as emergency, intensive care, coronary care, and neonatal intensive care, are now widely used for hemodynamic and vital sign monitoring, calculation of physiological indices such as peripheral vascular resistance and cardiac output, and environmental regulation of isolets. Sophisticated computerized ICU monitoring systems for management of patient data including patients' heart rates, arterial blood pressure, temperature, respiratory rate, central venous pressure, intracranial pressure, and pulmonary artery pressures are used around the world (Lyness et al., 1997). Automated approaches to patient monitoring free the nurses from the technician role of watching machinery and allow them to focus their attention on the patient, the family, and the nursing process. It is now widely accepted that computerized cardiac monitoring of patients dramatically increases the early detection of arrhythmias and contributes to decreased mortality of CCU patients. Additionally, many of these monitoring systems are integrated into decision support systems (Hughes, 1995; Tierney et al., 1995).

## *Assessment Data from Other Departments*

Detailed discussion of computer systems designed for use in special diagnosis (e.g., laboratory, x-ray), support (e.g., pharmacy, dietary), or special treatment (e.g., radiation therapy, dialysis) is beyond the scope of this book. However, patient data from many departments form the basis for computerized patient care plans and many decision support systems. Nurses must be able to retrieve and use these data to provide quality patient care.

## Nursing Generated Assessment Data

Source data capture is the key to useful nursing generation of patient data. As discussed in Chapter 6, source data capture means gathering data and information about patients where it originates, that is, with the patient. By entering data wherever the patient is, the reliability of the data is increased. There is less chance of transcription errors than if the nurses copy data that they have written on their hands (or on pieces of paper towel) into the patient chart.

For source data capture to be feasible, nurses must be able to enter patient data from many places other than the nursing station. This need has required a revolution in computer hardware. The local nursing station terminal of the hospital mainframe computer is no longer adequate. Computer data entry must occur wherever patients are found. This is called a "point of care" information system. Goals for moving to point of care systems are identified as follows:

- To minimize the time spent in documenting patient information
- To eliminate redundancies and inaccuracies of charted information
- To improve the timeliness of data communication
- To optimize access to information
- To provide information required by the clinician to make the best possible patient care decisions (Hughes, 1995)

Source data capture is the first step in reducing the time nurses spend charting and in eliminating redundancies and inaccuracies. When information can be entered directly into the patient's electronic health record at the point of care, either by the health care professional or by a medical device such as hemodynamic monitors, infusion pumps, or ventilators and made immediately available to others involved in the patient's care, then time is saved and data have been accurately transformed into usable information (Hughes, 1995). Point of care systems use a variety of computer hardware. Ideally, a portable, real-time communication device with many input options such as touch, pen, or voice, able to display patient information as needed, including graphics, an easy documentation method, and long battery life, would be preferred. Technology is fast moving toward this ideal. However, most point of care systems in existence rely on full-sized personal computers, workstations, bedside terminals, and some portable terminals (see Figures 7.2–7.4).

When considering the adoption of point of care systems, the following points should be evaluated.

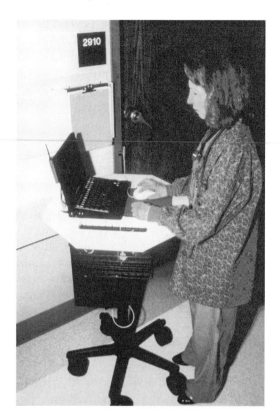

**FIGURE 7.2.** Portable terminal. (Photograph courtesy of Aironet Wireless Communications, Inc.)

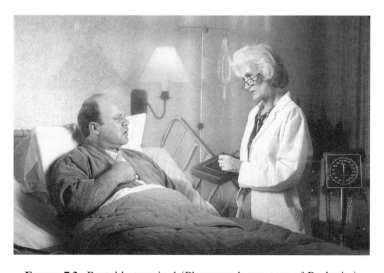

**FIGURE 7.3.** Portable terminal (Photograph courtesy of Prologix.)

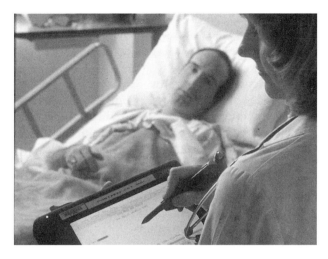

**FIGURE 7.4.** Portable terminal. (Photograph courtesy of Netwave.)

1. Point of care systems must allow the nurse to interact with the main information system. Systems that do not allow information to be extracted, as well as entered, are not useful to nurses.

2. Point of care systems must interface with the existing Hospital Information System. The nurse, at the patient bedside, must be able to access data that has been generated by the laboratory, or radiology, or pharmacy.

3. The open systems concept is valuable to nurses considering point of care systems. This concept allows machines from all vendors to communicate. Open systems allows the most appropriate type of machine to be selected for each nursing environment.

4. Point of care systems must have a very small footprint (take up a small amount of floor space). Not all hospitals have the opportunity to completely configure a new building from the ground up. Most hospitals are trying to fit new technology into "old skins." Early examples of bedside terminals took up a large amount of space in patient rooms. With limited electrical outlets, and no piped-in oxygen or suction, a patient room that had all the equipment necessary to care for seriously ill patients left no room for the nurse!

5. Point of care systems must be easy to use and must adapt to a variety of nursing environments. Patient contact occurs 24 hours a day. For example, bedside terminals must allow the nurse to access and input data without turning on the lights or disturbing the patient. The annoying little "beeps" that a computer makes when you have made a mistake in data entry have no place in bedside terminals.

6. Point of care systems must be easily disinfected and cleaned between patients. Many bedside keyboards should have a membrane keyboard or a protective "skin" over the keyboard to protect it from liquids.

7. For source data capture to be easily accomplished, nurses require a variety of ways for entering data. Keyboards require some typing skills. Other devices include bar code readers (Figure 7.5) for scanning ID bands and medications, physiological probes, microphones for voice input, light pens and touch screens, digital cameras, and natural speech input devices. The touch screen illustrated in Chapter 2 uses icons (pictures) rather than words. Icon menus are easier to use, especially if the exact key word is not known.

8. For effective source data capture, the nurse must go wherever the patient is. If that is the visiting lounge or the coffee shop or the outside deck, a fixed bedside terminal is not appropriate. Notebook technology and pen-based portable systems offer the best choice for mobility.

9. Information to be retrieved on the point of care system must be represented in ways that can be quickly used and easily understood by nurses. Traditional nursing notes are voluminous. Trying to find key data in a narrative is too time-consuming when the information is urgently needed. Figure 7.6 illustrates a cardiac risk assessment tool. At a glance, the nurse can tell which factors must be addressed.

We have talked about the advantages of using source data capture through point of care systems. Alternatives to traditional charting have also been mentioned. However, a brief discussion of computer-mediated documenta-

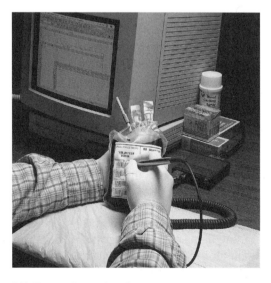

**FIGURE 7.5.** Bar code reader. (Photograph courtesy of Prologix.)

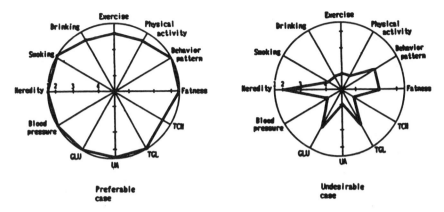

FIGURE 7.6. Cardiac risk assessment. (Reprinted with permission from Bakker, Ball, Scherver, and Willems. Towards New Hospital Information Systems. New York: Elsevier-North Holland, 1988.)

tion is necessary because it is the primary application of nursing informatics in many institutions.

# Documentation

Good nurses' notes are generally lengthy, narrative, handwritten, and unbiased observations. At their worst, they are inaccurate, inconsistent, incomplete, or consist of such trivia as "Had a good day." Automated methods for recording nursing observations are some of the most readily available nursing computer applications. Two approaches are predominate. In the first approach, a computerized library of frequently used phrases is arranged in subject categories. The nurse chooses the phrase or combination of phrases that best describes the patient's condition. For example, by selecting a primary subject such as "sleeping habits," a screen menu of standard descriptions would appear, allowing for additionally selected comments such as "slept through breakfast—voluntarily" or "awoke early at a.m." When completed, the nursing station printer immediately prints a standard, easy-to-read, complete narrative that could then be attached to the patient's chart. An example of an assessment screen is shown in Figure 7.7.

The second approach has been to develop a "branching questionnaire." The terminal displays a list of choices, the nurse selects her choice, and indicates it by pressing the corresponding number on the keyboard or touching the terminal with a light-sensitive input device (called a light pen). The terminal then displays a further list of choices appropriate to the original selection. Thus, the nurse is led through a series of questions that can be "customized" for each patient. For example, a question might be "SKIN INTACT—YES, NO." If "yes" was selected, no further questions in

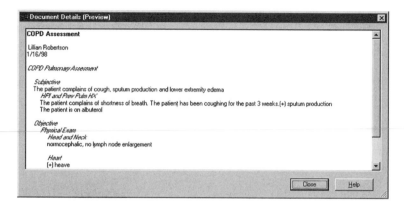

**FIGURE 7.7.** Example of an assessment screen. (Photograph courtesy of Health Vision.)

that set would be necessary. If "no" was selected, then other choices might appear such as a choice between "wounds" and "pressure sores," and so on. The option of free-form input is usually available via the terminal's keyboard. At the user's signal that the entry has been completed, the computer processes the information and provides a narrative printout for the patient's chart. In both approaches, the option of free-form narrative text input, using the keyboard, is usually also available.

Many advantages that have been claimed for automated documentation of nursing observations include these (Minda and Brundage, 1994; Walker and Prophet, 1997):

- Content standardization: increased charting completeness including increased numbers of observations because of prompting or forced recall and increased standardization, accuracy, and reliability of observations
- Improved standards compliance
- Increased efficiency: legible notes, which decrease reading time and increase accuracy of interpretation and elimination of repetitive data recording and resulting transcription errors
- Enhanced timeliness: less time spent writing notes, specifically end-of-shift charting
- Expanded accessibility: data available on-line immediately and access not limited to one person at a time as with paper record
- Augmented data archive: ready statistical analysis and easier nursing audit because of the use of standard terminology

Better observations—that is, increased number, accuracy, and reliability of observations—facilitate better assessment, planning, and evaluation of nursing care. Less time spent in writing notes provides more time for assessment, planning, implementing, and evaluating care. Increased use and accuracy when interpreting notes facilitates consistency and continuity of care. Statistical analysis facilitates research that ultimately will lead to refinements in the nursing process and improved patient care.

## Data Issues

Nurses spend a great deal of time and energy gathering data. Unfortunately, many of these data are probably for someone else's use, e.g., administrative or government statistics. Often these same data will be duplicated by the data-gathering activities of other health care professionals, e.g., how many times are patients, who are being admitted to your institution, asked by different categories of staff why these patients have presented themselves. Similarly, data are gathered ostensibly for nursing use but are never looked at again, e.g., the voluminous nursing histories gathered in many institutions. Nurses should only be gathering data that are essential for nursing decisions about patient care. The principle involved is to gather essential information, while avoiding replication and duplication of data that waste resources such as manpower, storage space, and memory. Although much research remains to be done in this aspect of nursing practice, the foundational work has been done that defines that essential information (see Chapter 6 for a detailed discussion of minimum data sets and nursing classification systems).

## Planning

### *Automated Care Planning*

In most health care settings, the kardex or some similar tool has been the repository of nursing care plans. This tool has had drawbacks similar to those encountered with nursing notes and other drawbacks that are unique to the kardex. Nursing care plans, if they ever get entered in the kardex at all, are usually outdated, illegible, inconsistent, and incomplete. Notations are made by all levels of nursing personnel from nursing aides to head nurses. Written patient care assignments are usually accompanied by verbal explanations that are often forgotten.

One alternate approach to the automation of nursing care plans is to design basic care plans or care maps for meeting patient needs, store them in the computer memory banks, and then adapt them to individual patients (Andolina, 1995; Catt et al., 1997). The resulting printout is unique for each patient's assessed needs for daily care. In all cases, it is the nurse who assesses, plans, and evaluates the plan for care, although auxiliary personnel might be involved in implementing the plan. The newer evolving approach is the development of decision support systems for nursing practice.

This concept is discussed in detail in Chapter 6 and in the following section of this chapter.

The following list summarizes the advantages of automated care plans over traditional nursing care plans:

- Time is saved by eliminating the necessity for daily handwriting of patient assignments and by decreasing the amount of verbal explanation required.
- Accountability is increased because personnel have printouts of care plans for each of their patients.
- Errors and omissions are decreased.
- Consistency of care from shift to shift and day to day is increased; quality of patient care improves.
- Judgments for nursing care are no longer delegated to whomever walks into a room to care for the patient; they are the responsibility of the professional nurse who now has tools available to help her in making nursing judgments.

There are many implications of these advantages for nursing practice (Sahlstedt et al., 1997). Time saved in the preparation and communication of care plans means more time available for the nursing process. Increased accountability for care improves nursing practice because documentation is available to evaluate the quality of care and thus the quality of practice. Benefits to patient care of decreased errors and omissions and increased consistency of care include more rapid diagnosis, more valid assessment, and more rapid recovery. These all reduce the cost of health care for the patient and open the system to more patients. Placing the responsibility for nursing judgments clearly on the shoulders of the professional nurse assists in defining nursing practice and helps the profession in its search for a clearly delineated identity.

## Decision Support Systems

Decision support systems help nurses to maintain and maximize their decision-making responsibilities and to focus on the highest priority aspects of patient care. The care planning systems previously described are not decision support systems. Standardized care plans, whether manual or computer based, only provide care for standardized patients. Standardized care plans do not enhance nursing decision making; on the contrary, their "cookbook" approach discourages active decision making by nurses.

A true decision support system allows nurses to enter their assessments at the bedside using source data capture technology (discussed earlier) and then use the computer to analyze those assessments and recommend nursing diagnoses. The nurse then accepts or rejects the recommendations. Having accepted a particular diagnosis, the range of interventions acceptable in that agency or institution can be retrieved and presented by the computer. The nurse then chooses those nursing interventions that are appropriate for the patient. Such a system provides a tailor-made personalized care plan.

Decision support systems are useful because each nurse's repertoire of interventions is based solely on previous professional experience. Each nurse's own repertoire is also influenced by a "forgetting" curve. If the nurse has not encountered a specific nursing diagnosis for a long time, the remembered interventions may not reflect the whole repertoire. The advisory system not only accumulates the experience of *all* nurses in the organization but also serves as a "reminding" function.

As you may have noted, decision support systems are not appropriate for all patient care settings or at all times. Emergencies such as cardiac arrest do not allow time for the nurse to scroll through suggested actions! Highly complex patient problems may also prove too great a challenge for the current types of decision support systems. In addition, decision support systems are usually designed to address nursing diagnoses one at a time, not in combination.

Decision support systems will never replace the need for nurses with expert clinical and decision-making skills. Brennan and McHugh (1988) stated that the "complexity and/or detail necessary in the decision making process are beyond human capacities, yet some human judgment is necessary either because all the information needed to make a decision is not available to the computer, or because the decision making process is too poorly understood to specify the steps in such a way that the computer can be programmed to make the decision" (p. 93). Therefore, the nurse is still required to exercise clinical judgment, whether or not a decision-modeling or expert system has been used. The fundamental idea that must be stressed is that decision support tools should *add* to the nurse's decision-making capacity and not attempt to replace it (Brennan and Casper, 1995).

## Implementation

Computers rarely help the nurse in the actual giving of care or nursing service. Generally, computers are used more in other phases of the nursing process. One example of how computers are used in intervention is the programmed administration of preloaded drugs in the ICU.

## Evaluation

Computers can be used for evaluating nursing care through real-time auditing and quality management activities. These uses are discussed in detail in Chapter 9.

# Conclusion

In summary, nurses must respond to the challenge to identify the data essential for decisions about patient care; "Nurses cannot leave the decision making about nursing's essential retrievable data to vendors and other health care professionals; those decisions are part of the responsibilities that members of an autonomous profession must assume" (Werley, 1988, p. 431). Nurses must also evaluate technology so that it better serves their needs and the needs of their patients. Last, now is the time to capture the immense collective knowledge of nurses to create the decision support systems that will lead to consistent, high-quality patient care and acknowledgment of our nursing expertise.

## *References*

Andolina, K.M. The automation of Critical Path/Care Map® Systems. In Ball, Hannah, Newbold and Douglas (eds.) *Nursing Informatics: Where Caring and Technology Meet.* Springer, 1995:167–183.

Brennan, P.F., and Casper, G.R. Modelling for decision support. In: Ball, M.J., Hannah, K.J., Newbold, S.K., and Douglas, J.V. (eds.) *Nursing Informatics: Where Caring and Technology Meet*, 2nd Ed. New York: Springer-Verlag, 1995:287–294.

Brennan, P.F., and McHugh, M. Clinical decision-making and computer support. *Applied Nursing Research* 1988;1(2):89–93.

Catt, M.A., Nagle, L.M., and Shamian, J.S. The patient care process: Pathways in transition, in Gerdin U., et al. (eds.) *Nursing Informatics: The Impact of Nursing Knowledge on Health care Informatics*, 1997:318–329.

Erb, P.S., and Coble, D. Vital signs measured with nursing system. *Computers in Health* 1995;10:32–34.

Hughes, S.J. Point-of-care information systems: State of the art. In: Ball, M.J., Hannah, K.J., Newbold, S.K., and Douglas, J.V. (eds.) *Nursing Informatics: Where Caring and Technology Meet*, 2nd Ed. New York: Springer-Verlag, 1995:144–154.

Lyness, A.L., Hravnak, M., and Martich, D. Nurses' perceptions of the impact of a computerized information system on a critical care unit. In: Gerdin, U., Tallberg, M., and Wainwright, P. (eds.) *Nursing Informatics: The Impact of Nursing Knowledge on Health Care Informatics*. Amsterdam: IOS Press, 1997:463–468.

Minda, S., and Brundage, D. Time differences in handwritten and computer documentation nursing assessment. *Computers in Nursing* 1994;12(6):277–279.

Sahlstedt, S. Adolfsson, H., Ehnfors, M., and Kallstrom, B. Nursing process documentation: Effects on workload and quality when using a computer program and a key word model for nursing documentation. In: Gerdin, U., Tallberg, M., and Wainwright, P. (eds.) *Nursing Informatics: The Impact of Nursing Knowledge on Health Care Informatics*. Amsterdam: IOS Press, 1997:330–336.

Tierney, W.M., Overhage M., and Takesue, B., et al. *Computerizing Guidelines to Improve Care and Patient Outcomes: The Example of Heart Failure.* JAMIA, 1995;2:316–322.

Walker, K.P., and Prophet, C.M. Nursing documentation in the computer-based patient record. In: Gerdin, U., Tallberg, M., and Wainwright, P. (eds.) *Nursing Informatics: The Impact of Nursing Knowledge on Health Care Informatics.* Amsterdam: IOS Press, 1997:313–317.

Werley, H.H. Research directions. In: Werley, H.H., and Lang, N.M. (eds.) *Identification of the Nursing Minimum Data Set.* New York: Springer, 1988:427–431.

# 8
# Clinical Practice Applications: Community Based

## Introduction

Community-based care is the fasted growing segment of health care. Health reform in all parts of the world has meant a decrease in numbers of hospital beds and increases in home care. Community-based health promotion and illness prevention programs are also increasing. Surveillance programs must also be maintained. Informatics are playing an integral role in facilitating community-based care. Many community-based organizations have information systems that mirror those of hospital facilities. Systems are typically used for tracking, scheduling, billing, and human resources functions. Because of health reform reorganization, many community-based care providers and organizations are now incorporated into regional health systems. Often the information systems are also combined.

Patient appointment-identification systems are found in many community-based settings. At this level of computer support for nursing, three functions are performed by the automated system. The patient appointment system helps the scheduling of a patient's clinic visits to minimize waiting time, smooth the clinic load, and establish patient priorities for appointments along carefully delineated guidelines. The second function is to maintain the patient registry and determine the extent to which the patient must pay for services and establish billing procedures for third-party liability for each individual patient. The third function of this system is to maintain security and guarantee the privacy and confidentiality of the remainder of the patient record. Access is limited to authorized personnel— nurses and physicians have total access, secretaries and laboratory technicians have limited access. This type of system frees the nurse from many tedious clerical chores. By restricting access to the patient record, this system maintains the confidentiality of the patient record and thus increases the credibility of the professional staff by assuring the patient that his confidences are truly confidential. This fact is particularly important in such areas of distributive nursing as mental health clinics and venereal disease clinics, where the risk of social stigma is a significant factor in an individual's decision to seek care.

The greatest gains in applying informatics to the community setting have come from the linkage with telecommunications. This chapter describes the concepts of telehealth and provide examples of applications in a variety of settings.

# Telehealth

The nurse in the community and the hospital-based nurse require similar information to deliver required patient care. Both practitioners require patient demographic data, past medical history, diagnosis, laboratory and radiology test results, and a treatment and/or care plan. Additionally, whether in the hospital or community setting, delivery of patient care is facilitated by the availability of patient teaching materials, policies and procedures, drug and treatment information, technical data, community services listings, and current contact directions. The point of care is in the community or the patient's home. However, traditionally, the patient's medical record, policy and procedure manuals, teaching materials, and clinical reference books are inaccessible because they are kept in the agency offices. Another key missing link in community-based care, yet traditional in the hospital setting, is collaboration with a multidisciplinary health team during the delivery of patient care (Hassett and Farver, 1995). Telehealth offers technological and information systems solutions to many of the challenges of community-based nursing practice.

There have been many definitions of telemedicine in the literature, but few definitions to aptly define telehealth, an integrating and more holistic term encompassing all the telematics applications in health and healthcare. In Europe, the field is referred to as *health care telematics*. Also in Europe, Telenursing is not related to telecommunications applications specifically, but is the name of the European Community (EC) classification and nomenclature project. Telehealth is defined as "the use of communications and information technology to deliver health and healthcare services and information over large and small distances" (Picot, 1997). Telehealth is born of the confluence of information technology and telecommunications (IT&T), health care, and medical technology. Each of these three sectors is undergoing transformations, although in quite different directions. The first, IT&T, is enjoying accelerated growth with rapid technological and regulatory changes. Health care and medical technology, however, have lately been subject to downsizing and restructuring in many parts of the world. Several factors are influencing the development of telehealth:

• An aging population: the needs of aging health care consumers have initiated efforts to develop and adopt better telehealth systems outside institutional walls, systems that would be better geared for home-based applications.

- Cost containment: telehealth systems are facilitating redistribution of health care services, reducing duplication, reducing numbers of drug interactions and inappropriate prescriptions, and reducing patient and professional travel.
- Access: demand is increasing for equitable access to health care services for inhabitants of isolated geographic areas (e.g., in sparsely populated areas of Canada's north, and in many parts of Latin America, China, and Africa).
- Technology: ever more powerful technologies and communications bandwidth are becoming available at decreasing costs.
- Demand: the increasing consumer demand for wellness and health information of all kinds has fueled increased access to the Internet and World Wide Web.
- Information explosion: the exponential increase in medical and health information has given rise to demands for better information management systems, faster and more efficient electronic access, and better on-line research networks.

Telehealth encompasses practices, products, and services bringing health care and health information to remote locations. Remote can mean across the street or across the globe. Telehealth extends the arm of the health care system for people at home and provides health services direct to consumers. It offers continuing medical, nursing, and health education and assists consumers in obtaining emergency assistance wherever they may be. Health informatics and telematics applications are incorporated, using communications technologies in association with monitoring and medical devices, emergency systems, health, medical, and computer systems to transform and transfer health content and deliver health services, education, and assistance at a distance. An overview of possible applications is found in Table 8.1 (Picot, 1997, p. 8). Specific applications are described next.

The technologies and systems used for telehealth vary greatly from one application to another, but each application, even the simplest, contains at least three components:

1. A device or means to capture, process, and store content (*input*)— whether sound only, electronic or digital images, tracings, alpha-numeric data, or a combination
2. Content and a means to transfer or exchange the content (*throughput*)— communications, telecommunications, or network technologies of all kinds and their associated software
3. A means for receiving, storing, and displaying the content (*output*)—this could be a video monitor, a computer file server, or a recorder of some kind

**TABLE 8.1.** Telehealth applications that can facilitate health care procedures

| Health care procedure, process | Possible telehealth application |
|---|---|
| Telephone-based or face-to-face consultation between specialists and general practitioner | Videoconferencing, IATV, computer-based e-mail |
| Physical transfer of medical image for specialist opinion on radiographs, ultrasound, CT scans, pathology slides | Electronic transfer of images to specialists via any number of networks. Comparison of images against banks of stored electronic slides and images for comparison |
| Handwritten, paper-based patient files and charts | Palmtop pen-based computer tablets, desktop workstations, computerized patient records |
| Handwritten, paper-based prescriptions | Electronic ordering of the prescription using a CHIN, HIN, or pharmanet |
| Consulting CPS for information regarding drug being prescribed | Drug interaction software, drug information database on line |
| Home visits unassisted by technology | Laptop or portable computer with modem to communicate with physician or health care institution |
| Home care, elder care | Telemonitoring from the home; assisted devices, and technologies |
| Visits to the emergency room of the local hospital | Telecare, tele-assisted triage, 1-900 telephone calls to obtain assistance, video visits |
| Referrals from general practitioner | Appointments by e-mail, by electronic scheduling from general practitioner's office |
| Patient traveling from remote location if requiring specialized counselling, diagnosis, or treatment | Videoconsultation with specialist from afar |
| Literature search in medical library for current literature on new procedures, clinical trials, etc. | Electronic search from home or office using Medline or other medical information management and database retrieval service |
| Travel to another location for grand rounds, CME, conference, meetings, seminars | Attendance from home or office via audio-, video-, or computer conferencing, or IATV |
| Clinical trials | Clinical trial management systems, expert advice on line |

The different technological systems are used to transfer the different kinds of information, such as epidemiological, clinical, research, or educational. Users range from health care professionals and administrators to patients and consumers. Settings for telehealth include pharmacies, hospitals, clinic, physicians offices, remote nursing stations and private homes. The following table categorizes telehealth applications and users (Picot, 1997). This categorization is used to structure the following discussion of more specific telehealth applications (Table 8.2).

1. All forms of healthcare at a distance: teleconsultations, telepathology, teleradiology, telepsychiatrty, teledermatology, telecardiology

The Telemedicine Exchange Database (http://tie.telemed.org) reports more than 200 telemedicine projects worldwide that include dermatology, oncology, radiology, pathology, surgery, cardiology, and psychiatry. Echocardiograms, frozen sections, ultrasounds, CT scans, and mammograms are routinely sent by telemedicine applications between remote centers and receiving institutions and between researchers requiring more than the written word. Many of these applications have implications for nurses in both remote and urban areas. In remote areas, videophones, digital medical imaging (X-rays) and ECG monitors transmitting over a regular telephone line can be used to provide information for a consultation with a physician or hospital (Miyasaka, 1997; Nordrum, 1996). In the same way, in urban areas, it is often the nurse who uses the technology to gather patient information that is transmitted to medical facilities.

The U.S. military operates one of the largest telemedicine organizations and is especially active in researching new applications and technologies

TABLE 8.2. Categorization of teleheath applications and users

| Category | User |
|---|---|
| 1. All forms of health care at a distance: teleconsultations, telepathology, teleradiology, telepsychiatrty, teledermatology, telecardiology | Physicians<br>Nurses<br>Psychologists<br>Other health care professionals<br>Health care institutions |
| 2. Interinstitutional patient and clinical records and information systems: electronic health and clinical records and databases accessible by network | Health care institutions and organizations<br>Health care professionals<br>Researchers<br>Physicians offices and community health centers |
| 3. Public Health and Community Health Information Networks (CHINs) and multiple-use health information networks | Government (including policy makers)<br>Epidemiologists<br>Public health professionals<br>Pharmacies<br>Health care providers' offices and clinics |
| 4. Tele-education and multimedia applications for health professionals, and patients, and networked research databases. Internet services. | Health care professionals<br>Patients and consumers<br>Universities and colleges |
| 5. Telemonitoring, telecare networks, telephone triage, remote home care and emergency networks. | Consumers<br>Elderly<br>Chronically ill<br>Telenurses<br>Call center users and operators |

(Zajchuk and Zajchuk, 1996) With its military personnel located in 70 geographic locations worldwide, telemedicine provides medical personnel in the field with 24 hour tertiary care capability. The MERMAID (Medical Emergency Aid Through Telematics) system uses the full range of telecommunications technology, including two-way transfer of live images to maximize the effectiveness of medical assistance to sailors at sea (Anogianakis and Maglavera, 1997). Several areas use telemedicine in correctional facilities to decrease transfers of inmates, thereby improving the safety of health care personnel and the public (Picot, 1997; TRC, 1997).

2. Interinstitutional patient and clinical records and information systems: electronic health and clinical records and databases accessible by network

In this category, telehealth covers the use of networks to link care providers and their institutions. Regional Health Networks and Community Health Information Networks (CHINs) often include pharmanets, which link clinics and physicians' offices to pharmacies for the transmission of information regarding prescriptions. At the basis of the CHIN and the Community Health Management Information System (CHMIS) is the Electronic Health Information System (EHIS) or computerized patient record (CPR) (see Chapter 5 for more detail). A major trend in telehealth applications is the integration of health networks, including institution-based and community-based systems. The major benefits are realized from avoiding duplication, timely provision of information, reducing unnecessary multiple diagnostic procedures, and optimizing resources.

3. Public Health and Community Health Information Networks (CHINs) and multiple-use health information networks

Surveillance systems and registries are increasing used by policy makers, and funders to measure progress and compare delivery systems. Population health networks permit epidemiologists, health policy makers, and governments as well as public health officials to exchange information regarding the health status of entire populations. This type of information has become all the more valuable in recent times because of the prevalence of certain diseases believed to have environmental causes. The WHO makes increasing use of the Internet to disseminate population health information widely (http://www.who.org).

Disease surveillance networks are designed to identify epidemics and emerging diseases. National governments have supported such networks to support disease prevention efforts and to monitor and control risks to health. It will be some years before fully operational *Global Emergency and Disease Prevention Networks* become a reality. There is a growing realization that such networks are essential in light of the high volume of travel and exchange between countries and the growing number of senior and frail travelers.

4. Tele-education and multimedia applications for health professionals, and patients, and networked research databases, Internet services

Tele-education, not telemedicine, constitutes the principal content in many telehealth networks. Mediated distance education for health professionals has been ongoing since the 1930s, when radio was the main communication medium. Many universities and colleges worldwide offer credit and noncredit courses by distance, using all forms of telecommunications, from videoconferencing to the Internet. Virtual nursing education for postbasic degree programs is available across North America and Europe from a variety of universities. Continuing medical education (CME) and continuing nursing education (CNE) are increasingly offered via telecommunications and computer-based networks. In many institutional settings, the teleconferencing facilities used for telemedicine applications are also used for tele-educational purposes.

Patient education remains a growing field. The advent of the Internet and the World Wide Web (WWW) have had a substantial impact on tele-education for consumers. Consumers now have access to health information that previously was unavailable to them, even in public libraries. Web sites offering medical advice are popular as are newsgroups, electronic medical forums, virtual hospital, and even disease control networks, such as Housecall and Global Health Network from the United States and Globalmedic from Canada. The WWW is also a source of wellness information, although with quackery as a potential hazard, there is rising demand for guarantors granting legitimate status to the content published by various information providers.

5. Telemonitoring, telecare networks, telephone triage, remote home care, and emergency networks

It is difficult to discuss each of these applications separately as many overlaps occur in reality. The rise of ambulatory care, shorter hospital stays, and the care of the elderly and chronically ill in the home setting have all generated community care needs that can be effectively met, in part, with video visits or tele-monitoring devices. New products such as cardiac monitoring and haemodialysis systems complete with telephone coupling mechanisms have been developed to serve this need. Videoconferencing systems, including the use of videophones for home care video visits, are gaining in popularity. Examples include the use of videophones to monitor home-ventilated children (Miyasaka, 1997) and cystic fibrosis patients (Adachi, 1997). Videophones are becoming widely available and, as the cost decreases, will be used increasingly in health care. Videophones do not require a computer, use standard telephone lines, and the technology is as simple as making a phone call. Videophones include a wide range of features to facilitate telehealth applications including electronic pan, tilt, zoom, self-view, and autoanswer.

Telecounseling using videoconferencing or videophone technology has been reported as having high user satisfaction and reducing travel costs to both patient and professional. Some patients actually prefer the television monitor or videophone to the face to face experience (Elford, 1997; Elford and House, 1997; Hawker, 1997). Telepyschiatry and tele-counseling applications are expected to rise as practitioners are increasingly located in large urban areas where the majority of patients are located. Relocating psychiatric and mental health professionals to rural areas may not be feasible because of the lower numbers of patients in rural or remote areas.

Another outgrowth of the telecounseling application is the advent of on-line support groups, either sponsored by an organization specifically for its patients (Brennan, 1997) or open to the general public. ComputerLink projects serving persons living with AIDS and caregivers of persons with Alzheimer's disease provide information organized in an electronic encyclopedia, electronic communication including public bulletin boards and private mail, and a decision support service. Comments from users indicated that the ComputerLink served as a "support system without walls" (Brennan, 1997, p. 522).

In-home monitoring is available for ECG, blood pressure, heart rate, and peak-flow spirometer readings (Carthy, 1997). In many instances the facility receiving the transmissions speaks directly to the patient while the information is being transmitted. Immediate feedback can be given to the patient and, if necessary, ambulance services or mobile intensive care units can be summoned. This approach removes the intervention of third parties that have traditionally taken the ECG and transmitted it to the physician, and reduces the number of unnecessary visits to emergency departments. Natori et al. (1997) has reported on a program for low risk pregnant women to transmit their own cardiotocograms via e-mail and thus reduce routine physician visits.

Video and telecommunications technology, sometimes but not always coupled with tele-monitoring, has spawned the development of many remote home care programs for the elderly (Roman, 1997; Yoshio et al., 1997). Benefits to this type of program are identified as

- Empowerment and independence of the elderly patient
- Return to the comfort of home with the security of flexible health care for an estimated 5% of those currently in nursing homes
- Great savings to our nations (Roman, 1997, p. 79).

Some additional home care services that can be tele-assisted, partly replacing and augmenting home care visits, include the following: wound management; oncology patient management via home infusion; electronic and tele-house calls; remote programmable infusion; blood glucose meters with telecommunication capabilities; tele-monitoring of haemodialysis; use of laptop computers by home care nurses to note and check medication and progress on patients' electronic health record and to electronically communicate with home care teams; and emergency or alert systems linking homes to clinics or hospitals (Picot, 1997) (Figure 8.1).

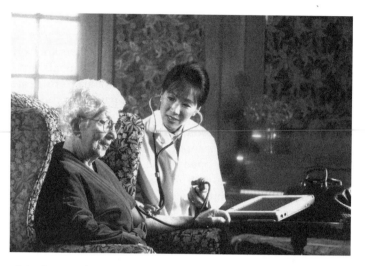

**FIGURE 8.1.** Community-based nursing informatics. (Photograph courtesy of Prologix.)

The health care sector is increasingly using the concept of call centers in the delivery of services. Many jurisdictions and managed care organizations have implemented toll-free numbers and call centers to handle health-care queries and problems. Nurses are providing emergency or first level information and triage and advice over the telephone. In the province of Quebec, at *InfoSante*, nurses managed more than 660,000 calls in 1997 (Picot, 1997).

## Challenges Related to Telehealth

Although the potential for telehealth applications to contribute to health care is unlimited, several challenges remain to be addressed:

- Obsolescence: Many of the technologies have a short shelf life. Rapid obsolescence is a major concern for managers and administrators be-cause most information technologies come in 18- to 36-month cycles, each bringing significant increases in processing speeds, flexibility, and storage capacity and decreases in price.
- Access: Even with user acceptance and available funding, telehealth is not accessible to any and all who need it. Technical infrastructure dictates at least in part the if, how, where, when, and what of telehealth technolo-gies that can be implemented.
- Health information infrastructures: The creation of a health information infrastructure requires the integration of existing and new architectures and application systems and services. A core element of this infrastruc-

ture includes patient-centered care facilitated by computer-based patient record systems (electronic patient record).

- Provider reimbursement: The issue of physician and other provider compensation for telehealth services has yet to be resolved in most jurisdictions.
- Interdisciplinary and interinstitutional collaboration: Jurisdictional conflicts between institutions and between physicians, nurses, pharmacists, radiologists, and nuclear medicine specialists must be resolved.
- Documentation standards: Telehealth documentation standards must be developed for use by all providers to ensure a useful and usable patient record.
- Data security: Confidentiality, privacy, and security issues related to the collection, storage, and transmission of patient information must be resolved to the satisfaction of professionals and consumers alike.
- Liability issues: Medical and nursing responsibility issues related to continuing responsibility for a patient's care, liability of consultants' opinions, and licensing for cross-jurisdictional consultation must be resolved.

## Conclusion

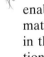

The development of inexpensive, reliable telecommunications technology enables health professionals, patients, and consumers to access health information, health care resources, and health service delivery directly from and in their homes. Telehealth applications exist as discrete nursing interventions (Brennan, 1997), and provide pathways for nurses to reach patients and provide nursing interventions. Nurses can use technology to assist them in providing home care and in-home monitoring. Networks serve as educational vehicles whereby nurses can reach patients and clients with health promotion, disease and prevention, information and illness management nursing interventions. Telehealth applications hold great promise for extending the ability of nurses to reach individuals in communities and the communities themselves.

## *References*

Adachi, T. How videophones affect patient's families. In: *Proceedings of the 3rd International Conference on the Medical Aspects of Telemedicine*, Kobe, Japan, 1997:58.

Anogianakis, G., and Maglavera, S. MERMAID—Medical emergency aid through telematics. In: *Proceedings of the 3rd International Conference on the Medical Aspects of Telemedicine*, Kobe, Japan, 1997:154.

Brennan, P.F. The ComputerLink projects: A decade of experience. In: Gerdin, U., Tallberg, M., and Wainwright, P. (eds.) *Nursing Informatics: The Impact of Nursing Knowledge on Health Care Informatics*. Amsterdam: IOS Press, 1997:521–525.

Carthy, Z. Commercial implementation of homecare telemedicine—The Shahal experience. In: *Proceedings of the 3rd International Conference on the Medical Aspects of Telemedicine*, Kobe, Japan, 1997:136.

Elford, D.R. Telemedicine in northern Norway. *Journal of Telemedicine and Telecare* 1997:25.

Elford, D.R., and House, A.M. Telemedicine Experience in Canada 1956–1996. Presented at Medicine 2001 Conference, Montreal. 1996, June. Cited in Picot, J. *The telehealth industry in Canada*. Industry Canada, Ottawa, 1997.

Hassett, M.M., and Farver, M.H. Information management in home care. In: Ball, M.J., Hannah, K.J., Newbold, S.K., and Douglas, J.V. (eds.) *Nursing Informatics: Where Caring and Technology Meet*, 2nd Ed. New York: Springer-Verlag, 1995:155–166.

Hawker, F. Telepsychiatry to rural and remote South Australia: an established telemedicine service. In: *Proceedings of the 3rd International Conference on the Medical Aspects of Telemedicine*, Kobe, Japan, 1997:127.

Miyasaka, K. Videophone system for pediatric home care. In: *Proceedings of the 3rd International Conference on the Medical Aspects of Telemedicine*, Kobe, Japan, 1997:56.

Natori, M., Kitagawa, M., and Akiyama, Y. A preliminary study of home nursing for low risk pregnancy. In: *Proceedings of the 3rd International Conference on the Medical Aspects of Telemedicine*, Kobe, Japan, 1997:81.

Nordrum, I. Telepathology: Is there a future? *Telemedicine Today* 1996;4(2):24–26.

Picot, J. *The telehealth industry in Canada*. Industry Canada, Ottawa, 1997.

Roman, L.I. Caring for the elderly at home. In: *Proceedings of the 3rd International Conference on the Medical Aspects of Telemedicine*, Kobe, Japan, 1997:79.

TRC. What is telemedicine? Telemedicine Research Center (TRC), 1997. Online. Available: http://tie.telemed.org

Yoshio, M., Kunihiko, D., Masayuki, N., and Eisuke, F. A report of telecare for the aged at home via ISDN. In: *Proceedings of the 3rd International Conference on the Medical Aspects of Telemedicine*, Kobe, Japan, 1997:80.

Zajchuk, J.T., and Zajchuk, R. Strategy for medical readiness: Transition to the digital age. *Telemedicine Journal. Special Issue on Telemedicine and the Military.* 1996;2:3.

# 9
# Administration Applications[1]

## Introduction

Managers and caregivers throughout the health care system are being asked to increase the efficiency and effectiveness of patient care while simultaneously reducing or at least maintaining levels of resource consumption. A principal strategy being used to achieve these goals is to consider information as a corporate strategic resource and provide enhanced information management methods and tools to caregivers and managers across the health sector. The idea is to use information to enable managers to most effectively utilize available resources.

Administrative uses of information systems in nursing can be classified in two ways: those that provide nurse managers with information for decision making and those that help nurse managers in communicating decisions. In this chapter, those administrative uses of information systems that help nurse managers in decision making are called "management information systems." Those applications of information systems in nursing administration that help nurse managers to communicate their decisions are called "nursing office automation systems." This chapter defines management information systems and describes the nursing information needs related to the management of nursing units. The chapter also includes discussions of word/text processing, electronic document distribution, and electronic mail, group ware, and scheduling. The chapter concludes with the nursing role in the management of information and obstacles and issues in management information systems.

---

[1] Parts of this chapter are based on material originally published, as Hannah, K.J. 1992. Nursing management of information. In: Ogilvie, M., and Sawyer, E. (eds.) *Managing Information in Canadian Health Care Facilities*. Ottawa: Canadian Hospital Association Press. It is used here with permission of the publisher.

# A Definition of Management Information Systems

The idea of management information systems was developed in the business and industrial sectors. It has been studied, analyzed, and evaluated in detail by management scientists for a considerable time. In those sectors, there are many definitions of the concept of management information systems (MIS). Some definitions place an emphasis on the physical elements and design of the system while others focus on the function of an MIS within an organization. In this book, MIS refers to, the classic notion of "a method of collecting, storing, retrieving, and processing information that is used or desired by one or more managers in the performance of their duties" (Ein-Dor and Segev, 1978). Although this definition could include both manual and computerized systems, we discuss only computerized management information systems in this book. Figure 9.1 illustrates a simplified management information system.

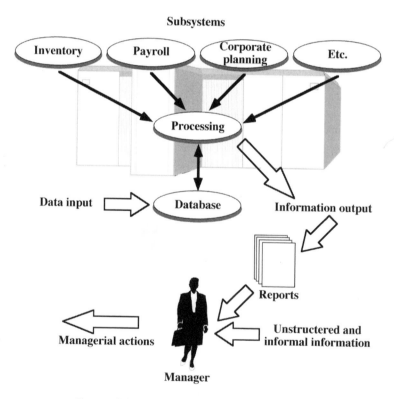

FIGURE 9.1. Management Information System.

# Nursing Information Needs for the Management of Nursing Units

This aspect of information need focuses on the information that the organization (as represented by its nurse managers) needs to fulfil that aspect of its mission related to providing patient or client care. Management information systems help nursing in the areas of quality management, unit staffing, and ongoing reporting. Such systems also support nurse managers in their responsibilities for allocation and utilization of the following resources necessary to accomplish the nursing function in the patient/client care environments: human resources, fiscal resources (including payroll, supplies, and materiel), and physical resources (including physical facilities, equipment, and furniture).

## *Quality Management*

Total Quality Management (T.Q.M.) has superseded the previous quality assurance movement. T.Q.M. is an important process for staff nurses and administrators alike. It is useful to staff nurses in two ways: it provides them with feedback about the nature of their individual practice and it provides them with opportunity to influence patient care in their organization. Nurse administrators use it to assess the general quality of patient care provided within their institutions and use it as a process to receive and communicate opportunities to enhance patient care and organizational effectiveness.

T.Q.M. is the process of establishing and maintaining the organizational effectiveness, i.e., the quality of care provided to patients. T.Q.M. is an institutional plan of action to establish a process for empowering staff to influence corporate achievement of the highest possible standards for patient care. The delivery of patient care is monitored by all staff to ensure that these standards are met or surpassed. Implicit in the concept of T.Q.M. is the ongoing evaluation of the standards themselves, thus ensuring that they reflect current norms and practices within health care. Institutions use a variety of formal and informal means to gather information to evaluate the quality of care provided to patients. The formal means are encompassed in a quality assurance program. Information needs associated with quality assurance might include patient care databases, patient evaluations of care received, nurses' notes on the chart, patient care plans, performance appraisals, and incident reports. These sources of information are reviewed by either a concurrent or retrospective audit. Concurrent nursing audits occur during the patient's stay in the hospital while retrospective nursing audits occur after the patient leaves the hospital. Audit reviews are a major tool for any T.Q.M. program.

Originally, the impetus for the establishment of quality assurance programs came in the 1970s as the result of rising consumer awareness, increasing health care costs, and the growing professionalism of nursing. An additional factor was the desire of the U. S. government to monitor the cost and quality of care associated with its Medicaid program. Almost simultaneously, three things happened: professional standards review organizations were established in the United States, the American Nurses Association published its standards for practice, and the American Joint Commission on Accreditation for Hospitals established the requirement for medical and nursing audits. These events added pressure to the entire quality assurance process. The established quality assurance programs were dependent on reviewing and evaluating massive amounts of data. These reviews and audits consumed enormous amounts of nursing time. As these audits were done, nurses gained an increased awareness of their professional accountability. This greater awareness, in turn, prompted nurses to produce more documentation in the form of nursing care plans and patient records. This further increased the volume of information to be reviewed and evaluated in the nursing audits.

As the pressure from nursing audits was building, integrated hospital information systems made their timely entry to the health care delivery system. Quality assurance programs in nursing needed two things to really succeed: standardized terminology and standardized care plans. These two things were also required if information systems were to be any help to nurses. The standardization of terminology required in computerized documentation of nurses' notes, and the development of standardized care plans for use in generating computerized patient care plans, coincided with the need for standardized terminology and quality assurance standards.

The ability of a computer to rapidly retrieve, summarize, and compare large volumes of information has proven very useful for nurse administrators charged with the responsibility of implementing quality assurance programs. Unfortunately, only a few hospitals have integrated hospital information systems that provide the capacity for concurrent on-line data retrieval for nursing audit purposes. The first obstacle to use of computers for this purpose is the lack of widespread availability of integrated hospital information systems. The second obstacle is the lack of a widely accepted method of coding nursing problems.

Both obstacles may be on the verge of being overcome. The lack of widely available integrated hospital information systems is being resolved by the decreasing cost of such systems and their greater sophistication. The North American Nursing Diagnosis Association (NANDA) is addressing the matter of standardized nomenclature for describing nursing diagnoses. Other initiatives are underway to develop taxonomies for nursing interventions and nursing contributions to patient care outcomes (Grobe, 1992). McCormack and Zeilstorff (1992) have advocated the development of a Unified Nursing Language. Unfortunately, much of this work has not yet received widespread support in the nursing profession and has not yet been incorporated as a framework for the organization of nursing databases by developers of information systems. Figure 9.2 attempts to summarize the interrelationships between clinical practice, informatics and computer technology.

Another problem associated with computerized quality assurance programs is the quality of the tools used in providing input to the program. The validity of even the most widely used audit tools and criteria is largely unsubstantiated. Consequently, much effort has been focused on the process aspects incorporated in the T.Q.M. concept. Unfortunately, the vendors of computer software have not given high priority to the information needs related to T.Q.M. or the development of clinical software pack-

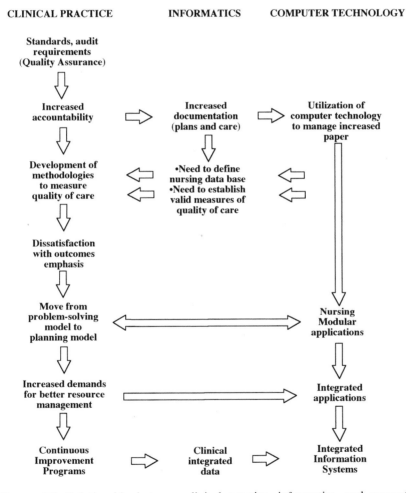

**FIGURE 9.2.** Relationship between clinical practice, informatics, and computer technology.

ages for health care institutions. This situation has created a major barrier to the effective and widespread use of information systems for quality monitoring in hospitals. Several institutions have developed sophisticated T.Q.M. programs that incorporate procedures for conducting concurrent chart audits. These institutions use a manual concurrent audit conducted by staff nurses (with special training in concurrent auditing) on the nursing units. The data from the completed audit forms are then put into the computer for tabulation, analysis, and summarizing. This combination of manual and computer methods partially reduces the labor-intensive process associated with totally manual audits.

There is a growing emphasis on patient care outcomes as the major focus of nursing T.Q.M. programs. Similarly, there is a growing trend away from the problem resolution model to a planning model as the major criterion for measuring quality assurance. Simultaneously, there is an increasing demand from the public for better resource management within the health care sector, and the public has an increasing awareness of quality as a cost component of health care. These factors are creating a demand for the most sophisticated computerized information handling in the form of relational database software.

## Patient Classification, Nursing Workload, and Unit Staffing

In the past, innumerable head nurses and supervisors in health care institutions and agencies around the world spent countless hours each day "doing the time." Even when master rotation plans were used, manual scheduling of personnel work rotations could not eliminate all the problems: vulnerability to accusations of bias in assigning days off or shift rotation, difficulty in establishing minimum staffing to avoid wasting manpower, and depending on an individual's memory within the nursing administrative structure. Consequently, automated staff scheduling is a highly desired component of a management information system for nursing administration. Frequently, when an institution has limited resources and no other computerized nursing management information system, it will mobilize resources to set up a computerized staffing system.

Researchers at many health care institutions have developed many diverse systems for personnel time assignment. The complexity of these systems varies greatly. Some merely use the computer to print names into what was formerly a manual master rotation schedule; others adjust staffing interactively and dynamically on a shift-to-shift basis by considering patient acuity, nursing workload levels, and the expertise of available personnel. To develop complex, sophisticated systems for automated personnel scheduling, a great deal of planning and data gathering is required: nursing workload must be identified within the institution; the various levels of expertise of staff members must be categorized and documented; criteria for determining patient acuity and nursing workload must be established; personnel policies must be clearly defined; and the elements of union contracts must be summarized. When all this information is available, a computer program is designed to schedule nursing staff on nursing units. The capacity of the computer to manipulate large numbers of variables consistently and quickly makes personnel time assignment an excellent use of this technology.

Documented advantages of automated scheduling of personnel include the following:

- Easier recruitment and increased job satisfaction because schedules are known well in advance
- Less time spent on manual scheduling, thus providing more time for nurse managers to carry out other duties
- Advance notice of staff shortages requiring temporary replacements
- Unbiased assignment of days off and shift rotation
- Workstation printouts available for staff inspection and for ward assignment lists
- More effective utilization and distribution of personnel throughout the institution or agency
- Capacity to document the effect of staff size on quality of care
- Ability to relate quantity and quality of nursing staff to patient acuity

Workload measurement systems add to the ideas of automated scheduling. Nursing Workload Measurement Systems (NWMS) are tools that measure the number of direct, indirect, and nonclinical patient care hours by patient acuity on a daily basis. In 1931, the U. S. government brought in legislation requiring all hospitals to record and return data relating to hospital activity. Since then, NWMS have evolved to focus on providing uniform and reliable productivity information to help in staffing, budgeting, planning, and quality assurance. NWMS have become a valuable management tool for nursing unit managers, nursing department heads, hospital administrators, and governments alike. As health care costs and demands continue to escalate, the appropriate and effective utilization of scarce human resources becomes increasingly onerous. There are many NWMS on the market. All differ in one or many respects, and the criteria used to choose such a system ultimately depend on the specific institution's needs. The three most widely used NWMS are considered here: PRN, Medicus, and GRASP. For more detailed information, the reader is advised to refer to the excellent book *Workload Measurement Systems in Nursing* by Claire Thibault, published by the Quebec Hospital Association in 1990.

PRN (Project Research in Nursing) was developed by the province of Quebec in 1976. It is composed of the Patient Care Plan, the Evaluation Form, and the Measurement Module for Staffing. PRN is based on the contents of the care plan in which 154 nursing activities are identified according to patient needs. Each activity or factor is given a time value in minutes that is then totaled. These total times required by the patient then determine the staffing requirements of the unit. This system is widely used in Canada and Europe.

Medicus was designed in Chicago to measure patient needs as an indicator of projected nursing workload. Medicus involves the implementation and development of a Patient Classification System, a Quality Monitoring System, a Staffing Framework, Variable Staffing Procedures, Analysis and Data Processing, and a Management Reporting System. It is based on 37 patient indicators that are assigned point values. The points illustrate the ratio of care required in one of five types of acuity. Depending on the number of points, the total workload can be calculated for each acuity class that, in turn, can determine the unit workload. This system is used extensively in Canada and the United States.

GRASP (Grace-Reynolds Application and Study of PETO) originated in North Carolina between 1973 and 1976. It was designed as a system for balancing admissions and care available. GRASP is based on three assumptions. First, no two patients require the same amount of care, whatever the medical diagnosis. Second, measurement of patient care needs for budgeting and staffing must identify the care the patient should receive, not the care actually received. Third, if the hours of care required equal the hours of patient care available, then there is greater potential for quality care, personnel satisfaction, and cost containment. GRASP identifies 120 patient care activities that are then assigned time standards. Patients are evaluated daily and the time required for care is converted into a PCU (Patient Care Unit), which is equivalent to 1 hour of nursing care. The total number of PCUs can then determine nursing workload. The GRASP system is used extensively in the United States and the United Kingdom.

None of the three systems identified here produce the same result for the same patient population (O'Brien-Pallas, 1987). PRN produces significantly higher care hours than GRASP or Medicus. GRASP and Medicus produce approximately the same number of care hours. GRASP and PRN are task-oriented systems whereas Medicus considers critical indicators related to patient needs. In terms of implementation and modification, GRASP and PRN are user dependent whereas Medicus is vendor dependent. With respect to quality assurance, all three interrelate the Nursing Care Plan and the Quality Assurance Program. PRN goes so far as providing its own unique care plan format.

Increased job satisfaction, easier recruitment of staff, unbiased rotation assignment, workstation printouts, and advance notice of temporary shortages—all contribute to improved staff morale and thus indirectly result in better patient care. Administrative time saved and more effective utilization and distribution of personnel have also been suggested as factors influencing quality of patient care within the agency or institution. Documentation of the relationship between staffing and quality of patient care gives the nurse manager strong data to justify staffing requests and decisions to senior hospital management.

# Reporting

In most hospitals, nursing costs represent upward of 40% of the entire hospital budget. Management information systems collect, summarize, and format data for use in administrative decision making related to the nursing component of the hospital budget. Nurse managers are familiar with periodically produced budget summaries that allow monitoring of the budget, adjustments between overcommitted and undercommitted categories and help in the planning of next year's budget. A variety of retrieval modules have been designed and are being refined to provide similar decision-making support in areas ranging from the nosocomial infection rate to sickness and absentee abuses by staff members. The emphasis in these reports is on graphic displays (histograms, time series charts, map plots, etc.). The advantages for nurse managers with this level of support lie mainly in the speed with which data can be retrieved, compiled, summarized, and presented in a meaningful and comprehensive form. Another major advantage is the ability to tailor reports to each nurse manager's information needs. This facilitates the ongoing monitoring of activities within the institution and the preparation of reports by the nurse manager to superiors or outside agencies.

# Human Resource Management

Management of people on a nursing unit is a complex and time-consuming task. In the increasingly decentralized administrative structures that characterize modern hospitals, nurse managers need information related to all aspects of the allocation and utilization of staff on nursing units. For example, the nurse manager must have immediate access to such information as this:

- The skills and education of all nursing employees
- Job classification and salary level for all staff on the unit
- Dates for performance appraisals
- Dates for recertification of medically delegated and transferred functions
- Dates for annual inservice education sessions, whether required by contract, by organizational policy, or by accreditation standards (e.g., back care, CPR, fire and disaster response, restraints)
- The format of letters of offer used in the hiring of nursing employees on the nursing unit
- Annual vacation schedule summary for the unit

- Statutory holiday schedules
- Labor relations contracts for all collective bargaining units representing employees employed on the unit, including grievance procedures
- Sick time records for each employee

The management of this and other human resource-related information by nursing managers is accomplished using either an incredible memory, a superb filing system, or a shoe box filled with scraps of paper! It is even possible that some lucky nurse managers have access to databases on personal computers in their offices! These types of information are used regularly by nurse managers in combination with nursing workload measurement systems to develop staff schedules and duty rosters.

## Fiscal Resources

Hospitals are gradually moving toward the implementation of modern, business-oriented management information systems. These systems identify, define, collect, process, and report the information necessary for the planning, budgeting, operating, and controlling aspects of the management function. The current demands for fiscal responsibility in hospitals exceed all previous experience in the health care sector. Increasingly, nursing managers are expected to understand the contextual challenges of their organizational environment. To respond to internal and external factors influencing the corporate environment in which they function, nurse managers must do many things:

- Understand their fiscal responsibilities and situation
- Identify the issues and opportunities
- Generate solutions
- Monitor progress toward unit and organization goals
- Evaluate the effectiveness of the solutions or the achievement of goals and objectives

These activities require the management of financial and statistical data. The ultimate objective is to relate the cost of resources consumed to patient outcomes. To effectively manage information related to their responsibilities for fiscal accountability, nurse managers need financial information (including payroll, supplies/materiel, and services) and statistical information (such as patient length of stay or nursing hours per patient day). This information needs to be timely, accurate, relevant, comprehensive, complete, consistent, concise, sensitive, and comparable. In Canada, the MIS guidelines are establishing national standards for the structural framework, data definitions, and accounting guidelines necessary to provide nursing managers with the appropriate financial and statistical information. In the United Kingdom, similar data standards exist through the use of the Körner data set. In the United States, such data standards are established by the Health Care Finance Administration (H.C.F.A.)

## Physical Resources

Nursing managers are also responsible for overseeing the care and maintenance of the physical facilities of their patient care unit. They are responsible for equipment and furniture on their units and ensuring that it is in good working order. Although the actual inventory may be conducted by another department (such as materiel management), nursing managers are accountable for budgeting, ordering, and retaining capital assets on their units, and for initiating maintenance or replacement procedures. Consequently, nursing managers need access to capital asset inventory for their unit. In addition, they should also conduct regular systematic inspection of the workplace for physical hazards such as faulty electrical equipment or loose floor tiles. These inspections must document identified hazards, the date on which corrective action was requested or initiated, and the date that the hazard was repaired or removed from the workplace. Such information must be stored on the nursing unit in an easily retrievable format with a calendar to bring forward reminders of follow-up items.

## Office Automation

Nursing office automation is the integrated electronic technology distributed throughout the nursing administrative office. The purposes of nursing office automation are to improve effectiveness, efficiency, and control of nursing office operations. This technology can have application in nursing administration, nursing education, continuing nursing education, and nursing research. Office automation affects the filing and retrieval of documents, text processing, telephone communications, and informal meetings. Some economic factors that are demanding the move to nursing office automation are the following:

- The cost of computing is decreasing. The computer capability that cost $4,000,000 in 1972 could be purchased for $15,000 in 1982, and in 1992 that same power could be purchased for less than $5,000.
- The demand versus supply. Office support workload is increasing, and there is a shortage of skilled workers. All indications are that the problem will become worse. The supply of skilled workers will not grow as fast as needed, and the demand for a skilled pool of secretaries will increase.

Nursing office requirements are demanding more skills in transcription or dictatyping, word processing, spreadsheets, and electronic filing. Offices will have special printers and eventually teleconferencing, voice response systems, and voice mail systems. An entire book could be devoted to the various facets of nursing office automation. The authors have chosen to limit the detailed discussion to word or text processing, electronic document distribution, and electronic mail.

## Word/Text Processing and Electronic Filing

### Word Processing

A little paperless typewriter with a glowing face and a silicon chip in its heart has touched the world, and the world is quietly being changed. Word processing is a misnomer. To say that we are processing words suggests that we are blending them chemically and that they are not flowing from our brain. Perhaps this is why people who should be using word processors seem to avoid them. Word processing is writing just as we always have done, except that we sit at a keyboard and see what we have written appear on a CRT screen instead of a sheet of paper. Indisputably, the word processor is a piece of equipment that has revolutionized running an office.

Support personnel have been doing word or text processing since the invention of the first typewriter. So the reader may wonder, What is the big deal? The use of the term word or text processing in the automated office means that the typed material is entered onto some form of magnetic media. Of course, there have been devices around for some time (e.g., memory typewriter) that have this capability. The new generation of equipment has the capability of easily moving sentences, paragraphs, or entire pages to a different part of the document or to an entirely different document (see Figure 9.3). The document can be processed against automatic spelling and grammar checker programs that can highlight any errors. Also, the document can be automatically paginated, thus relieving the operator from tedious work. Most current generation equipment provides for a "user-friendly" environment, which enhances the productivity of the support staff or the manager. As a part of this function, the completed document is "filed," or stored, on a central memory or on a diskette at the workstation. This enables the document to be retrieved later for further revision or to produce additional copies. If the automation effort is properly planned, the hard copy will not have to be manually filed and the material will be stored on magnetic media for as long as is useful.

Managers can now do much of their own work, for example, composing, spell-checking, and grammar checking, and when the document is ready, transfer it electronically to their assistant for final formatting, transmission, and storage.

### Electronic Filing

On some equipment it is possible to search for documents by keywords, titles, originator's name, or date of preparation. This is a productivity tool

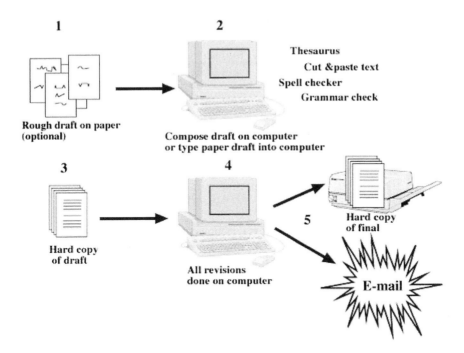

**FIGURE 9.3.** Word/text processing and electronic filing/distribution.

that helps with the day-to-day administrative chores. Because manual filing of paper documents is a burdensome task and usually relegated to the newest person in the office (which usually results in having documents misfiled), the electronic filing system offers many advantages.

## *Electronic Document Distribution*

In light of slow mail and lost letters, the ability to easily send a complete document electronically is a bonus. With some systems, it is possible to send the completed document to one or many locations with ease. The receiving location can see the document on a monitor or print it for further distribution.

Many large hospitals are regularly using Electronic Document Distribution (EDD) for transmitting weekly cash reports, drafts of contracts, questionnaires, routine correspondence, and other administrative documents. The ability to communicate between the various locations on multiple sites has improved the productivity and timeliness of decision making. For example, one of the academic campuses of this system uses EDD to transmit copies of the academic catalog to the deans' offices for review and to return comments to the sending office. With this approach, several offices can work on the same document without the need for retyping, photocopying, or cutting or pasting efforts. Similarly, as hospitals merge to create multisite organizations, administrative staff find such systems essential to their productivity as they have office hours and hold meetings in diverse locations.

## *Electronic Mail*

Electronic mail is the name given to unofficial electronic communications among individuals or offices. Generally speaking it replaces several telephone calls that would be required to impart the same message (see Chapter 4 for more detail).

"Telephone tag" is a problem that is present in all administrative environments. It is a waste of time and creates much lost motion. In case the reader is not familiar with the term, it means that you call someone for the answer to a question or to pass on some information but, for any number of reasons, the person is not available. You leave word (or a "tag") for the party to call you. The person returns your call and you are unavailable, and he or she leaves word (another "tag") that they returned your call. This can go on for days and sometimes does. It is quite possible to have forgotten the reason for the initial call by the time both parties are on the line at the same time! Some executives use several mail systems (electronic mail, express mail, federal mail system, fax, voice mail), and it has increased their productivity. There is a good feeling in being able to compose the question or statement, send it, and forget it. Their desks are not cluttered with little notes or telephone call slips, as they were before electronic mail.

At this point, the reader is probably saying, "I would never use this new technology because I am used to doing it the traditional way." We also hear comments like, "I don't type" or "I need to talk to the person to really get the message across." We have learned from experience that the old saying "Try it, you'll like it" applies to nursing office automation. Once a person begins to use the tools, it is hard to revert back to using the telephone or handwriting material.

## Implementation Tips[2]

In the event the reader is faced with the challenge of implementing some level of office automation, the following points need to be understood:

1. Be prepared to implement change within change.
   - Personnel change
   - Organizational change

---

[2] This section was contributed by Gary L. Hammon, Superior Consulting, San Antonio.

- Technological change
2. Most automation requires economic justification.
   - Deal with dollars saved in salaries
   - Look for highest impact areas
   - Look for 2-year payback
   - Calculate investment per person
3. All groups will demand something immediately.
4. Be prepared to violate some classic principles now and then.
5. Develop and implement in phases.
   - Start with a "friendly" organizational unit
   - "Fly before buy"—use the equipment on a trial basis
   - Learn from the mistakes of others
6. Anticipate that software will be a problem area.
   - Buy, do NOT build office automation software
   - Do not be a testing ground for new software
   - "Not invented here" (NIH) and "we're different" issues abound
   - Uncoordinated programming efforts breed like rabbits
7. Be aware of the automation paradox.
   - Demand for automation will exceed supply (information begets information)
   - Full automation capabilities will not be used (the imagination gap)
8. The biggest challenge is the people challenge.
   - Grab support where you can
   - Light some fires
   - Harness some zealots
   - Invest in training
   - Do a lot of handholding (get the feedback and let the people know you care)
9. There will always be something you did not think of.
   - Known-unknowns are threats
   - Unknown-unknowns are show-stoppers
10. Establish standard software and communication protocols for your organization's equipment.
11. If at all possible, use vendor-provided maintenance services.

# Nursing's Role in Managing Information in Health Care Facilities

Nursing's role in managing information in health care facilities is, of necessity, related to the role of nursing within the organization. In most hospitals, nurses manage both patient care and patient care units within the organization. Usually, nurse clinicians manage patient care and nurse managers administer the patient care units within the organization. Therefore, for some time, nursing's role in the management of information generally has been considered to include the information necessary to manage nursing care using the nursing process (see Chapter 6) and the information necessary for managing patient care units within the organization, e.g., resource allocation and utilization, personnel management, planning and policy making, and decision support.

Concerning the nursing management of patient care, nursing practice is information intensive. Nurses handle enormous volumes of patient care information during every tour of duty. In fact, nurses constantly process information mentally, manually, and electronically. In every aspect of patient care, nurses are continually carrying out the nursing process, i.e., assessing; identifying nursing problems, nursing diagnoses, or nursing hypotheses; determining appropriate action or interventions; evaluating; and reassessing and communicating. Nurses have long been recognized as the interface between the patient and the health care organization. Nurses integrate information from many diverse sources throughout the organization to provide nursing care and to coordinate the patient's stay in the hospital. They manage patient care information for purposes of providing nursing care to patients. There is also a long-standing tradition that during hospitalization the patient's information resides at the nursing station where nurses have the responsibility for maintaining that information on behalf of other caregivers and users of patient information. A classic study of three New York hospitals found that registered nurses spend from 36% to 64% of their time on information handling, with those in administrative positions spending the most time (Jydstrup and Gross, 1966).

A major factor that influences nursing's role in managing patient care environments is the patient assignment methodology used in the hospital or on individual nursing units. While there are variations and modifications, most patient assignment methodologies fall into one of four major categories: functional, team, primary, or case management. Functional nursing focuses on the tasks (or functions) to be carried out on a nursing unit to provide nursing care for patients on that unit. Team nursing focuses on coordinating the nursing staff available on a unit to work together in small groups (or teams) to provide nursing care for geographic clusters of patients on a nursing unit. Primary nursing links a patient and a principal (or primary) nurse care provider who plans and coordinates the patient's nursing care throughout the hospitalization, including discharge planning. Case management is a new system that emphasizes the nursing case manager's responsibility for coordinating and monitoring the care (including but not limited to nursing care) of an individual patient. This care is provided by a multidisciplinary team using predetermined critical or key incidents that must occur among patients with similar diagnoses in a predictable and timely order to achieve an appropriate length of stay. Each of these patient assignment methodologies requires a different nursing role in managing patient care information. Consequently, it also requires different information management skills for the nurses involved.

Similarly, nursing's role in managing information for purposes of administering patient care units is influenced by the role of the nurse managers within the organization, which, in turn, is influenced by the nursing care delivery systems in individual organizations. Variations in decision making, patient assignment, documentation protocols, and institutional governance style all affect nursing's role in information management for administrative purposes. Nursing care delivery systems vary widely among hospitals. Some of the elements of nursing care delivery systems include organizational governance, resource allocation and utilization, patient classification and workload measurement systems, patient assignment methodology, information handling methodology, documentation method, type of patient database, and nursing diagnosis. However, the single most important element that determines the nursing care delivery system, and consequently nursing's role in information management for administrative purposes, is the governance model being used in hospitals today.

A wide range of governance models for nursing delivery systems are being used, ranging from a highly centralized and bureaucratic model of hospital governance to a decentralized, shared governance model. For example, some models allow only central decision making by nurse administrators with only minimal staff input. Other models provide for unit policies to be made by staff and head nurses and allow the staff to have input into departmental policies through committees. In some cases these include membership on senior board committees such as the Board's Joint Conference Committee. In other models, there is a formal shared governance having nursing membership on hospital boards or even self managed units. As the role of staff nurses in organizational governance and decision making diversifies, their role and responsibility for information management to support these decision-making responsibilities will also change. One can envision a future environment in which current information related to organizational planning and policies, as well as resource allocation and utilization, will need to be much more widely available to nursing staff than in the past.

## Obstacles to Effective Nursing Management of Information

In most hospitals, the major obstacles to more effective nursing management of information are the sheer volume of information, the lack of access to modern information handling techniques and equipment, and the inadequate information management infrastructure. As the reader will have noted from reading Chapter 6 and the preceding sections, the volume of information that nurses manage on a daily basis, either for patient care purposes or organizational management purposes, is enormous and continues to grow. Nurses continue to respond to this growth with incredible mental agility. However, human beings do have limits and one of the major sources of job dissatisfaction among nurses is information overload, resulting in information-induced job stress.

Antiquated manual information systems (e.g., handwriting an order, a requisition, a medication card, and a kardex entry for each medication) and outdated information transfer facilities (e.g., nurses hand-carrying requisitions and specimens for stat blood work to the lab on nights because the pneumatic tube system and the portering system are not available between the hours of 2400 and 0700) are information-redundant and labor-intensive processes, to say nothing of an inappropriate use of an expensive human resource. Modern information transfer and electronic communication systems allow rapid and accurate transfer of information along electronic communication networks (see Figures 9.4 and 9.5).

The lack of the software and hardware for modern electronic communication networks is only one aspect of an information infrastructure. The other major aspect lacking in most hospitals is appropriate support staff to facilitate information management. Information systems support

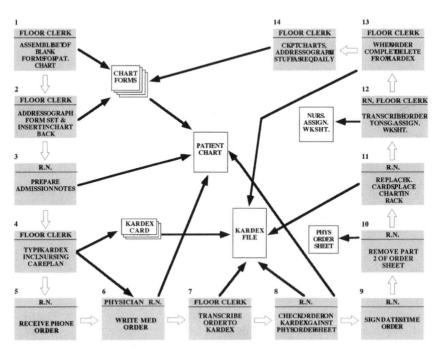

FIGURE 9.4. Manual preparation of new chart and processing of new medical order.

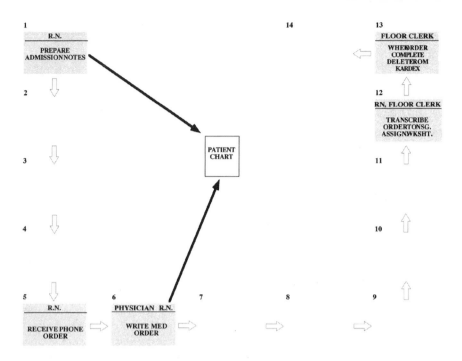

**Figure 9.5.** Electronic preparation of new chart and processing of new medical order.

staff require preparation in health information science (e.g., as offered by the School of Health Information Science at the University of Victoria, British Columbia) to gain expertise in both information systems and a solid understanding of the functioning of the health care system, its organizations and institutions. Similarly, financial and statistical support staff are necessary to help nursing managers appropriately interpret information.

## Issues Related to Effective Nursing Management of Information

Primary among the nursing issues regarding information management is the lack of adequate educational programs in information management techniques and strategies for nursing managers. Presently, there are only a few courses in preservice nursing education programs offering a course in modern information management techniques and strategies related to nursing. At a minimum, such a program must include advanced study of information management techniques and strategies such as information flow analysis, the use of spreadsheets, databases, and word processing packages. Ideally, such courses would also introduce concepts and provide hands-on experience related to the use of patient care information systems.

Nursing involvement and participation in the selection and installation of patient care information systems and financial management systems is imperative. Regrettably, many senior nurse managers fail to recognize the importance of this activity and opt out of the process. They then complain when the systems do not meet the needs of nursing. Senior nursing executives must recognize the importance of allocating staff and money to participate in the strategic planning process for information systems in their organizations. Other senior management personnel must also recognize the importance of nursing input into the strategic planning process for information systems. In any hospital, nurses are the single largest group of professionals using a patient care system, and nursing represents the largest part of the budget requiring financial management. Nursing, therefore, represents the single largest stakeholder group related to either a patient care information system or a financial information system.

The final major issue that nursing must address regarding information management in hospitals is the patient discharge abstract. The patient discharge abstracts prepared by medical records departments across Canada and the United States currently contain no nursing care delivery information. Therefore, the abstracts fail to acknowledge the contribution of nursing during the patient's stay in the hospital. This is important because the abstracts are used by many agencies for a variety of statistical purposes including funding allocation. Presently, much valuable information is being lost. This information is important in determining hospitalization costs and the effectiveness of nursing care. As the importance of national health database increases, it is imperative that a minimum number of essential nursing elements be included in that database. Such a set of data elements would be similar to the Nursing Minimum Data Set currently being tested in the United States (see Chapter 5). The purposes of the Nursing Minimum Data Set are "to establish comparability of nursing data across clinical populations, settings, geographic areas, and time; to describe the nursing care of patients and their families in both inpatient and outpatient settings; to show or project trends regarding nursing care needs and allocation of nursing resources according to nursing diagnoses; and to stimulate nursing research" (Werley et al., 1988, p. 1652). Such data are essential to allow description of the health status of populations with relation to nursing care needs, establish outcome measures for nursing care, and investigate the use and cost of nursing resources. The nursing profession must provide leadership when defining appropriate nursing data elements that must be included in the patient discharge abstract. There is definitely a need to extend the use of the Nursing Minimum Data Set.

# Summary

It should be clear that management information systems and nursing office automation systems will be part of the nursing "world." It is important that nursing education, nursing administration, and nursing research be in the forefront of applying this new technology.

## References

Ein-Dor, P., and Segev, E. *Managing Management Information Systems*. Toronto: Lexington Books, 1978.

Grobe, S. Response to Bulechek and McCloskey's paper. CNA Nursing Minimum Data Set Conference, unpublished paper, 1992.

Jydstrup, R.A., and Gross, M.J. Cost of information handling in hospitals: Rochester region. *Health Services Research* 1966;1:235–271.

McCormack, K.A., and Zeilstorff, R. Building a unified nursing language system. CNA Nursing Minimum Data Set Conference, unpublished paper, 1992.

O'Brien-Pallas, L.L. Analysis of variation in nursing workload associated with patient's medical and nursing diagnosis and patient classification method. Ph.D. dissertation, University of Toronto, Ontario, 1987.

Thibault, C., David, N., O'Brien-Pallas, L.L., and Vinet, A. *Workload Measurement Systems in Nursing*. Montreal: Quebec Hospital Association, 1990.

Werley, H.H., Devine, E.C., and Zorn, C.R. Nursing needs its own minimum data set. *American Journal of Nursing* 1988;88(12):1651–1653.

## Additional Resources

Ball, M.J., Douglas, J.V., O'Desky, R.I., and Albright, J.W. (eds.) *Healthcare Information Management Systems: A Practical Guide*. New York: Springer-Verlag, 1991.

Burke, L.J., and Murphy, J. *Charting by Exception: A Cost-Effective, Quality Approach*. New York: Wiley, 1988.

Fitzpatrick, J.J., Kerr, M.E., Saba, V.K., Hoskins, L.M., Hurley, M.E., Mills, W.C., Rottkamp, B.C., Warren, J.J., and Carpenito, L.J. Translating nursing diagnosis into ICD code. *American Journal of Nursing* 1989;89:493–495.

Hammer, P.S. The next generation in computerized patient classification/acuity systems: Nurse staffing based on actual care delivered. In: Hovenga, E.J.S., Hannah, K.J., McCormick, K.A., and Ronald, J.S. (eds.) *Proceedings of the Fourth International Conference on Nursing Use of Computers and Information Science*. New York: Springer-Verlag, 1991:238–241.

Harsanyi, B., Middlemiss, C., Lehmkuhl, D., Myers, S., and Alig, B. The quest for nursing productivity and quality: Technological tools for nursing administration. In: Hovenga, E.J.S., Hannah, K.J., McCormick, K.A., and Ronald, J.S. (eds.) *Proceedings of the Fourth International Conference on Nursing Use of Computers and Information Science*. New York: Springer-Verlag, 1991:382–386.

Henry, S., Holzemer, W.L., Tallberg, M., and Grobe, S. *Informatics: The Infrastructure for Quality Assessment and Improvement in Nursing*. San Francisco: University of California Nursing Press, 1994.

Hurley, M.E. *Classification of Nursing Diagnoses: Proceedings of the Sixth Confer- ence.* Toronto: C. V. Mosby, 1986.

Kiley, M., Halloran, E.J., Weston, J.L., et al. Computerized Nursing Information Systems (NIS). *Nursing Management* 1983;14:26–29.

Lampe, S.S. Focus charting: Streamlining documentation. *Nursing Management* 1985;16:43–46.

Management Information Systems (MIS) Project. Guidelines for Management Information Systems in Canadian Health Care Facilities. Ottawa: Management Information Systems Project, 1985.

Porter-O'Grady, T. Creative Nursing Administration. Rockville, Md.: Aspen Systems Corporation, 1986.

Wake, M. Changes in Hospital Care Delivery Systems: Implications for Nursing Information Systems. Milwaukee, Wis.: National Commission on Nursing Imple- mentation Project, 1989.

York, C., and Fecteau, D.L. Innovative models for professional nursing practice. *Nursing Economics* 1987;5:6–10.

Zander, K. Nursing case management: Strategic management of cost and quality outcomes." *Journal of Nursing Administration* 1988;18:23–30.

# 10
# Education Applications

RICHARD S. HANNAH

## Introduction: Impact of Computers on Education

Technological change has placed a strain on the educational system. In trying to keep pace with the information explosion associated with the technology revolution, educators have had to devote more time and energy to simple information transfer, leaving little time to help beginners apply information.

Historically, three eras, or "waves," of education can be identified. The "first wave" of education preceded the printed word. Education was a controlled, tutorial process, available for the very few under special circumstances. It was reserved for the literate elite: the clergy and nobility. The "second wave" was ushered in by the Gutenberg press. With the printed word, a centralized education process evolved. Colleges and universities multiplied and became the focal points of learning. Their libraries served as the repositories of existing knowledge. The first two waves of education relied on approaches to learning that remain the cornerstones of today's educational system. These two traditional approaches are academic education and training. Academic education encompasses the conceptual learning process. It is subject driven. Credit is given for learning achievement, and the application of knowledge gained is usually deferred. Achievement is decided by examination. Training is task and skills oriented. Application of knowledge is immediate and achievement is demonstrated by performance and behavior.

Computer-based multimedia may be the "third wave" in education. Computer-based multimedia aids in the knowledge and information transfer process, provides feedback to students about the efficiency of their learning processes, provides access to a vast warehouse of electronic databases, and enables students to problem solve and apply their learning. Ultimately, computer-based multimedia will free teaching staff to concentrate on helping students with their individual learning needs, with emphasis on the "art" rather than the "science" of nursing. The computer applications in this chapter can be applied to the initial education of nursing students, to staff development (continuing education), and to patient education.

In education of health care professionals, as in all areas of education, the traditional modes of learning are straining under the requirements of technological change. The good news is that although technology has created problems within the traditional educational system, it has also provided the solutions for resolving them. Computer-based multimedia has the potential to help educators create a new order from current confusion. With computer-based multimedia, education can move from an era of scarce resources into an era of abundant learning resources. Computer technology has moved faster than the ability of educational and health care systems to assimilate it. The integration of technology-assisted information gathering and learning into the educational system will take time. Three basic stages of assimilating technology can be described as follows:

- Stage 1: Replacement. New technology replaces old technology, but outcomes are not altered. An example is the use of computers to do accounting functions. Stage 1 data-processing functions such as automated record keeping, drill and practice, and machine-scored multiple-choice exams, have been successfully introduced into health care education. Search systems are used by universities for accessing library information, student records, and other types of data.
- Stage 2: Innovation. The capabilities of technologies are combined with traditional functions to create new tasks. For example, increased computing speed and the establishment of wide area networks have created new home banking services. CD-ROM technology, which allows storage and retrieval of vast amounts of information, makes literature searches fast, feasible, and complete.
- Stage 3: Transformation. Innovations accumulate, transforming the way we live. For example, telecommunications and computers have transformed the life and work of travel agents who can give us travel services that would have been impossible, at any cost, a decade ago. In health care, CAT and MRI scanning have transformed X-ray departments into diagnostic imaging departments.

Current applications of computer technology within the education system are concentrated in stages 1 and 2 of development. In many areas, computer technology has been adapted to the established approaches of academic education and training.

The remainder of this chapter focuses on the use of computer technology in health education. This is not imply that other technology (e.g., television, two-way audiovisual communication, videotext) are unimportant, merely that they are beyond the scope of this book. Large central computer systems, minicomputers, and personal computers, video disks, and other modes of interactive learning provide a means for individualizing learning even within a centralized learning system. The traditional modes of academic education and training will always have their place. However, they will be augmented by the power of individualized learning systems to act as information and knowledge transfer vehicles, freeing faculty members to do what only people can do: develop understanding, skill, judgment, and wisdom (Jenkins et al., 1983). The use of computers in Nursing education dates back to 1966 when Bitzer and Bitzer (1973) reported using CAI via the PLATO system, to teach Nursing courses. In 1971, the earliest forms of simulated patient management problems were instituted (Harless et al.). There has been a trend in the past two decades toward the increasing use of technology in nursing education. This is the result of the need to individualize instruction in nursing education and the availability of the technology to do so. Many factors have contributed to the development of this trend: among them are influences arising from general education and nursing practice factors.

## *General Education*

- Tremendous growth in human knowledge and the resulting increase in the amount of information to be learned
- Increased understanding of the teaching-learning process and greater sophistication in identifying the learning styles of individual students with diverse abilities and rates of learning
- Financial retrenchment and budgetary restraint internationally in postsecondary educational institutions, which has produced a need to maximize effective use of limited human and financial resources. Increased wide-scale availability and affordability of educational hardware (e.g., microcomputers, television, video players, CD ROM players, and videotext)

## *Nursing Practice*

- Increased diversity in the settings where nursing is practiced. The focus of nursing practice ranges from the highly technical and largely physical nursing care required by individuals in acute critical care areas (such as emergency, intensive care, coronary care, or neonatal intensive care units) to the predominantly psychosocial nursing care provided to families in communities (such as family counseling, health maintenance, and health promotion)
- Need for nurses to have greater skills in independent decision making
- Need for nurses to have skills that allow them to continue learning throughout their professional careers

## What's in a Name?

The term computer-assisted learning (CAL) and its subdivisions, computer-assisted instruction (CAI) and computer-managed instruction (CMI), have been in existence for some time. Initially, CAI involved using video display terminals (monitors) linked to mainframe computers where the student was asked a series of questions and the computer responded with statements like "Yes that is correct" and suitable feedback for wrong answers such as "No that is incorrect because . . . try again." Students quickly learned to answer incorrectly to view all the feedback responses placed in the program by the instructor. When personal computers became available they were still very primitive by today's standards, and CAI slowly evolved to include text-based lessons with a few images and colors added but was still referred to as CAI. Because the computer has become a much more multipurpose tool since these terms were defined, how do we rationalize this older terminology with what the computer is capable of today? During the past 5 years, the addition of words such as interactive and multimedia to the existing terminology has resulted in a taxonomic nightmare. A brief survey of the literature resulted in the following list of synonymous terms, which is by no means all inclusive:

- Computer mediated multimedia
- Interactive multimedia instruction
- Interactive multimedia
- Learner controlled instruction
- Learner controlled computer assisted instruction
- Interactive computer assisted instruction
- Multimedia computer assisted instruction
- Multimedia computer based training

This inconsistent terminology is confusing to the novice and expert alike.

## So What Is Multimedia?

In general, multimedia refers to computer-based technologies that permit an integration of traditional forms of communication to allow seamless access or interaction by users. It also implies that the computer-based technologies go beyond a single computer to include national and international networks such as the Internet. Because the field is evolving so fast, with so many diverse interest groups, a more concise definition is not possible at this time. The primary advantage of a multimedia approach over more traditional forms of communication is based in the freedom it allows for the creative and innovative expression of ideas and the opportunity it provides for interactive student teacher dialogue through one common tool, that being the computer. How well multimedia will be able to fulfill its enormous potential remains to be seen.

The many traditional forms of communication that form the "pieces" comprising multimedia are summarized in Figure 10.1. These include textual material, graphics, video (both still and motion), animation, and sound. Future advances in technology will soon see virtual reality capabilities being

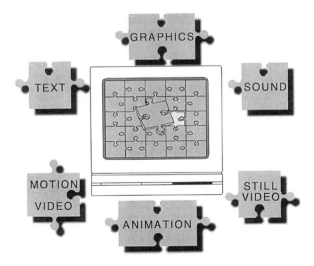

**FIGURE 10.1.** The "pieces" of the multimedia puzzle.

added to this list. Who knows when the senses of taste and smell will also be accommodated?

Just as there are many diverse tools that come together to make up a multimedia program, so there are many different ways in which this thing called multimedia can be used. The major hurdle to overcome lies in making sense of the multiplicity of terms and categories that abound in the literature. As demonstrated in Figure 10.2, there are many different flavors of multimedia but only two basic or primary goals:

- Information gathering activities: information gathering programs provide the user with information and are controlled by the user
- Learning activities: learning activities programs generate learning through exercises and developing skills and are controlled by the system

Information gathering programs can currently be divided into three types: hypermedia/hypertext, multimedia books, and multimedia databases.

- **Hypermedia/hypertext** programs use highlighted text or terms that the user selects to receive more information such as a definition, graphic, or animation about that term or to link to another area or topic. The World Wide Web, for example, is an experimental hypermedia/hypertext system.
- **Multimedia books** are electronic versions of conventional textbooks. In addition to text and images, they contain video and audio clips and allow the reader to dynamically interact with the content.
- **Multimedia databases** are set up as records and fields like the conventional textbased databases you are probably already familiar with but

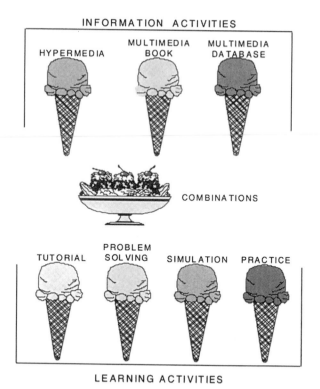

FIGURE 10.2. The many "flavors" of multimedia.

with user controlled access to all the "pieces" that comprise multimedia such as graphics, video, etc.

Learning activities programs fall into four basic categories, tutorials, simulation, practice, and problem solving.

- **Tutorials** is the category where one would place classic computer-assisted instruction (CAI). Historically, the user was presented with some information followed by an activity such as a question, with appropriate feedback for a wrong response. CAI has evolved so much over the years that some use this term to mean multimedia or refer to it as multimedia CAI. However, because of the negative connotation associated with the term CAI, meaning merely drill and practice format, which was all early computers were capable of doing, the term has fallen into disfavor. A modern multimedia tutorial attempts to mimic a live lecture that takes the user through a series of objectives but allows the user to undertake the operation at their own pace and still provide the option of interactivity with the "Teacher". The main difference is an emphasis on thinking and motivation rather than a simple stimulus response. Some national organizations such as the National Council of State Boards of Nursing (1997) in the United States are developing computerized testing programs to measure competence as a potential component of licensure examinations.

- **Simulations**, in the health sciences, are usually of patients. The simulation attempts to provide the user with the same type of experience with patients that they would encounter, for example, by learning to fly using a flight simulator. Health related examples are programs such as "Ethical Dilemmas in Nursing" by the *American Journal of Nursing*.
- **Practice programs** allow the user the develop skills by using repetition and somewhat overlap simulation programs.
- **Problem solving** programs present the user with a problem, provide a number of resources to solve the problem, and let users come up with the correct answer on their own.

Several resources discuss the process of authoring and delivery of multimedia material (Hannah, 1998; Jerram and Gosney, 1996; Kristof and Satran, 1995; Locatis, 1992; Lopuck, 1996). It should be noted that many available programs are so varied in content and presentation that they use combinations of these categories. An excellent example is the program "Learning and Using ICNP" (http://www.omv.la.se/icnp).

## *"Learning and Using ICNP"** *

This is a prototype of a web based environment for learning to navigate within the International Classification for Nursing Practice, ICNP. It is also an interactive tool for nurses in practice, research and nurse students around the world to share their experience of nursing and contributing to the continuing development of a unifying classification. Nurses can participate and contribute to this ongoing process of development to make sure that the ICNP continues to be developed as an international and practice based instrument for nurses.

This application is designed to acquaint the user with The International Classification for Nursing Practice, Nursing Phenomena, alpha version. Different interactive procedures according to learning needs and requirements are built into the application. These will facilitate the learning and training within the classification of Nursing Phenomena. There are possibilities in each module to make comments, statements and/or suggestions and submit these to a database for retrieval. For learning environments there are opportunities to create various kinds of exercises and assignments with this functionality.

---

* This paragraph provided by Gunilla Nilsson and Lars Rundgren Lund University, Lund, Sweden.

TABLE 10.1. The modules of the application "Learning and Using ICNP"

| Module | Contents |
|---|---|
| Data Entry Forms | Learning material with focus on working "physically" with the terms. There are also explanations of important key words to better understand a classification. |
| Hierarchies of Terms | Focus is on hierarchies and how a term is structured in a hierarchy, principles of division, criteria for a term. |
| Terms and Definitions | Focus is on the specific term and it's code, name and definition. It is possible to review, make comments about the term and it's criteria, submit the comments and share the comments about the term. |
| Update/New Terms | Choose a specific term and it's criteria, review, make proposals for updating terms or propose new terms to a proposal database. Review the proposals. |
| Two Languages | Combine two languages and get an immediate translation of a specific term and oppurtunity to compare the original English version of the ICNP with different translations of the ICNP, Nursing Phenomena. |

For the time being, the application is composed of 4 modules, and limited to Nursing Phenomena, alpha version (Table 10.1).

## Nursing Education Settings Using Computers

Whether used for information gathering or learning, the computer is being used in all facets of nursing education. Their use in basic nursing education at both the diploma and baccalaureate and graduate levels is widely reported. In addition, their use in continuing education programs and in inservice education is growing at a logarithmic rate. Most educational institutions and many hospitals and clinics now provide Internet access. An excellent source of information on the Internet can be found in "The Internet for Nurses and Allied Health Professionals" (Edwards, 1997).

## Effectiveness of Multimedia Technology

Many studies of learner achievement using classic CAI have been conducted in undergraduate nursing education. These studies consistently conclude that classic CAI is at least as effective as other teaching strategies in effecting behavioral changes in students (Nyamathi et al., 1989). Substantial reductions in the time spent learning subject matter have been shown in studies of classic CAI (Chang, 1986). Similarly, when classic CAI was compared with traditional strategies, significant cost benefit in favor of CAI was shown. These findings, regarding the effectiveness of nursing CAI with respect to learner achievement, time savings, and cost benefit, are consistent with findings in the health professions collectively, and with findings in general education. The consensus among findings from a variety of disciplines, however, lends support to the generalization that classic CAI is at least as effective as other means of teaching (Belfry and Winne, 1988; Gaston, 1988).

The development of multimedia computers and software and the resulting enhanced capabilities have led to yet another round of comparison studies. The time has come to finally accept that computers are now as effective as any other traditional teaching tool, no better or no worse. Several factors are involved with determining the effectiveness of computer instruction. These are the quality of the programs, environment of use (location and accessibility of computers), and characteristics of the learner (anxiety, level of computer knowledge, etc.) (Khoiny, 1995). Future research should be aimed at developing tools for evaluating new programs and determining how students learn with computers so that existing programs and new programs can be improved rather than this continual comparison with other teaching methods.

## Limitations of Multimedia Technology

Limitations that emerge from detailed study of computer usage in nursing education include the following:

- Cost factors: The initial time investment in developing good programs is extensive. For example, to author 1 hour of effective, terminal-tested tutorials requires 120 to 150 hours. Once instructors become more adept at design strategies, the time required is reduced. However, extensive analyses of cost benefit and detailed studies of cost figures for the development and operation of nursing CAI programs are unavailable. While the cost of the hardware may be dropping consistently, software development costs are not. Hopefully, in the future, institutions will enter into joint development projects to control costs.
- Content control: Unless more nurse educators become knowledgeable in the area of multimedia, there could be a tendency to abdicate the preparation of computer programs for nursing to educational computer software firms. Decisions about nursing and nursing education could slip out of nursing hands. Nursing educators must monitor their own learning programs to ensure that decisions related to nursing remain in the hands of nursing content experts. Conversely, without a firm foundation, sophisticated computerized nursing curriculum will instead become a patchwork coverage of course material.
- Altered professorial roles: Teachers who have felt secure in their role as dispensers of information may feel uncomfortable as they find their role

changing to that of facilitators, moderators, and coordinators. In addition, active involvement by faculty members in computerized instruction requires that a reward structure exists which places value on published instructional design efforts to the same extent that it values research and other publication activities.

- Technology: The dominance of the Windows and MacIntosh personal computer operating systems, along with Internet access, has greatly facilitated the sharing of programs within, and among, institutions. However, many programs are still locked into a single computer language and hardware system. Translating an existing program from one computer operating system and language to another may require more programming time than was required to produce the original. This is an impediment to wider dissemination of nursing material. For this reason, there is probably a redundancy of lessons among nursing users.

- Large central computer systems: These place the nurse user at the whim of the individual or group controlling the system. The autonomy and control provided by personal computers has removed this limitation. Nursing multimedia is now dominated by the personal computer world. However, with number of programs available on the Internet increasing at a dramatic rate and with the huge potential of distance education via the Internet soon to be realized, nursing institutions must consider developing a balance between personal computers and large computer systems.

- Lack of formal communication among users: In North America the vast majority of information about multimedia in nursing education is communicated among nursing educators who meet at annual conferences such as the Symposium on Computer Applications in Medical Care, Association for the Development of Computer Based Instructional System, or the American Nurses' Association Council on Continuing Education. International exchanges, such as Medinfo and the International Symposium on Nursing Informatics, also permit formal and extensive exchange of information about the quality and quantity of available nursing programs.

## Summary

The objective of this chapter has been to provide a macroscopic perspective and conceptual framework concerning the place of computers in nursing education. The "third wave" requirements of education are here. The deficits in the existing system and the capability of using the computer to resolve those deficits must be acknowledged. Taking advantage of these capabilities will mean changes for educators, learners, and health care professionals, as well as changes in work processes and the educational system. The potential of multimedia technology offers education and health care professionals the opportunity to move out of the reactive positions into which they have been forced. Success will be achieved when these professionals contribute their efforts to these phases:

1. Adapt the technology to the needs of the professions
2. Provide users with quality, professionally validated educational resources
3. Develop, update, and monitor multimedia resources
4. Support the utilization of multimedia technology by health care professionals.

Commitment to these efforts will lead to innovation and transformation in learning. While education will surely continue in the classroom, it will also expand beyond it and into every area of professional life. Indeed, far from making traditional approaches obsolete, multimedia technology can become a source of revenue for institutions now hard pressed to make ends meet. The demand for effective learning resources is great.

Computer technology is an exciting addition to the repertoire of teaching strategies available for use by nurse educators. However, its use must be based on substantive content expertise, and success will be dictated by the imagination and creativity of nurse educators who author multimedia materials.

## *References*

Belfry, M.J., and Winne, P. A review of the effectiveness of computer-assisted instruction in nursing education. *Computers in Nursing* 1988;6(2):77–85.

Bitzer, M.D., and Bitzer, D.L. Teaching nursing by computer: An evaluative study. *Computers in Biology & Medicine* 1973;3:187–204.

Chang, B. Computer-aided instruction in nursing education. In: Werely, H.H., Fitzpatrick, J., and Traunton, R. (eds.) *Annual Review of Nursing Research*, Vol. 4. New York: Springer, 1986:217–233.

Edwards, M.J.A. *The Internet for Nurses and Allied Health Professionals*, 2nd Ed. New York: Springer, 1997.

Gaston, S. Knowledge, retention and attitude effects of computer-assisted instruction. *Journal of Nursing Education* 1988;27(l):30–34.

Hannah, R.S. *Designing Multimedia for Health Education*, New York: Springer, 1988 (in press).

Harless, W.G., Drennan, G.G., Marxer, J.J., Root, W.G., and Miller, G.E. CASE: A computer-aided simulation of the clinical encounter. *Journal of Medical Education* 1971;47:443–448.

Jenkins, T.M., Ball, M.J., and Bruns, B.M. The state of the art in technology assisted learning. *AAMSI Proceedings*, 1983.

Jerram, P., and Gosney, M. *Multimedia Power Tools*. New York: Random House, 1996.

Khoiny, F.E. Factors that contribute to computer-assisted instruction effectiveness. *Computers in Nursing* 1995;13(4):165–168.

Kristof, R., and Satran, A. *Interactivity by Design*, Mountain View, CA: Adobe Press, 1995.

Locatis, C., Ulmer, E., Carr, V., Banvard, R., Lo, R., Le, Q., and Williamson, M. Authoring Systems [web page], Jan 1992; http://wwwcgsb.nlm.nih.gov/monograp/author/. [Accessed 28 Jan 1998.]

Lopuck, L. *Designing Multimedia: A Visual Guide to Multimedia and Online Graphic Design.* Berkeley, CA: Peachpit Press, 1996.

National Council of State Boards of Nursing. Computerized clinical simulation testing [web page], Sept. 1997; http://www.ncsbn.org/files/programs.html#cst. [Accessed 28 Jan 1998.]

Nyamathi, A., Chang, B., Sherman, B., and Grech, M. Computer use and nursing research: CAI versus traditional learning. *Western Journal of Nursing Research* 1989;11(4):498–501.

# 11
# Research Applications

With Contributions by Ann Casebeer

## Introduction

The use of computer applications to facilitate research is now an inherent part of most research efforts. Computing hardware and software comprise useful timesaving tools and information gathering sources that are used regularly by researchers of all kinds (e.g., Axford et al., 1996). This chapter focuses on some of the ways in which nursing research can be enhanced by computer applications and the analytical tools they provide or the research information to which they provide access.

Nursing, as a profession, must continue to develop a research-based body of nursing practice knowledge. Therefore, the focus in this chapter is on clinical nursing practice research rather than on research related to nursing education or nursing administration, although many of the principles discussed apply equally well to these areas. Clinical nursing researchers need to exploit all available tools to aid the development of empirically based nursing practice. The purpose of this chapter is to provide an overview of the use of computer technology as one tool available to support clinical nursing research. It is not, however, our purpose to provide a comprehensive discussion of clinical nursing research.

The beginnings of clinical nursing research can be traced to Florence Nightingale. In *Notes on Nursing*, Nightingale states her firm belief in applied nursing research: "Devotion is useless without ready and correct observations. While statistics inform us what percent of the population may die," she writes, "observation tells us which one will die" (Seaman and Verhonick, 1982, p. 8). Unfortunately, much of nursing practice has been founded on intuition-based apprentice training programs. Much of that intuition was experiential, either the nurse's or the nursing teachers', and was passed on to new learners using practitioner authority as validation. The nursing profession has begun to make a concerted effort in its quest for empirical knowledge that will develop a scientific structure for the practice of nursing. To know the true effectiveness of nursing actions, practice-oriented research grounded in sound theoretical concepts is essential (Polit and Hungler, 1995). Nursing must continue to challenge and examine its traditions, experiences, and intuitive actions by actively engaging in nursing research. Training and practice in the use of critical appraisal (Crombie, 1996) and systematic review (Chalmers and Altman, 1995) will ensure that nursing research, like all sound health research, is rigorous, valid, and trustworthy (e.g., see Peckham and Smith, 1996).

## Searching the Literature

Nursing research is predicated in part on the ability of the nurse researcher to carry out a comprehensive review of the relevant literature and, in turn, to critically appraise this literature. This task used to be conducted manually by spending untold hours in the library thumbing through the cumulative indexes and journals. This time-consuming task might or might not result in the researcher locating relevant material.

The advent of computerized databases of literature in the 1960s allowed researchers, initially with the help of librarians, to search rapidly and to retrieve abstracts of literature immediately. University and college libraries as well as the libraries of many large teaching hospitals continue to provide this mediated literature searching to their staff, faculty, and students. In recent years, many databases that were formerly available only from on-line vendors have been mounted locally by hospitals, colleges, and universities, either as standalone CD-ROMs or networked, enabling end-users to search these datbases themselves, either via a telnet connection or via the World Wide Web. Many less commonly used databases are still available only through the on-line vendors, requiring library staff to mediate the search. A list of databases of primary interest to nurses conducting literature searches is found in Appendix D.

In mediated literature searching, a professional librarian works with the researcher to identify appropriate keywords and subject headings to generate a printout of citations and abstracts related to the topic. With the abstracts, the researcher can determine the relevance of a particular article to the research question before attempting to locate the article in a local library or ordering it through an interlibrary loan system. Researchers who choose to conduct their own searches should seek the advice and assistance of a professional librarian first. Library staff can provide guidance in the selection of keywords and subject headings, as well as the correct search protocol for a given database, saving the user hours of frustration. The capacity of a researcher to personally search the literature provides the opportunity for browsing and the serendipitous discovery of information, which might appear unrelated to another researcher or librarian but is important to the particular research question or problem being pursued. Another innovation that helped researchers was the development of on-line full-text information services. For example, Ovid Technologies Inc.

provides enhanced electronic full text to more than 350 of the leading scientific, academic, and medical journals (http//www.ovid.com). Ovid is available through libraries and also as an individual subscription. Ovid includes six separate collections:

- Ovid Care Biomedical Collection
- Ovid Biomedical Collection II
- Ovid Biomedical Collection III
- Ovid Biomedical Collection IV
- Ovid Mental Health Collection
- Ovid Nursing Collection

Once the researcher has searched appropriate literature databases, identified potentially useful citations, located and read the articles, and determined which are relevant to the research question, there is the matter of indexing and filing the information that has been so laboriously gathered. While it is still possible to use a manual system involving index cards or photocopied pages covered with highlighter pen, general-purpose database software packages are available for both office and personal computers. Bibliographic packages have undergone many changes and improvements in the past several years. These packages allow the researcher to set up a personal database of bibliographic references. Further, most of these packages allow reformatting of entries automatically with only one command. If, for example, the researcher has entered all the references in a personal bibliographic file in APA format but the journal to which a paper is being submitted requires Terabian format, the researcher selects the appropriate references, issues a command, the computer automatically reformats the selected references, and they are ready to be printed out. Commonly used programs in biomedical/nursing research are Reference Manager, ProCite, and EndNote (Nicoll et al., 1996).

## Preparation of Research Documents

The bane of every researcher's existence is the paperwork! Grant proposals, correspondence with funding agencies, consent forms, data-gathering forms and instruments, ethics applications, consent forms, progress reports, grant renewals, manuscripts for publication, all require multiple copies of essentially the same information with minor modifications or slight revisions. The advent of electronic text editing facilities and word processing equipment has been a boon to all researchers when preparing research documents. The speed and ease of computer use is well established, assisting in the preparation, revision, and formatting of research documents and reducing the time spent on the paperwork associated with research. An early study by one nurse researcher (Degner, 1986) using a text editing facility on a large university computer observed, during a 4-year period, an estimated 20% saving in writing time required to generate essential research documents.

Text editing facilities today are a regular component of all word processing software available for computers. Standard software packages (such as Microsoft Word or Word Perfect) have become increasingly sophisticated and easy to use. Centers of nursing research and learning resource centers now include computers with appropriate word processing and other software packages as required equipment for their researchers. As publishers move toward increased use of technology, manuscripts are typeset directly from the word-processing diskette prepared by the nurse researcher. For example, *Research in Nursing and Health* provides authors with the option of submitting manuscripts for review either on computer diskettes or via electronic data transmission. Similarly, book publishers, including this book's publisher, Springer-Verlag, are typesetting books directly from diskettes prepared on personal computers by the authors.

The benefits of computerized methods of producing research documents include reduced costs and fewer errors resulting from repeated retyping of the manuscript, increased control of the document by the author, faster production of the finished work, and greater ease of revision. In other words, speed, accuracy, flexibility, and control are the result. The costs incurred are the investment of the researcher's time in acquiring keyboarding skills, locating appropriate software, and in learning to use the available software tools. Additional costs are purchase, lease, or rental of appropriate equipment and software. All these are one-time costs that provide long-term benefits. Access to and ability to use computerized word-processing packages has become essential.

## Data Gathering

There has been an explosion in the range and scope of increasingly accessible data of potential value to nursing researchers. To avoid information anxiety or overload (Wurman, 1989), researchers need to use technology in a helpful manner, improving the ease of data-gathering requirements. Facts (or data) originate with the patient. Nurse researchers who seek to gather reliable and accurate facts should ensure that the data capture occurs as closely as possible to its source, i.e., the subject/patient. Nurse researchers are increasingly using a variety of input devices including digital photography (McGuiness and Axford, 1997), microprocessors, and probes (Reilly, 1985), and bar code generators and readers for source data capture in physiological nursing research studies.

Nurse midwives in the obstetrical department at King's College Hospital Medical School (University of London) in London, England, are using bar code generators and reader interview schedules. These nurse midwives have been instrumental in developing a computer system that generates an interview schedule with each answer option printed in English and accompanied by a unique bar code. The nurse midwife then conducts the interview with the prepared interview schedule in one hand and a bar code reader (which looks like a pen) in the other. As the patient responds, the interviewer locates the appropriate printed response and then passes the bar code reader over the corresponding bar code. The data are then automatically and directly entered into a database on a microcomputer. There are far fewer opportunities for coding or transcription errors with this system.

Principles of source data capture can also be applied to computer-assisted interviewing methods. Computer-assisted interviewing methods allow the researcher to capture the data immediately in the computer in a usable format. Using computer-assisted interviewing methods eliminates the step of data entry. This has the potential to improve data quality as errors are commonly found in the transcription from code sheet to computer. There are three types of computer-assisted interviewing:

- Computer self-administered interviewing (CASI): Research subjects answer on-screen questions by selecting their response with a keyboard, light pen, or touch screen. This method has been used in areas such as lifestyle risk assessment, nutritional surveys, and health behavior studies.
- Computer-assisted telephone interviewing (CATI): In using CATI, a telephone interviewer reads each question from a computer screen. The answer to the question is entered through the keyboard. The answer is immediately placed in the correct preprogrammed row/column position. The captured data are then already in the final form necessary for analysis.
- Computer-assisted personal interviewing (CAPI): Laptop computers allow the researcher to use the CATI process in a face-to-face setting. Questions are posed on the screen. Answers are entered immediately in a form ready for analysis. Both open-ended and closed-ended questions can be posed with these systems.

## Advantages of Computer-Assisted Interviewing

- Automatic branching can be programmed. This decreases error resulting from incorrectly followed skip patterns.
- Text can be inserted into later questions. For example, if current nursing diagnosis or patient problem has been previously entered, a subsequent question would replace "patient problem/nursing diagnosis" with the answer given. This personalizes the interview.
- Question order and response categories can be automatically randomized. When long lists of choices are given, particularly in telephone interviewing, respondents tend to select from those at the end of the list. Random reordering of the responses is one way to address this problem.

- On-line editing and consistency checking allow the interviewer to check data captured while still interviewing. Many programs do not allow out-of-scope answers to be recorded. This also increases the precision of the data gathered.
- Typing is faster than writing when capturing answers to open-ended questions. Software resident spellcheck programs can then clean the captured data. Content analysis of captured data is facilitated because the information does not have to be entered from written notes.

## Considerations in Using Computer-Assisted Interviewing

- Each question is restricted to the size of the computer screen. If a question scrolls to a second page, then the speed of screen redisplay is very important. Each new screen must be immediately useful.
- Provision must be made for nonstandard movement through the questionnaire. The interviewer or respondent must be able to go back to a previous question and check or change an answer.
- A major consideration is the up-front cost in both time and money to initially acquire the hardware and develop the software and questionnaires.

Much clinical nursing research is still at the stage requiring descriptive studies, i.e., the initial gathering of a database from which inferences and conclusions are drawn. With the introduction of computerized information systems in health care institutions, nurses' opportunity to access large databases of nursing practice documentation has become a reality in many institutions. Hospital information system databases provide unique possibilities for retrospective studies generating nursing research questions and descriptive nursing research. However, not all systems are equally suitable for the storage or manipulation of data relevant to nursing research. From a nursing research perspective, there are several considerations and problems associated with the data currently being accumulated in many computerized hospital information systems. Too often such data are formatted and retrievable merely as patient record data rather than with any view to retrieval for research purposes. The introduction of relational database management systems has been most supportive of achieving the goal of simultaneously gathering clinical documentation for the purposes of both legal records and nursing research.

The technology is now available to allow interfacing among computers within one institution as well as between computers in different institutions or facilities. For example, it is possible to use the computer in one site via a modem and telephone lines to merge existing data with data entered on, and processed by, a computer at another location. This technology of intercomputer communication or networking allows creation of larger, more diverse databases. Random sampling, large samples, and control groups may be easier to delineate using the database linkage provided by computer networking.

Furthermore, networking also makes possible collaboration with colleagues in widely separated geographic locations by using electronic mail. Messages can be composed on a personal computer, the personal computer is linked by a modem or Internet connection, and the message is sent and instantly available for reading whether the recipient is in Washington, D.C., Amsterdam, London, England, or the office next door. This enables rapid communications at affordable prices. No longer are researchers dependent on very slow mail service, nor are they plagued by problems that arise when collaborators live in a variety of time zones in widely separated parts of the world. Moreover, "telephone tag" is virtually eliminated. Whenever the recipient next signs on to his or her computer, the message is immediately delivered. Researchers now have the means at their disposal to collaborate with colleagues having similar research interests and expertise, regardless of the fact that they may live and work in locations that are widely separated geographically.

Using electronic means of communications, dialogue and exchange of ideas, refinements in protocols, and interpretations of data can occur in a timely fashion. Previously, these types of interactions among investigators have not been possible unless the investigators lived and worked in close geographic proximity to each other. The advent of listservers on specific topics of use to the nurse researcher (Lakeman, 1997) alongside electronic mail via computer networking and telecommunications now makes multisite research feasible. The regular interactions and contact that are vital to the outcome of any research study are fully available to all investigators working on a project, independent of location. Thus, both data gathering and data analysis are enhanced by the use of computer networking and telecommunications.

## Data Analysis

A critical part of any research process involves analyzing data. Research data can include numerical information of a quantitative or statistical nature or take the form of narrative text providing qualitative information. Computerized software packages can assist both types of data manipulation.

Most experienced nurse researchers are familiar to a greater or lesser degree with the use of computers in statistical analysis. There were hundreds of software packages for use in carrying out statistical analysis on computers. The best known and most widely used include BMDP (programs for statistical analysis of biomedical data), EPINFO (Epidemiological Information), SAS (Statistical Analysis Software), and SPSS (Statistical Packages for the Social Sciences). Institutions in which research is being conducted have at least one of these packages available through their main computing facility. These particular software packages are widely available internationally and on the Internet, possess demonstrated consistency and stability, provide a wide variety of statistical treatments, and are fairly easy to learn and use. These programs are powerful enough to handle quite large volumes of data.

Statistical software packages are increasingly designed for use on personal computers. Some packages, such as EPINFO, are available free of charge on the Internet (http://www.cdc.gov/epo/epi/epiinfo.htm). Francis (1981) has identified five fundamental criteria for the novice to use when evaluating the utility and quality of statistical programs: capabilities, portability, ease of learning and use, reliability, and cost. Although they are not as powerful as the statistical packages available on larger computer systems, researchers may, for a variety of reasons, wish to carry out data analysis on a personal computer. If so, in addition to the criteria just mentioned, researchers must consider the compatibility of their hardware and operating system with what the software package requires, as well as the quality of the documentation provided by the software distributor regarding how to use the system, and availability of upgrades when the software is modified. Other important considerations would be limitations in the volume of data that can be manipulated and stored as well as the constraints in the number of statistical functions that can be performed.

One of the more innovative applications of computers in data analysis is the use of text editing programs in qualitative research. Any researcher who has conducted qualitative studies is well aware that the volume of field notes and interviews to be transcribed is enormous, costly, and frequently overwhelming. Qualitative data analysis packages, such as Ethnograph or NUDIST, provide for entering these data into computer files. This method also provides the capacity to have the machine search the text for occurrences of particular words or phrases indicative of data related to a specific category or cluster. Using these types of programs for qualitative research permits illustrative blocks of text to be copied and moved easily into another file for use in composition of the final report.

## Graphics

Remember the old phrase, "A picture is worth a thousand words"? Before the advent of computer graphics, researchers were confronted with mounds of paper containing the outcome of statistical processing of their data. As they attempted to aggregate and interpret this mound of paper, researchers often sketched graphs and charts of the results. These rough sketches were useful when summarizing data and reducing it to manageable scale. Eventually these sketches were refined and given to an artist, who produced the formal published versions that were used in research reports to illustrate the findings. Computers have the capacity to rapidly and inexpensively produce a wide variety of graphs, scattergrams, histograms, and charts simultaneously with the numerical data analysis. People (and researchers are people, too!) can only retain a limited number of figures in their heads at one time. These pictorial representations greatly assist the investigator's progress in interpreting the data. At the same time, the use of computer graphics to prepare illustrations to accompany research publications also is accelerating the rate and reducing the cost at which findings can be prepared for publication.

## Summary

The advantages of computers to researchers are speed, accuracy, and flexibility. In common with most researchers today, nurse researchers must know how to use automated information systems to their advantage to provide them with better information at all phases of the data gathering, data analysis, and communication of research findings. These computer applications must be combined with well-developed critical appraisal and research method skills. This trend will allow increased creativity and aid the development of the body of scientific knowledge upon which nursing theory, practice, and education are based. Nurse researchers and practicing nurses alike must become proficient in the application and uses of computer technology so as to forward the development and use of an empirical base for nursing practice.

## *References*

Axford, R., Grunwald, G., and Hyndman, R. Information technology in research. In: Hovenga, E., Kidd, M., and Cesnik, B. (eds.) *Health Informatics: An Overview.* Melbourne, Australia: Churchill Livingstone, 1996.

Ball, M.J., and Hannah, K.J. *Using Computers in Nursing.* Reston, Va.: 1984.

Chalmers, I., and Altman, D.G. (eds.) *Systematic Reviews.* London: BMJ Publishing Group, 1995.

Crombie, I.K. *The Pocket Guide to Critical Appraisal.* London: BMJ Publishing Group, 1996.

Degner, L.F. The application of computers in clinical nursing research. In: Hannah, K.J., Guillemin, E., and Conklin, D.N. (eds.) *Nursing Uses of Computers and Information Science.* Amsterdam: North-Holland Elsevier, 1986.

Francis, I. *Statistical Software: A Comparative Review.* Amsterdam: North-Holland Elsevier, 1981.

Lakeman, R. Using the Internet for data collection in nursing. *Computers in Nursing* 1997;15(5):269–275.

McGuiness, B., and Axford, R. Exploring nursing knowledge by using digital photography. In: Gerdin, U., Tallberg, M., and Wainwright, P. (eds.) *Nursing*

*Informatics: The Impact of Nursing Knowledge on Health Care Informatics.* Amsterdam: IOS Press, 1997:281–287.

Nicoll, L.H., Ouellette, T.H., Bird, D.C., Harper, J., and Kelley, J. Bibliographic database managers: A comparative review. *Computer in Nursing* 1996;14(1): 45–56.

Peckham, M., and Smith, R. (eds.) *Scientific Basis of Health Services.* London: BMJ Publishing Group, 1996.

Polit, D.F., and Hungler, B.P. *Nursing Research: Principles and Methods,* 5th Ed. Philadelphia: J.B. Lippincott, 1995.

Reilly, S.M. Infants and colic. Unpublished study, 1985.

Seaman, C.C.H., and Verhonick, P.J. *Research Methods for Undergraduate Students in Nursing.* Norwalk, Conn.: Appleton Century-Crofts, 1982.

Wurman, R.S. *Information Anxiety.* Toronto: Doubleday, 1989.

## *Additional Resources*

CINAHLdirect
   http//www.cinahl.com

International Health Care Research Guide
   http//www.health.ucalgary.ca/

National Institute of Nursing Research (NINR)
   http//www.nih.gov/ninr

National Institutes of Health: Scientific Resources
   http//www.nih.gov/science

SVR Nursing Connections Links to Nursing E-Journals
   http//home1.inet.tele.dk/box4280/nursedk/journ.htm

Research Institutes
   http//pie.org/E21224T3783

Newsgroups
   Usenet newsgroup:sci.research

# Part IV
# Infrastructure Elements of the Informatics Environment

# 12
# Defining Information Management Requirements

Steven C. Ball

## Introduction

Computers were first used commercially for numeric processing, for example, tabulating a sequence of numbers. Later, computers became widely used in transaction processing (e.g., in order entry systems), as well as for results reporting to and from the lab. Computers currently are used extensively to perform even more complex types of processing. For example, by using tables of rules to analyze data, they can help people use information to make higher level decisions. As a result, the manipulations that computers perform on data are becoming increasingly intricate. The people who build or buy computer systems must have an accurate understanding of end-user requirements for the system. It is during a Requirements Definition phase that these requirements are determined.

It is important to note that no single installation exists in which an information system incorporates all the possible functions currently available for use in health care facilities. Integrating all these modules into one system should be the ultimate objective of a total health information system. As the systems developers design and refine future systems for use in health care, nursing will have to play a more prominent role. In the past, nursing needs have been sadly neglected as the result of both vendor ignorance and lack of nursing involvement. There is no doubt that now is the time for a nursing presence in information systems planning and development.

## Stages in System Development/Acquisition

Figure 12.1 shows the major stages in developing, or acquiring, a system. Note that regardless of the option chosen, whether to build or buy, it is the Requirements Definition phase that determines, in detail, the kind of system which the end-user will receive.

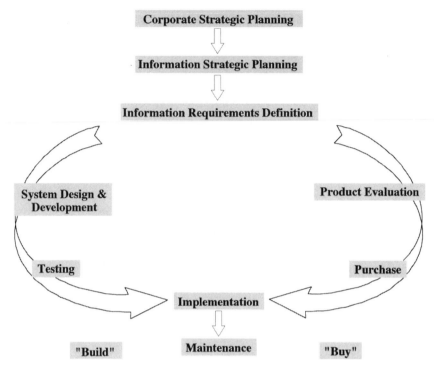

FIGURE 12.1. Stages in system development/acquisition.

## Requirements Definition

During the Requirements Definition stage, system analysts and business experts construct blueprints of the proposed system for the end-user. The end-user reviews the blueprints to ensure the system will meet end-user needs. This is much like a prospective homeowner reviewing an architect's blueprints. The blueprints determine what the system will do, and how. The blueprints also describe how the system will interact with other systems. Traditionally, this has not been a consideration during the Requirements Definition phase. The current situation in most large organizations is a testament to this: computer systems operate independently and redundantly, and interact with each other very clumsily, if at all. For example, it is not uncommon for a nursing unit to have three different terminals, each connected to a different computer system.

Blueprints developed during Requirements Definition can take many forms:

- *Verbal agreements* are the simplest means of defining an end-user's needs. The end-user describes the information requirements directly to an analyst or programmer, and a system is coded based on these conversations. The risk of misunderstanding is substantial, however, given the number of details and level of precision necessary to define information requirements. In reality, only the most rudimentary of systems can be developed in this fashion.

- *Text documents* describe detailed end-user information requirements. However, a language such as English lacks the precision of a computer language and can easily be misinterpreted. Also, while a text document may appear to users to clearly describe their needs, it often misses many important details necessary for the development of an information system.

- *Detailed functional specifications* are text documents that try to overcome these problems. In an attempt to exactly describe end-user requirements, they employ technical language. Highly detailed, they are structured specifically to address the needs of systems developers. Their drawback, however, is their size. The detailed functional specifications for even a moderately sized system can take the form of several weighty volumes. End-users rarely have the time or the inclination to review such documents thoroughly.

- *Information models* are pictures of the end-user's information requirements, along with a glossary that describes the objects in the pictures. They provide the accuracy and comprehensiveness of detailed functional specifications, while eliminating much of the textual volume. In addition, they are effective in eliciting feedback from end-users, and they have the ability to hide unnecessary detail so that a particular property or scope of the requirements can be highlighted for benefit of user-reviewers. There are two primary types of models used during Requirements Definition: function models and data models.

- *Prototypes* are mock-ups of the end-user's information system. They are only shells of a system and cannot perform any real work, but they provide the end-user with an example of what the final system may look and feel like. While they cannot define an end-user's information requirements completely, they are very useful in prompting questions from the end-user regarding what the proposed system will do and how it will work.

## Benefits of Requirements Analysis

There is increasing recognition among systems developers regarding the importance of requirements analysis. Statistics have shown that the single greatest cost of a system over its lifetime is from the maintenance stage. Most computer systems currently in operation are continually being maintained. This maintenance can take many forms: a modification in response to a new end-user requirement (or to a requirement that was finally understood properly by the developer); a correction to allow the system to run properly; a revision to permit a link with another system, etc. The value of requirements analysis is that it is generally much less costly to modify a blueprint than it is to modify an implemented system.

## Function Models

A function model reflects pictorially what an organization does. It breaks down, or decomposes, each of the organization's functions into their respective component functions. A blueprint for a computer system can use the functions from the function model to describe the tasks that the system proposes to automate. Consider the function model shown in Figure 12.2. The parent function, Operate Hospital, is decomposed into five functions. Each of these functions (in relation to their parent they are called subfunctions) describes, in detail, one component of what the parent function does. Together, the five functions completely describe their parent.

In turn, each of the five functions is itself decomposed into subfunctions. This process continues until the lowest level (or leaf-level) functions are identified, and they describe the work done by the organization in sufficient detail for the purposes of the analysis. The functions shown in Figure 12.3 are leaf-level functions; note that these functions are often given reference numbers.

Associated with each function in the model is a textual description, which can include a definition and real-life examples of the function. These descriptions are usually kept together in a glossary. For example:

**2.2.4.3.2 Develop Treatment Plan**. *Based on the specific needs of a patient, a detailed treatment plan is established. This may include referral, enrollment in new treatment activities and services, discontinuance or change of existing treatment activities and services, and/or discharge planning.*

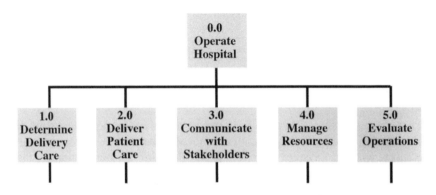

FIGURE 12.2. High-level function model.

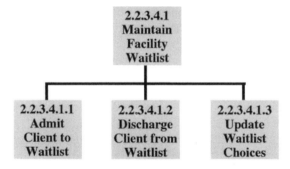

**FIGURE 12.3.** Leaf-level function model.

There are four essential areas for an end-user to consider when reviewing a function model: completeness, accuracy, leveling, and redundancy. A function model must be internally complete in the sense that subfunctions must be able to substitute for their parent. If any aspect of the work done by a function is not reflected in one of its subfunctions, the function model is incorrect. A function model must be accurate regarding descriptions in the glossary. Often, real-life examples can serve to most accurately describe a function for an end-user reviewer. Functions at the same level in the model should be roughly equal in detail. Higher functions represent broad activities, while lower functions represent more detailed activities.

Any activity performed by the organization should appear only once in the function model. A model with activities represented redundantly is incorrect.

## Data Models

A data model pictorially reflects the data an organization need to run its business. It describes these data using a series of pictures, along with a text glossary describing each object in the pictures. A blueprint for a computer system can use the objects from the data model to describe the data which the system will store and use. The data model pictures show how the organization groups its data; these groups are called entities. The pictures also show how the entities interact with each other; these interactions are called relationships. In the data model shown in Figure 12.4, the entities are Patient and Specimen, while the relationship is "supplies."

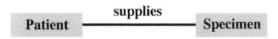

**FIGURE 12.4.** Entity relationship diagram.

These entities and the relationship should be described in the text glossary. The glossary might also contain the pieces of information kept about each entity, called attributes. For example, the Patient entity might have a set of attributes including name, date of birth, and gender. Note that the entity defines a category of data. A piece of real data is called an *instance* of the entity. An instance of the Patient entity, for example, might have attribute values "Moira Halley," "May 31 1958," and "female."

There are five essential criteria an end-user should consider when reviewing a data model: comprehensiveness, accuracy, redundancy, the existence of derived data, and the degree to which it anticipates requirements. A data model must be comprehensive: it must comprise all the information categories (as represented by the entities and their attributes) necessary to satisfy the data requirements of an organization or project. A data model should be capable of accommodating anticipated or impending changes to an organization's business information needs. These might include impending government acts or regulations, changing relationships with stakeholders from changes in the social or economic environment, or the growth or downsizing of programs.

A model should contain no redundant information across different entities. If an Employee entity captured hire date, for example, no other entity in the model should capture the hire date of an employee. The data model should contain no entities or attributes that are derived. If the model contained date of birth, for example, it should not also contain age, because this can be derived from date of birth. A data model must be accurate in terms of its descriptions in the glossary. Like the glossary of a function model, real-life examples can often serve to most accurately describe an entity, relationship, or attribute for an end-user reviewer.

## Summary

As increasing amounts and varieties of automated data become available to end-users, requirements for computer systems have become increasingly sophisticated. Translating these requirements accurately into detailed blueprints is essential for buying or building the appropriate computer system. In fact, an emphasis on defining accurate requirements is almost always cost-effective, given the savings that result later in maintaining the system.

There are several methods for translating requirements into blueprints. Verbal agreements, text documents, and detailed functional specifications are possibilities, but in each case they either lack the necessary precision or are unwieldy for the end-user reviewer. Information models do contain the requisite precision, and are effective in eliciting end-user feedback. Prototypes are also valuable tools for prompting feedback. Blueprints are useful in integrating the development of systems. They help coordinate systems development, preventing redundant systems, and ensuring that systems can interact with each other.

Function models represent the work done by an organization. They consist of pictures that describe how each organization function is made up of component functions. Each function is described in the model's glossary. The system blueprint uses functions from the function model to describe what it is going to do. In reviewing a function model, attention must be paid to completeness, accuracy, leveling, and redundancy. Data models represent the data needs of an organization. They reflect how the organization groups its data, and how these groups (called entities) are related to each other. Descriptions of each entity and relationship, along with the kinds of data important about each entity (called attributes), are kept in the data model's glossary. The system blueprint uses objects from the data model to describe the data of the proposed system. In reviewing a data model, attention must be paid to comprehensiveness, accuracy, redundancy, the existence of derived data, and the degree to which the data model anticipates requirements.

## *Additional Resources*

Barker, R. *CASE Method Entity Relationship Modeling.* Reading, MA: Addison-Wesley, 1989.

Fleming, C.C., and von Halle, B. *Handbook of Relational Daabase Design.* Reading, Mass.: Addison-Wesley, 1989.

# 13
# Selection of Software and Hardware

WITH CONTRIBUTIONS BY CHERYL PLUMMER

## Selection Process and the Role of Nursing

The installation of a computerized hospital information system (HIS) does not just happen. It proceeds from its earliest conception, usually by a senior hospital administrator or board member, through an elaborate decision-making and selection process that finally culminates in an evaluation of the chosen system. This process is summarized in Figure 13.1. It is imperative that nursing be actively involved in providing input at every stage in the process from beginning to end (Manning and McConnell, 1997; Mills, 1995).

The first step in the installation process occurs when the institution, usually the manager of information services on behalf of the chief executive officer, distributes a Request for Information (RFI) to as many vendors as possible. An RFI provides some general information about the institution and requests a general response from vendors regarding the types of products that they manufacture and market. The purposes of an RFI are twofold: first, to announce to vendors that the institution is in the preliminary phase of considering installing an HIS, and, second, to provide the institution with a quick, albeit superficial, educational overview of commercially available equipment. The RFI makes it easier for the search committee to eliminate companies that cannot possibly respond to the more detailed Request for Proposal (RFP).

Often, at the time the RFI is issued a committee of users is established. This committee is usually composed of various department heads (including nursing) within the institution or their designates. One of the first tasks addressed by a user committee is to gather detailed information and statistics about the institution. For example, this baseline description includes information about the type of hospital, daily patient census, number of staff, number of meals served, number of prescriptions dispensed, specialty units, level of patient acuity, institutional design, administrative structure, and geographic area served. This important exercise is frequently coordinated by the data processing computer information services department or, in some situations, independent consultants have undertaken this task. The

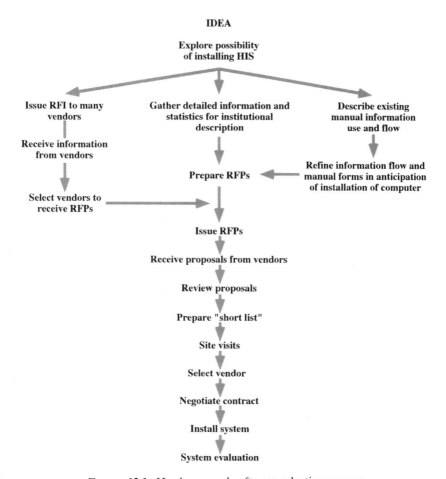

**IDEA**

**Explore possibility
of installing HIS**

**Issue RFI to many
vendors**

**Gather detailed information and
statistics for institutional
description**

**Describe existing
manual information
use and flow**

**Receive information
from vendors**

**Prepare RFPs**

**Refine information flow and
manual forms in anticipation
of installation of computer**

**Select vendors to
receive RFPs**

**Issue RFPs**

**Receive proposals from vendors**

**Review proposals**

**Prepare "short list"**

**Site visits**

**Select vendor**

**Negotiate contract**

**Install system**

**System evaluation**

**FIGURE 13.1.**  Hardware and software selection process.

objective is to gather as much information as possible. This information will be used for many purposes: by the user committee to define the specifications necessary in a computerized information system, by vendors to propose solutions, and by the selection committee to evaluate vendors' proposals, implement the chosen system, and evaluate the effectiveness of the system after installation. Obviously, in this phase, the nursing department has a great deal of information to provide.

While gathering the descriptive information about the institution, an examination of the existing manual information flow and usage should be undertaken. Often an existing manual system is cumbersome and inefficient. There is no point in computerizing such a system. Early self-evaluation will reveal areas needing minor improvement, modification, or major revision. Often time and cost savings can be realized by simply refining the manual information-handling procedures in preparation for installation of a computerized information system. This self-evaluation and documentation may be conducted by the user committee, the data processing computer services department, or a hired systems analysis consultant. The better the initial information handling system and the better its documentation, the better is the final product of a computerized patient information system. In addition, self-evaluation facilitates early identification of gaps or inequities in the existing information management methods. This knowledge permits initiating remedial action. For example, when patient care plans are to be included in the computerized information system, the information analysis may reveal that there is no standard format for patient care plans within the institution or that there is a standard format but it is not used consistently by all patient units.

Using the information received from the RFIs, the institutional description, and the documentation of information use and flow (see Chapter 12), the Request For Proposal (RFP) is prepared. An RFP is sent to selected vendors inviting them to submit a detailed response (proposal) as to how they would meet the needs of the institution. The format for an RFP varies depending on the institution and the author(s). However, the document should provide all available, detailed information to give vendors an accurate description of the institution and its information needs. The more detailed, specific, and precise the RFP is, the more accurate the responses will be. The RFP may be assembled by the chief executive officer, the information systems department, or an independent consultant based on decisions and specifications provided by a user committee representative of every hospital department. Every area reviews the final document before it is issued because clearly no department in a hospital can work in isolation. For example, admitting must work with medical records and they, in turn, with nursing and they, in turn, with the various ancillary areas. To best address the nursing input in developing an RFP for a hospital information system, an actual example is shown in Appendix A. The following paragraphs, however, present a brief abstract of the areas that the nursing member of the user committee should be prepared to address during this stage of the decision-making specifications for the RFP.

The order entry, result reporting, and communications system should allow physician or nursing order entry from all areas of the hospital. This should be done through the installation of remote terminals in all nursing units, patient care areas, and ancillary departments to provide the users in these areas with data entry and inquiry capabilities. Outstanding or queued orders should be approved and verified against a written order before their release to the system for processing. A generalized communication system should provide a standard interface that any future subsystem can use to obtain all required patient demographic and medical information captured by some other subsystem. Additionally, the communications system should allow each subsystem to transmit captured data, whether medical or financial in nature, to a central patient-oriented database for the purpose of storage or transmittal to the financial system. The capability of a future problem-oriented medical record must be displayed.

The second major area that the nursing section of the RFP should address is result entry, or result reporting. The system should provide the ability for on-line result entry by selecting the patient and then entering the results for that patient. Other systems requirements that are detailed in the appendix are a nursing scheduling system and a patient scheduling system. The patient scheduling system should schedule appointments for ancillary services and various treatments within the hospital so that a complete agenda exists for each patient. This eliminates conflicts in appointments between such services as x-ray and physical therapy or laboratory. The system must be able to schedule at least 7 days in advance with reschedule capability by authorized personnel only.

Vendors naturally have a strong self-interest in this process, and therefore institutions should not accept any vendor's offer of assistance with the preparation of an RFP, no matter how apparently innocent and well intentioned the offer. After all, one would not ask the manufacturer of blue socks what color socks to buy! The cost of preparing an RFP rests in the cost of gathering and compiling information. Nurses should be aware that the time involved is often four person-years (the equivalent of one person working for 4 years) or more, depending on the size of the institution.

Vendors interested in competing for the opportunity to sell their product to the institution submit bids in response to the RFP. Such bids specify the vendor's proposed means of meeting the specifications outlined in the RFP. For example, bids include such details as hardware and software descriptions, including number, type, location, and specifications; installation including location, wiring, delivery times, and staff training requirements; and a multiplicity of other specifics including a breakdown of total costs into unit costs. Purchasers should be aware that it will cost each vendor as much as $50,000 to properly prepare a response to an RFP for a total HIS.

When all the bids have been received from the vendors, the institution must select those vendors whose bids they wish to pursue. The bids from the competing vendors are reviewed and evaluated, usually by the user committee. It is imperative that the nursing department have membership on this selections committee so as to participate in the decision making. Some (among many) criteria that are considered in the evaluation process are as follows:

- Soundness of the vendor's technical approach
- Degree to which the proposed solutions for each area meet the evaluation criteria stipulated in the RFP
- Compliance with systems specifications stated in the RFP
- Total system costs over the expected system lifetime
- Past and current experience of the vendor with similar installations

- Qualifications of proposed implementation staff and consultants to be provided by the vendor
- Financial stability of the vendor
- Cost–benefit ratio

Clearly, the nursing perspective is crucial, because the effectiveness of an information system depends to a great degree on the satisfaction of the nursing staff with the system from patient care, clinical, and administrative perspectives. The outcome the evaluation process is a committee consensus on rank ordering all bids submitted based on comparison across all the evaluation criteria. This rank ordering identifies the two to four vendors whose solutions seem most acceptable on paper. These are often referred to as the "short list" of vendors competing for the business.

The next phase of the evaluation usually involves visits to locations where computer systems similar to the one being proposed by the vendor are installed and operational. The purpose of site visits is to inspect the systems being considered. Nursing should insist on being included in site visits. This is not a sightseeing tour. Each member of the site-visiting team is armed with a different structured interview schedule developed before departure with input from the total user committee. Manning and McDonnell (1997) provide a list of questions that should be asked about need, safety and security, effectiveness and efficiency, and economic and social impact. The purposes are to see the system, to clarify understanding of the system, and verify the vendor's claims. The site visiting team is usually composed of four to six members chosen from the senior administrators who are members of the user committee. Site visit locations are suggested by the vendor, but contacts and scheduling of visits are arranged directly by the prospective purchaser and the institution to be visited. Site visits should conform to a predetermined structure so that each system function or lack of function will be exposed and allow for fair evaluations across vendors (Staggers and Repko, 1996). In addition to looking for specific functional criteria, the team should also try to gain a general opinion of the system. Here are some things to watch for, or do, during the site visit:

- Observe the general state of cleanliness and order around the terminals: a smooth running system tends not to have dozens of little notes of "helpful hints" stuck to the walls or terminal.
- Observe the response time of the system, particularly when it is busy.
- Observe whether all staff use the system; in some cases, only clerks use it.
- Ask the staff if they would prefer to go back to a "traditional" method.
- Attempt to speak to staff other than the ones the vendor has arranged for you to see.
- Ask the staff what they do when the system "goes down," i.e., stops working: what you want to hear is "the system rarely goes down."
- Ask "who fixes the terminal when it stops working": this can clarify how many people really support the system.

This is also the time to ask about training, i.e., how long did it take the staff to learn the system and who trained them?

Chapter 16 outlines specific criteria to evaluate the usability of a proposed system. The criteria presented in Chapter 16 can be used in vendor demonstrations or site visits. The final selection of the vendor is based on information presented in the bid and on the site visit. A contract is negotiated between the vendor and the institution; the system is installed and evaluated.

## Suggested Selection Methodology

In summary, here is a methodology that is commonly used by many hospitals and is well supported in the literature. The aim is to minimize the time required to select a system and provide a structured means for all participants to contribute to the selection process.

- Phase I: Narrowing Process
- Eliminate all vendor proposals that fail to meet all mandatory requirements
  Distribute the vendor remaining responses to the RFP to all committee members. Each member should review the responses and decide whether a vendor's proposal appears to address essential requirements. The idea is to reduce the number of proposals to a workable number, from three to five.
  Correlate the member findings. Discuss the proposals where members held different views.
- Phase II: Telephone Survey
  A telephone survey can help determine what sites might be visited. Ask each hospital location about the system: does it meet their needs, why did they choose a particular vendor, what type of computer hardware and software is required to use the system, would they be willing to have a visit?
- Phase III: Site Visits
  Site visits, as we discussed, help to minimize the risk of a wrong choice of vendor or system. Use them.
- Phase IV: Performance Scoring
  Choose a number of factors that are important to the success of the system in your organization. Assign a "score" to each vendor or system.
- Phase V: Financial Analysis
  Remember to consider all the financial costs. There can be front end costs, such as installation, conversions from old systems, renovations to facilities, and training. There will be operating costs, such as hardware and software costs, maintenance costs, insurance, supplies, ongoing training, and staffing. The goal is to try to compare the proposals objectively and consistently.

- Phase VI: Price–Performance Comparison
  Bring together all the price vs. performance and financial information. Try to identify the vendor or system that gives the most results for the least investment. However, keep in mind that price should not be the overriding consideration: it just happens to be one that is in everyone's mind.

## Selecting a Consultant

All nursing directors or administrators during the course of their administrative responsibilities must, at times, make the decision to consider various forms of assistance. Because the history of computers is so brief, virtually no nurse in practice today has grown up with computers as part of her education or environment. The thrust of this book is to provide nurses with a means of learning about computers and information systems. However, not all nurses, now or in the future, need to be computer experts. Those nurses in decision-making positions may choose to seek advice from a health care computer consultant.

## *What Is a Health Care Computer Consultant?*

In choosing a health care computer consultant, a nursing director or administrator should be aware of the several options available. The choice is based on who will be capable of giving the precise help that is being sought. One option is an internal consultant who is a member of the organization and who is most knowledgeable in a certain aspect of the institution's (either patient care or nursing education) problem. The second option is to use the expertise of a computing vendor in the field of health care data processing or educational computing. The third option is an independent professional consultant.

In many cases, the internal consultant can be a good liaison with a consultant brought in from the outside because the internal consultant is intimately involved and knowledgeable in the present state of affairs. While there is no doubt that there is a place for each of the three types of consultants, and it is up to each nursing director or administrator seeking help to choose from the various alternatives on the basis of need, expertise offered, and financial resources.

## *When Is a Health Care Computer Consultant Needed?*

There are a number of specific reasons for bringing in additional assistance in the form of consultants.

- It is often advisable for a nursing director or administrator to seek the advice and support of an outside consultant to justify or modify the current operation of a department.

- The nursing director might have a very specific management or technical problem that needs an expert opinion of a very specialized nature.
- In major equipment decisions, reorganizations, or financial commitments, a consultant might be needed to help management see different points of view to assist them in making the best decision.
- Employing a consultant would also be a step in the process of reviewing the current health care, hospital, or clinic situation with a view toward developing a long-range plan for the organization.

It is important to note that a good consultant very rarely makes the definitive decisions but rather presents for the client a set of viable alternatives. The role of the consultant can be viewed in the broad context, not only as a specialist who might be called on for specific advice, but also as a generalist to whom the nursing department can turn to at regular intervals for the purpose of preventing unanticipated problems.

There are three additional reasons for bringing in a health care computing consultant:

- To provide a state-of-the-art evaluation of the current information system
- To analyze current operations with the intent of providing recommendations for improvement
- To perform a rescue operation, usually at the request of the board of trustees, in the areas of management replacement or cost reductions. This reason is applicable when drastic action is required.

## What Is a Good Health Care Computer Consultant?

One of the most difficult tasks for the nursing administrator or director is defining what a good health care computer consultant is. Such an individual will meet the following criteria (Concordia and Hammon, 1995, p. 96):

- Relevant professional preparation
- Significant experience
- Recognition in the field
- Recommendations tailored to needs of the client
- Reports delivered on time and within budget
- Ability to accomplish change
- Good communication skills
- Fees comparable to those of similar organizations

## Where Can a Good Health Care Computer Consultant Be Found?

One of the best ways of assuring competent consulting assistance is to check with colleagues who have already worked with a consultant who they feel comfortable recommending. Second, the credentials of computer health care consulting firms should be checked by the prospective employer. Another avenue is to work through the various national professional organizations who are often quite willing to suggest several private consultants who might be in business for themselves or affiliated with major universities.

At this time, it is relevant to point out that it is up to the individual who is hiring the consultant to precisely define the parameters of the contract. It is often most valuable to have a preliminary meeting with the consultant in question. At that time financial arrangements and the duration of the consultant's employment should be discussed. In addition, a written agreement about expected outcomes should be reached. In the overall consideration, the employer should be aware of what can and cannot be expected from a consultant. A competent information systems consultant will be able to review the present information system and anticipate future needs; will usually suggest alternative solutions for various organizational, technical, and system problems; and will offer advice about how the system can be integrated with other information systems in the organization.

One might think that a consultant can solve all the problems encountered in the organization. However, a consultant cannot, or at least should not, make basic decisions for the administrator. A health care computer consultant can hardly be expected to solve fundamental management problems in your organization; this is a job for a different type of consultant. Finally, a health care information system consultant cannot legitimately assist you in fighting your private internal political battles.

## Importance of a Good Computer Contract

The definitive legal document that defines the hospital information systems (HIS) or the standalone computer system in the nursing department, laboratory, pharmacy, and so on is the contract. This contract is the legal umbrella that defines every step from the needs assessment document, the request for proposal (RFP), the implementation plan, and evaluation criteria. Given the importance of this document and its consequence, it follows that the contract must be precise and comprehensive, because it will serve both user and vendor for the duration of their relationship.

The points discussed here are broad in nature and are meant only to kindle an awareness in the reader regarding the importance and consequent implications of a computer contract. The objective of this section is to point out the need for a good legal document and the importance of good advice before contract signing. The following is a list of items that have been compiled to help the first-time purchaser of computerized health care systems. These tips are offered to avoid major problems that have been encountered by current users after the contract was signed and could not be amended.

- Involve an attorney at the beginning of the contract negotiation—not just any lawyer, but a lawyer who understands the technology.
- Be a firm negotiator.
- Be demanding of special items your institution has defined as essential while you negotiate the contract with the vendor.
- "It is not so much that the buyer beware, but that the buyer should always be aware."
- Avoid signing a vendor's standard contract. It is his contract and is protecting his interest primarily. You have rights too. Do not hesitate to change the contract to protect yourself.
- Make sure everything is in writing; do not accept verbal promises.
- Read the fine print.

Several key steps can be taken before entering a contractual relationship:

- Prepare the request for proposal (RFP) as clearly as possible, paying specific attention to the fact that those requirements stated in the RFP will become part of the final contract.
- Ask the vendor to attach to their response to the RFP "all agreements they expect to tack onto the computer contract."
- When comparing systems and while doing the final systems evaluations, keep in mind that your choices will be a major part of the final contract.
- A reference check on vendor performance and a check on the financial stability of the vendor(s) being considered is crucial.

After having a broad idea of what a contract should address, the user or purchaser must have some notion of how to negotiate a good contract. Certainly, the overall purpose of a contract is to have a comprehensive document that provides the nursing director or the hospital administrator with the flexibility to monitor the satisfactory performance of the vendor. It is very important to remember that the final contract must be signed before the actual purchase of the system. If the hardware or software is installed before contract signing, additional problems are introduced.

It is to the buyer's disadvantage if only one vendor is being considered in the final negotiation period. At least two vendors should be considered until the contract is signed. The contract is also much more effective if top level management from both organizations are present in the final phases of the contract negotiations. By this time the hospital, including the nursing department, should have clearly defined its needs and be able to document their requirements in the contract.

Try to evaluate the vendor's position throughout the negotiation. Every computer company has its own "standard contract" that has been carefully written by their lawyers to the best advantage of the computer company. Your lawyers must help you to implement your contract needs and protect you from the vendor's lawyers who will undoubtedly try to implement their standard contract.

Ask your legal counsel to define the element of profit for the vendor. What will the effect be on the vendor of having you as a user? Consider the time and other resources invested in the proposal, site visits, and demonstrations by the vendor. Is the vendor strictly a provider of the health care computer services you need or is it a larger company marketing many health care or even general computer services? This will give you some idea as to how the vendor values your business.

All these points can help you develop a strong negotiation strategy. A few more logistic points that might be of interest are:

- It is advantageous for the buyer to maintain control over what is being negotiated and how it is being negotiated.
- The buyer should have an agenda and set the times and locations of negotiation.
- The buyer should decide the chronological order of items to be negotiated.
- A healthy two-way negotiation of give and take should be established to reach the desired goal.
- The buyers should always have a set of alternatives, but it is essential that a position statement be developed from which no compromise is possible (the bottom line).
- To draw an analogy, when bidding at an auction, have a set price on each item over which you will not bid. Working with a contract is very similar. There must always be limits or the game is lost before you start!

The ultimate purpose of contract negotiation, however, is to produce a workable arrangement that satisfies the buyer and can be carried out by the vendor. Compromise is almost essential even on key issues of importance to the buyer. The buyer must remember that if the contract becomes too restricting or burdensome for the vendor, the relationship can end up in legal friction to the point of nonperformance. Negotiation is an art—in a good contract, both parties feel they have won.

A sensible contract will differ according to the objectives of the purchaser. One basic similarity remains, however, that the contract is the written document of mutual consent made between the buyer and the seller. The contract will stand as the written testament of the legal obligations of both parties. It should be written to anticipate problems and should establish an ordered mechanism as to how these problems will be remedied. In addition, the contract should deal with the following:

- Acceptance listings
- Ownership of software source code
- Payment plan
- Ownership
- Warranties and liabilities

- A detailed set of descriptions of responsibility for both parties including software, maintenance, and support functions
- Technical and legal standards to measure success or failure of the implementation

## Linking Nursing and Health Care Information Systems

The object of this section is to impart an understanding and recognition of the importance of nurses being educated about computers as a way of ensuring the success of computerized information systems.

One of the essential aspects of a successful information system project is establishing good communication between and among the various professionals, technicians, consultants, and administrators within a health care organization. This section emphasizes a few basic rules that have been effective in closing the communication gap between nurses and the computer systems department. In other chapters, basic computer concepts and details of information systems have been expanded upon, but the emphasis here is to make the reader aware of the importance of basic conceptual understanding between these two professional groups.

Hostility toward computerization produces definite obstacles in the course of system implementation. It is, therefore, vital that nursing management be fully committed to the changeover so as to make a smooth transition and sustain the morale of the nursing staff. Given the fullest commitment by all parties, it is still hard to computerize effectively. One of the most difficult problems encountered in the relationship between the nurses and the data-processing professional is the establishment of a communications link. Most tasks in the health care computing field require the expertise of both disciplines. An effective working relationship is a prerequisite for the accomplishment of these complex tasks.

The basic characteristics of the average health information professional are that he or she is energetic, anxious to help the user, wants to be creative, is convinced that the computer can help solve the problem, and is totally unaware of the user's real problem. The willingness and technical capabilities of these individuals must not be underestimated. The question is "How can the health professional best utilize these highly motivated, specially trained individuals who are most eager to lend their talents to the improving of health care delivery?"

Moreover, to effectively work with clinical information systems, it is essential to recognize the principles and methods of modern information processing. Nurses should grasp the basic concepts, such as design of computer-compatible records and transformation of English statements into logical computer-compatible systems, as well as the benefits and risks of electronic storage of medical information. On the other hand, to achieve a mutually beneficial working relationship, the computer professional must learn the terminology and practice of modern nursing. The following suggestions will be most helpful in integrating computer systems into the various areas of nursing practice.

1. Have the operation of your department well defined in your own mind (Mills, 1995). One must know what is happening in the nursing department before one can undertake the task of creating a computerized system. All activities of the operation must be documented, and the sources and recipient of all transactions must be identified (see Chapter 12). The smallest detail must be explainable. If you do not know what is going on, there is no way of making the computer help you. If anything, you will have a more serious problem on your hands. You must precisely define the input to the new system to begin the task of developing a useful tool.

2. Know what you want to do. One must know what is desired as output; the end result must be well defined. If you want nurses' notes in a certain format, be able to explain to the computer professional why you want it that way. Do not worry, at the design stage, about how the data are manipulated by the computer; be more concerned with what you want to get out of the system. Draw a detailed picture of your desired report.

3. Be aware of all the exception conditions. This is the most difficult part of designing any system. Finding out and satisfying all the exceptions that can arise during the implementation of a new system will eliminate most of the traumatic situations that might occur. The more precise the identification of exception conditions during the design phase of the project, the smoother and more well accepted the final system will be.

4. Ask questions. No one enjoys talking about their work more than a dedicated computer professional. Get explanations about the purpose of each device that your application is using. "Oh, you wouldn't understand" is a response that should not be accepted. Unless you understand what facilities the computer has available and what their functions are, the mystique of "DO NOT FOLD, SPINDLE, OR MUTILATE" will inhibit you from taking full advantage of the computer's capabilities. It is wise to remember that "a little knowledge is dangerous." Make sure you understand the answers to your questions.

5. Get explanations of the computer solution. The computer user must understand how the computer is maintaining the data for the system. Nurses must be able to compare the computer data flow with the data flow that occurs in the manual system. The computer person typically thinks very logically, and many of the techniques implemented within a computer system could also be valuable if adapted to the manual system. It has been said that the best method of developing a good manual system is to plan for a computer. Develop a complete computer system and design a manual backup system that emulates the computer system, then install the manual backup system. This may be a bit extreme, but it does emphasize the fact

that much can be learned by comprehending the computer solution to your problem.

6. If you are not getting what you need, speak up. Once the computer system is installed and running, keep the data processing or information services people informed about what they need to do to make the system better fit your requirements. If all you do is complain to your coworkers about how bad the computer is, then it will never work satisfactorily. You have to tell the people who can do something about it. A good system is never quite complete and must be maintained and changed to stay up to date.

7. Make constructive suggestions. Do not limit your criticism of the computer system to "the dumb computer doesn't work." Tell the computer programmer or analyst, specify the problem, and participate in solving the problem. A successful well-received computer system is a partnership between the end-users and the data-processing people who implement the system (Clough, 1997). Good communication between these groups is essential for the realization of a successful system.

8. Do not be overly impatient. It took a long time for your system to evolve to where the decision to use a computer was made. Computer systems are not created in a day. Extensive work must be done in system design, programming, and interfacing to have a current operational system. Ask the information systems people for their time estimates to implement the new system, then double the time because data-processing people are habitually overoptimistic about how fast they can accomplish a task. Keep thinking about the benefits of the system once it is operational, but maintain sufficient pressure on the computer people to be sure the system gets implemented. However, do not be too impatient. If you force a "quick and dirty implementation," the system will not be what you really want and will require a great deal of your time to correct.

9. Be considerate of the computer professional's problems. Computer professionals are human beings and, therefore, have all the emotional conflicts, problems, and stresses to which any other human being is subject. A family member may get sick, or their computers can be out of order, and that impacts implementation schedules. They are not immune to the frustrations of everyday life because they work with sophisticated machines and speak in computer buzzwords. Treat the computer programmers and systems analysts as you would any other valued coworker, and the world will be more pleasant for everyone involved.

10. Understand the system's limitations. After you have a functioning system, it is very easy to escalate your desire to the unattainable. You have to understand the restrictions well enough to not make impossible requests. There are many reasons why a computer cannot fulfill all your desires. Talk to the information systems people about this, and perhaps there is an intermediate solution. Try to keep your dreams realistic and do not demand the impossible.

The total organization can derive significant benefits by the early establishment of an Information Systems Steering Committee (previously referred to as the user committee). This committee should represent every department of the health care institution. Find out if your organization has one and who the nursing member is. By defining the goals and objectives of the institution, the administration can make effective use of the catalytic characteristics of the information management professional.

## Summary

This chapter has considered various aspects related to the preparation required in anticipation of the implementation of computer applications in nursing practice settings. The focus has been on preparation for clinical applications, but the same principles apply for administrative, educational, or research applications. Guidelines for communications between nurse users and information systems specialists are provided.

The following "commonsense" guidelines might be of help during the selection process:

- Write down what is not clear.
- If you do not understand, say so.
- Keep the document simple. Do not try to "snow" others.
- Realize you cannot know it all.
- Assign responsibility for tasks.
- If someone else drops the ball, pick it up.
- Head off trouble before it happens.
- Two heads are sometimes better than one.
- Avoid distractions.
- Isolate tasks; do things one step at a time; use a time line.
- Be patient; involved problems take time to solve.
- Be willing to follow up.
- Do not be afraid to fail; we all learn from our mistakes.
- What you do will make a difference!
- Do not hesitate to ask questions!

The employment of a competent health care information systems consultant should be considered as one of the wisest decisions that nursing management can make when computerized patient information systems are being considered. What the organization is doing is hiring one or two people who have spent a lifetime in education and experience dealing with a question or a problem being posed by the organization. For what amounts to a minimal financial commitment, the nursing organization will have bought the most competent information, addressed specifically to their defined needs. However, as with any type of advice, nurse administrators must use the advice of health care information systems consultants with discretion; after all, consultants do not have to live with their proposed solutions. Consultants' advice must always be tempered by the nurse administrator's common sense, intimate knowledge of the institution, and a deep and abiding faith in personal knowledge of the nursing discipline.

To prepare nurses for the widespread use of information systems in health care, there is a strong need for continuing education, inservice education, and undergraduate education programs that provide nurses with general knowledge about information systems. Some nurses require more advanced education about information systems to enable them to maintain their nursing focus and to enable them to serve as interpreters between information systems people and nurse users of information systems. A third group of nurses is required to be knowledgeable in both nursing and information system science. This latter group will participate in developing, implementing, and initiating new health care information systems.

## *References*

Clough, G.C. Getting the right system: The CHIPS experience. In: Gerdin, U., Tallberg, M., and Wainwright, P. (eds.) *Nursing Informatics: The Impact of Nursing Knowledge on Health Care Informatics.* Amsterdam: IOS Press, 1997:569.

Concordia, E.E., Hammon, G.L. How to select a nursing informatics consultant. In: Ball, M.J., Hannah, K.J., Newbold, S.K., Douglas, J.V. (eds.) *Nursing Informatics: Where Caring and Technology Meet,* 2nd Ed. New York: Springer-Verlag, 1995:95–98.

Manning, J., McConnell, E.A. Technology assessment: A framework for generating questions useful in evaluating nursing information systems. *Computers in Nursing* 1997;15(3):141–146.

Mills, M.E. Nursing participation in the selection of HIS. In: Ball, M.J., Hannah, K.J., Newbold, S.K., Douglas, J.V. (eds.) *Nursing Informatics: Where Caring and Technology Meet,* 2nd Ed. New York: Springer-Verlag, 1995:233–240.

Staggers, N., Repko, K.B. Strategies for successful clinical information system selection. *Computers in Nursing* 1996;14(3):146–147, 155.

# 14
# Data Protection

## Introduction

The issue of privacy is difficult. The individual has the inherent right to control personal information. However, to provide the best possible care and service to the individual, public and private organizations must know some of that information. The issue is further complicated because "privacy" has not been defined in a way that is widely and generally accepted. Actions such as collecting and storing unnecessary personal data, disclosing data to individuals or organizations that do not have a genuine need for it, or using private information for something other than the original purpose could be considered intrusive.

Since the 1960s, the widespread use of computers has led to concern about the large mass of data collected through sophisticated data linkage capabilities. The following sociolegal concerns are widespread among the public:

- How and what information will be collected
- How the collected information will be used; who will have access to it
- How the collected information can be reviewed and, if necessary, corrected

Within the nursing community, concern over data protection has always been present. The power provided by new technologies such as computers and the Internet has heightened the concern of nurses for these reasons:

- More data and information are available
- More possibilities exist for errors in the data
- Organizations rely on information systems for essential functions
- More data is shared between disciplines and organizations/institutions/facilities
- Public concern over possible abuse of information and privacy is strong

Until recently, terminology in the area of data protection has not been uniform. However, a standard is emerging, based on the headings used by

Working Group 4 of the International Medical Informatics Association (IMIA) (Hoy, 1997). In the area of data protection, then, Data Security is the overarching concept, with three subareas:

- Usage integrity, more commonly called confidentiality
- Data or program integrity
- Availability

This chapter provides a foundational understanding of the concepts contained in Usage Integrity (confidentiality), Data or Program Integrity, and Availability. The major focus has been on addressing usage integrity (confidentiality). As approaches to data usage integrity have been identified and implemented, more attention will be focused on data/program integrity and availability.

## Usage Integrity (Confidentiality)

Exchange of information is a cornerstone of the provision of health care. Nurses are continually asking patients to share information relating to their health, including work, home, and social life. When a patient shares something with the expectation that the information is for a limited audience only, that is called confidentiality. The formal definition for *confidentiality* is the respect for the privacy of information that is disclosed and the ethical usage of that information only for the original purpose. *Privacy* is the right of individuals and organizations to decide for themselves when, how, and to what extent information about them is transmitted to others.

Some degree of anonymity within the environment is necessary for mental and physical well-being. On the other hand, often the needs of society supersede the individual's right to privacy. As computer data banks proliferate, the public's concern rises. In a 1994 survey, 52% of respondents thought that computer records were more secure than written records. Surprisingly, when the same survey was conducted in 1995, only 42% thought this (McKenzie, 1996). The increased use of automated personal data systems creates a serious potential for abuse and for the "invasion of privacy." Today, systems abstract a uniform data set from medical records at the hospital level and forward it to local, state, and federal organizations. The exchange of medical records information between hospitals and third parties has been made easier because of computers. This exchange will increase in the future.

To date, these exchanges usually have the personal identifying data removed. The main problem with automated medical records is the *potential* for breach of privacy. Many health professionals, citizen groups, and other individuals directly affected by such systems consider them to threaten the basic rights of the individual. Underlying these attitudes is a deep concern for confidentiality. Data collection did not originate with the use of computers. In 1918, physicians began, as a matter of practice, to record information in a medical record. Today, the record is the vehicle for communicating information among health care professionals. A health team administering comprehensive care to the patient develops and uses the patient record. Health care professionals assume that a patient will fully disclose all information related to his condition so that proper care and treatment can be given. For an effective relationship to exist between the health care professional and the patient, the patient must believe that all information provided will be treated confidentially. Unless patients can feel assured that the highly sensitive and personal information they share with health care professionals will remain confidential, they may withhold information critical to their treatment. This need for assurance existed before computerized records. However, the introduction of computerized health care records has brought the issue of confidentiality and security to the forefront.

The capabilities of modern technology have created a public awareness regarding the loss of confidentiality inherent in the systems being developed and installed. People other than the direct caregivers have become responsible for the storage and safekeeping of records. Other uses of individual information—in accounting, administrative decision making, and biomedical research—are being explored now because the information is easy to retrieve. The flowchart in Figure 14.1 suggests the multitude of possible uses for health care data. The ability of computers to match data from diverse sources, to handle large quantities of data, and to maintain records over time has resulted in an unprecedented risk to personal privacy. Record keeping and record protection (i.e., data security) are only parts of the problem. It is access to records for "secondary" purposes that poses the major risk to maintaining confidentiality. Demands for computerized patient data in the health care setting, other than for the actual administration and delivery of an individual's medical care, include these:

- Utilization of facilities and standards reviews
- Epidemiological studies
- Program evaluation
- Biomedical, behavioral, and health services research
- Financial/billing purposes

In the United States, many third-party payers have access to patient information. For example, the Medical Information Bureau (MIB) has a computer data bank. The MIB is a trade association of more than 700 life insurance companies of which most of the insurers have computer terminals in their own offices and for 20 cents an inquiry can directly search the health records of 12 million persons. Health and accident insurance may be sold by member firms of MIB, and thus information secured for one purpose may be used for another. Attempts by third party providers to control costs by requiring prior approval of prescribed medical treatment using case

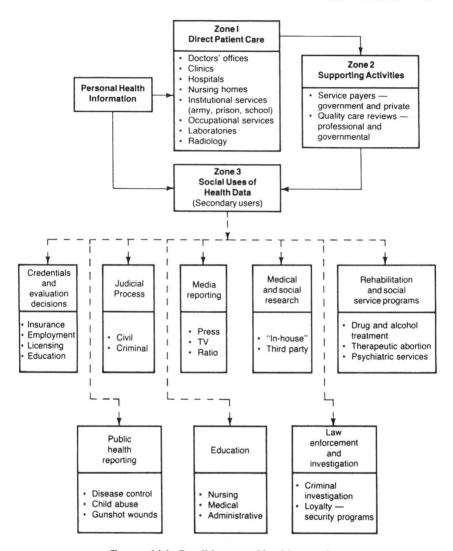

**FIGURE 14.1.** Possible uses of health care data.

management techniques provide the insurers with access to even more personal health data.

Putting private and personal information to "secondary" uses poses a major threat to patient privacy and creates complex social and ethical dilemmas in health care. Examples of misuse of confidential information, from old medical files left in the trash whatever to identification left on computerized health databases, are readily found in the newspapers. This sort of abuse does little to reassure the public. Possible linking of various databases and fast retrieval and distribution capabilities have increased concern over how private this information might truly be. The needs of users, that is, physicians, nurses, police, and insurers, to have easy access to medical information systems must be balanced with the needs of the individual for privacy.

## Data Security Breaches

There are many outcomes that can occur as a result of breaches in data security:

- Public embarrassment or loss of public confidence
- Personal safety
- Infringement of personal privacy
- Failure to meet legal obligations
- Commercial confidentiality
- Financial loss
- Disruptions of activities (Barber, 1997, p. 62)

Damage to patients is of vital concern; however, other types of damage can also be important. Legal cases, financial loss, and loss of public confidence can cause great damage to organizations. To address these concerns before problems occur, it is essential nurses be involved in formulating specific, documented policies related to data security. When such policies are in place, nurses are not left in the dangerous situation of having to make judgments about use of data without any regulations to assist them. The three areas identified here must be considered when defining data protection policies. Data protection policies will contribute to an overall organizational disaster plan as discussed in Chapter 17. A Confidentiality Risk Check-up questionnaire can be found at http://www.ahima.org/publications/1a/Jan-Feb.inconf.html

## Protecting Data Usage Integrity

Three approaches to protecting data usage integrity are suggested: hardware, software, and organizational.

### *Hardware Approach*

*Hardware security* is concerned with those protective features that are part of the architectural characteristics of the data-processing equipment. It also includes the support and control procedures necessary to maintain operational integrity of those features. Hardware security features include hardware identification, isolation features, access control, surveillance, and integrity. Specific protection could include physical barriers such as special doors, locks on individual machines, and control over the use of communication links to the system.

## Software Approach

*Software security* requires the operating system to provide the same features as the hardware security system. It must be able to identify and authenticate, to isolate, to control access, and have surveillance and integrity features. Security mechanisms designed to protect patient confidentiality generally rely on some combination of authentication, authorization and auditing (Bowen et al., 1997).

Authentication refers to the methods by which a system verifies the identity of a user, usually based on passwords or physical tokens. Passwords, although a useful approach, have many inherent problems. Users exchange passwords, passwords are left written down by the computer, common words are used, and passwords are not changed on a regular basis.

Authorization denotes access controls or other means used to provide specific information to a given user. Systems that implement authorization procedures generally attempt to determine whether a given user has need-to-know for the requested information. Some of the dimensions that are considered in formulating mechanisms for making such decisions include user roles, types of database interactions, and the purpose for which the information will be used. Commercial programs exist to aid this process.

Auditing is used to record and review a user's interaction with the system. These user records create an audit trail. Depending on the system, auditing may be unapparent to the user. Audit records can then be used to identify unauthorized attempts at access and patterns of access. The threat of sanctions is often sufficient to deter abuse of information access. However, such systems depend on users being aware of and sensitive to the consequences of abuse. Another problem associated with the use of auditing as a security approach is that it is retrospective (Bowen et al., 1997). Depending on the design of the processes to review auditing records, much time can pass, with the result of continued information security breaches, before the unauthorized usage is detected and confronted.

## Organizational Approach

The procedural considerations that bring together computing equipment, software, and data in an operational electronic data-processing environment are collectively called *operations security*. These procedures must provide for secure processing during data input, processing, storage, and output. The administrative and organizational component of privacy protection involves the development and dissemination of policies, procedures, and practices related to privacy of patient information. Administrative policies and procedures need to be put in place to protect the privacy and confidentiality of patient information. These should include disciplinary measures for violation. An initial concern is the question of which individuals or categories of workers should have access to what information in a hospital information system. These are difficult decisions to make. Each user's or department's needs must be considered, along with those of the patient. The committee who makes these decisions and the information systems staff will most likely know how best to access the entire patient record. Yet, even then, there is potential for violation of confidentiality. For example, some institutions employ data entry clerks to enter previously written data. These employees have access to the entire patient chart while the data are being entered, but are not bound by a "code of ethics" as are other health care personnel. This could be a strong argument against using these employees to enter data. It might be better to have all professionals enter and retrieve their own data. Other considerations include where terminals, printers, and data storage are located. Portable computers and bedside terminals are liable to theft and may allow the patient or visitors unauthrized access to the system. The organizational decisions about ways in which physical items are sited will influence the hardware and software approaches to security that must be taken.

## Data/Program Integrity

Data must be collected, stored, and transmitted in a manner that preserves the integrity of those data. Accurate collection of data along with mechanisms for reviewing and correcting specific information are essential to preserving data integrity. The use of source data capture technologies enhance the probability of collecting accurate data (see Chapter 6). A key concern of consumers is the ability to view personal data and correct it as required. Accuracy is the foundation for data integrity. Arduously protecting the storage and transmission of that which is fundamentally flawed is a strong possibility if attention is not paid to all three aspects of data integrity.

There has always been a concern about protecting the storage of data. In times past, the primary threat was from natural disasters such as fires, floods, tornadoes, or earthquakes. Electronically stored data are also open to these threats. However, the more common threats to data are storage integrity come from system malfunctions, either accidental or malicious. Computer viruses that corrupt individual data or the entire system are a major threat to the security and integrity of data storage. The viruses are commonly introduced into an organization's information system by users transferring infected files between their personal computers and the organization's computers. Another threat to the secure storage of data is the ability of users to copy data files onto personal computers to work at home. Confidential patient information may be left on diskettes that are then partially copied over and given to someone else, with identifiable data remaining accessible on the diskette. As part of an overall data security plan, organizations must develop and enforce policies related to the transfer of information between the organization's information system and an individual user's personal computer.

The transmission of electronic data both within an organization and with outside agencies provides another large opportunity for exposure to security threats. Many organizations have developed policies to deal with the security of data transmitted with the organization, for example, between departments. However, the exponential growth of the use of the Internet for secure data transmission requires a fresh look at transmission policies. The level of concern about Internet security depends on how an organization is using the Internet. Even organizations that have not connected their networks to the Internet are at risk as staff members use the organization's systems and networks to connect to the Internet using their personal subscriptions. Organizational use of the Internet can be roughly divided into three categories, each with specific data transmission security concerns (Miller, 1996).

1. Using the Internet as an information resource or on-line library, which includes searching the CINALHDirect database or other on-line databases for articles and downloading articles from a website. The risk here is not from inappropriate transmission of secure data but of downloading a virus along with the article. The installation and maintenance of antivirus software should protect data from corruption from an Internet connection.

2. Using the Internet as a communication vehicle. Sending and receiving e-mail, participating in mailing lists or discussion groups, and making information available to the public through a website are examples of the Internet's use as a communication tool. As a communications tool, the Internet should not be considered to be secure. Messages may be read by many other persons in addition to the intended recipient. The message may be stored on a variety of computers before delivery, or the recipient may make copies or forward the message to any number of people. Transmitting electronic patient data to other health care professionals via e-mail, for either consultation or research, must also be regulated for the reasons stated above. Communicating with patients via e-mail may pose risks to the patient's privacy and data security, especially if the e-mail is directed to the patient's employment e-mail address. Policies must be developed to govern communication using the Internet so as to preserve data transmission integrity.

3. Use of the Internet as an extension of the Organization's Network, including linking your computer systems to another organization's computer systems to participate in a joint research project, or providing remote access for staff members or transfer of files to other organizations. File transfers (FTP) should be used with caution. When FTP is used to transfer

files into an organization, there is a risk of downloading software in violation of copyright or infecting the organization's computers with viruses. Transferring files outside the organization runs the risk of disclosing confidential patient or proprietary information either in the file transfer itself or as a result of the way in which the information is handled in the receiving organization. Research and policy discussions about the secure transmission of electronic patient information are accelerating as the electronic health record becomes a reality in many jurisdictions.

## System Availability

A system must be available in the right place at the right time. Overloading may slow down a system's response, while other more serious problems may shut it down altogether. All computer users live in fear of their system becoming unusable because of failure of the machine or its power supply. Solutions may involve uninterruptible power supplies and backup hardware on standby, and certainly should include backup of patient data on a regular basis to ensure that no information is lost if a system problem occurs. Buildings that house computer equipment require precautions against natural and manmade hazards. Chapter 17 contains detailed information related to disaster recovery planning.

## Legislation and Standards

As health care institutions use computerized medical records in more ways and as demands for personal data increase, public concern will continue to rise unless fears regarding potential abuse of information are addressed. In an effort to strike a balance between institutional objectives and public concerns, legislators have proposed or enacted policies to control and regulate the creation and use of large databases. However, many of these proposals have created legal conundrums because of their conflict with existing laws or through the resulting division of power between different levels of government. Because of these problems, there has been greater emphasis on the voluntary establishment of standards and codes of ethics within the data processing and medical record management communities. Internationally, the Organization for Economic Cooperation and Development (OECD) (1981) held that

... although national laws and policies may differ, member countries have a common interest in protecting privacy and individual liberties, and in reconciling fundamental but competing values such as privacy and the free flow of information.

This belief led to the adoption by member countries of a set of guidelines that should be minimum standards for handling personal data relating to an identifiable individual. The eight guidelines are as follows:

- **Collection Limitation Principle.** Collection of personal data should be limited, done through lawful and fair means, and wherever possible with the knowledge and consent of the subject.
- **Data Quality Principle.** Data should be relevant to the proposed usage, accurate, complete, and kept up to date.
- **Purpose Specification Principle.** The intended use of data should be stated at the time of collection and subsequent usage should be limited to that purpose or such other that is not materially different from the stated intended purpose.
- **Use Limitation Principle.** Data should not be disclosed, made available, or used for purposes other than those specified without the consent of the subject or unless authorized by law.
- **Security Safeguards Principle.** Personal data should be protected by reasonable security safeguards against such risks as loss or unauthorized access, destruction, use, modification, or disclosure of data.
- **Openness Principle.** A general policy of openness should exist about developments, practices, and policies with respect to personal data. Means should be readily available for establishing the existence and nature of collected personal data and the main purpose of their use, as well as the identity of the collector of the data.
- **Individual Participation Principle.** An individual should have the right:
  1. To obtain confirmation as to whether or not data relating to himself or herself exists
  2. To have data relating to him or her made available to him or her within a reasonable time, at a reasonable cost, in a reasonable manner, and in a form that is readily intelligible
  3. To be given reasons for refusal of a request made under the first two rights
  4. To be able to challenge data relating to him or her and, if successful, to have the data erased, rectified, completed, or amended
- **Accountability Principle.** A data controller should be accountable for complying with measures that give effect to these principles as just stated.

The principles embodied in the OECD guidelines are evident in many privacy-related laws passed in member countries and in principles and guidelines adopted by national professional organizations.

In the United States, the *Health Insurance Portability and Accountability Act* of 1996 is intended to "Improve portability and continuity of health insurance coverage in the group and individual markets, to combat waste, fraud and abuse in health insurance and health care delivery, to promote the use of medical savings accounts, to improve access to long-term care services and coverage and to simplify the administration of health insurance" (CIHI, 1997, p. 13). As part of the administrative simplification provision, the Secretary of Health and Human Services is required to adopt security standards that take into account:

". . . the technical abilities of record systems used to maintain health information; the costs of security measures; the need for training persons who have access to health information; the value of audit trails in computerized record systems; and the needs and capabilities of small and rural health care providers." Within 18 months of the enactment, security standards must be adopted. These standards selected must have been developed, adopted or modified by a standards-setting organization accredited by the American National Standards Institute (ANSI), or have followed a formal consultation approach for those areas where no standards exist. The legislation also makes wrongful disclosure of individually identifiable health information an offense with penalties ranging from up to $50,000 or one year imprisonment or both to $250,000 or ten years imprisonment or both. The latter penalties apply when the person intends to sell, transfer, or use individually identifiable health information for commercial advantage, personal gain, or malicious harm (CIHI, 1997, p. 13).

In Canada, eight jurisdictions, including the federal government and seven provinces, have passed freedom of information and protection of privacy legislation to protect personal information in the public sector. Common provisions in these laws include guidelines for the collection, use, and disclosure of personal information. In Quebec, the legislation also extends to the private sector. In other Canadian jurisdictions, privacy protection in the private sector depends on sector-specific legislation, professional codes of practice, and voluntary acceptance of codes of fair information practice. The Canadian Organization for the Advancement of Computers in Health (COACH) advocates that its members use the following principles concerning confidentiality and security of computerized health records (1979):

- Automated health-related information records of an organization shall be subject to at least the same protocols of confidentiality as apply to the manually written records of that organization.
- Automated health-related information records shall be obtained, retained, and accessed only by ethical and lawful means.
- The purposes of automated health-related information systems shall be defined and the systems shall be operated in accordance with those purposes unless the purposes are formally amended.
- Facilities that process and store automated health-related information records shall be subject to regular independent inspection and audit of the physical and system safeguards.
- The management of organizations responsible for processing and storing automated health-related information records shall ensure that appropriate physical and system safeguards, along with written policies and procedures, are utilized to secure such records, and facilitate timely and accurate maintenance of such records consistent with requirements for which the information is intended.
- These principles and guidelines apply to organizations using centralized computing, distributed computing, standalone computing, and personal

computing. The key determinant in applying principles and guidelines is how results of various types of computing affect the entire operation.

Additionally, most provinces have incorporated privacy and confidentiality provisions in Mental Health Acts, Vital Statistics Acts, and other health-related legislation. In addition, some jurisdictions are also introducing broad health information protection legislation (CIHI, 1997).

In Europe, since the 1980s a convention of the Council of Europe has bound members to pass privacy legislation. A new data protection directive, Directive 95/46/EC, was passed in 1995 (http://www.echo.lu/legal/en/dataprot/dataprot.html). The Directive covers the processing of personal data and the free movement of the data. Several countries have moved to supplement this broad legislation with laws that provide strict privacy safeguards for medical data. In the United Kingdom, *the Data Protection Act* categorizes information relating to an individual's physical or mental health as sensitive data, requiring special efforts to protect its privacy (CIHI, 1997).

## Nursing Responsibilities

The components of privacy protection in a health care information system are not mutually exclusive but are highly interrelated and interactive. As patient advocates, nurses must be vigilant in protecting patient privacy. Nurses must initiate and participate in the evaluation of the privacy protection in new or existing computerized patient information systems. The following questions might be useful in guiding such an evaluation.

- What is the mechanism for restricting entry to main computer system areas?
- How are the terminals "locked"—that is, by card, key, or password?
- What security is provided for media storage areas? Will a librarian be available to control access? Will stored materials ever be allowed to leave the storage area?
- What provision is made to protect data in the event of fire, destruction of the area, and the like?
- What control will be used to establish who can view, enter, or alter data?
- Are certain terminals designated for access to specific data sets only (e.g., dietary)?
- Will the sign-on be done by department, unit, or individual? Are codes a combination of alphanumeric symbols?
- Will an audit trail be available through a transaction log to process the time and identification code of each log-on?
- What mechanism(s) exists for encrypting personal data?

- Is there a mechanism whereby a terminal is identified before information goes out?
- Do statistical reports identify individuals in any way?
- Is an oath of secrecy or a signed statement on ethical position necessary for staff who are not governed by a code of ethics (e.g., those who process and store the data)?
- Does the duty of confidentiality transfer from direct caregivers to data processors?
- How are data-processing personnel screened for jobs? How is their responsibility for confidentiality emphasized? What are the consequences for inappropriate release of data?
- When personnel leave, what happens to their password?
- What agency will be used to test security of the system?
- How will security breaches be reported (by whom, to whom)? Who has authority to take disciplinary action when security breaches occur?
- Who has overall responsibility in the institution for confidentiality of information?
- Who is responsible for keeping the public informed of the purpose, use, and existence of computerized records?
- Who is responsible for establishing, updating, and enforcing written policies and procedures?

Knowledgeable nurses will advocate their institution's or organization's compliance with the following criteria, which the literature identifies in relation to both new and existing computerized health information systems:

- The use of passwords and identification codes is essential. Controlled terminal access can be used in conjunction with the measures described here; however, by itself, it does not appear to be adequate. Passwords should be changed at regular intervals and as necessary. The same password should not be repeated to eliminate the employees using old passwords to gain access to wrong information.
- Limits on the collection and recording of information need to be established. Individual institutions will formulate policies in this regard. As individuals, nurses need to assess the relevance of the information they record.
- When entering data, we need to ensure that the information is accurate. This has always been essential, but because of the qualities of automated records, now the potential harm of inaccurate charting has an even greater impact on the patient.
- When developing policies regarding to privacy, confidentiality, and a system's security, the patient must be the prime concern. To facilitate this objective, a patient's rights representative is a great asset.
- Informing the public when implementing a new hospital information system is very important. A part of the public awareness campaign should include its impact on privacy. This method may cause unwarranted con-

cern, but the public will be aware of the system's implementation and potential, both positive and negative aspects. Also, the more introduction given to the public about the system, the more likely it will be accepted.

- Before the input of an individual's data into a system, the patient needs to be informed that computerized medical records are operational in the institution. To withhold this fact from a person is an invasion of the patient's privacy.
- When using information for research, a consent is absolutely essential. Information should not be identifiable.
- The system and its controls need to be reviewed at regular intervals, and audits must be performed by an independent party.
- The use of a "Bipartite Record" is a direction that has been taken by some institutions. One part of the chart contains compromising data and the other part confidential data. The confidential data area would contain highly confidential medical information such as an adolescent pregnancy or the use of drugs. This information may, or may not, be stored on computer and would be available to only authorized individuals. The "Bipartite Record" appears to be advantageous in theory, but difficult to implement.
- At present, in Canada, medical records are the property of the hospital. A study on personal privacy performed in the United States recommends that patients have a right to see their own records and, furthermore, be able to make amendments as necessary to maintain their accuracy. Legislation is necessary to change this policy. Making the medical record the property of the individual allows patients to have access to their own medical record. Access to the record should be available anytime and anywhere. The patient could then assess its accuracy. Provisions would have to be made enabling the individual to make amendments to his record. Patient ownership of records is an issue in itself, but is beyond the scope of this section and is not be addressed further.
- With the implementation of computerized medical records, an entire new department of staff has access to the patient's record. These are the information systems personnel. A "code of ethics" should be formulated for them regarding privacy and confidentiality of the information. The document should be signed by each employee to obtain its full impact in maintaining confidentiality.
- Government legislation is necessary in the area of database linkages to control data transfer from one system to another and to control data uses. As previously stated, because of the potential harm to the individual and the institution, strict policies need to be enforced in governing both the access and use of information.
- Education of all personnel in the area of patient privacy and confidentiality is imperative. It is especially important for those persons who are new to the health care system and involved with patient care records for the first time (e.g., information systems personnel). Education is an es-

sential part of the maintenance of privacy and confidentiality. Professionals who are traditionally critical of automated medical records will accept the system more readily if they are educated about how security is maintained. Regular intervals of inservice will need to be carried out to inform the staff of new developments in this area.

## *References*

Barber, B. Security and confidentiality issues from a national perspective. In: *Patient Privacy, Confidentiality and Data Security: Papers from the British Computer Society Nursing Specialist Group Annual Conference.* Lincolnshire, UK: The British Computer Society, 1997:61–72.

Bowen, J.W., Klimczak, C., Ruiz, M., and Barnes, M. Design of access control methods for protecting the confidentiality of patient information systems in networked systems. *Journal of the American Medical Informatics Association: Symposium Supplement.* Nashville: Hanley & Belfus, 1997:46–50.

Canadian Institute for Health Information (CIHI). *Working Group 3: Privacy, Confidentiality, Data Integrity, and Security, Background Document.* Ottawa, Canada: CIHI, 1997.

Canadian Organization for the Advancement of Computers in Health (COACH). *Guidelines to Promote the Confidentiality and Security of Automated Health Records.* Edmonton, Canada: COACH, 1979.

Hoy, D. Protecting the individual: Confidentiality, security and the growth of information systems. *Sharing Information: Key Issues for the Nursing Profession.* Lincolnshire, UK: The British Computer Society, 1997:78–87.

McKenzie, D.J.P. Healthcare trend improves security practices. *In Confidence.* 1996, May–June. 3 pg. Online. Available: http://www.ahima.org/publications/1a/May-June.inconf.html

Miller, D.W. Internet security: What health information managers should know. *Journal of AHIMA.* 1996, September, 4 pg. Online. Available: http://www.ahima.org/publications/2f/sept.focus.html

Organization for Economic Cooperation and Development (OECD). *Draft Recommendations of the Council concerning Guidelines Governing the Protection of Privacy and Transborder Flows of Personal Data.* Paris: OECD, 1979.

## *Additional Resources*

Dalander, G., Willner, S., and Brasch, S. Turning a dream into a reality: The evolution of the electronic health record. *Journal of AHIMA.* 1997, October. 6 pg. Online. Available: http://www.ahima.org/publications/2f/focus.2.1097.html

Dennis, J.C. Asking tough questions: Assessing top management support for confidentiality. *In Confidence.* 1997, Jan/Feb, 2 pg. Online. Available: http://www.ahima.org/publications/1a/inconf.1.1998.html

Miller, D.W. Current technology: Confidentiality risks and controls. *In Confidence.* 1997, July/Aug, 6 pg. Online. Available: http://www.ahima.org/publications/1a/july.inconfidence.html

Mills, M.E. Data privacy and confidentiality in the public arena. *Journal of the American Medical Informatics Association: Symposium Supplement.* Nashville, USA: Hanley & Belfus, 1997:42–45.

Murray, P.J. "It'll never happen to me." Revisiting some computer security issues. *Computers in Nursing* 1997;15(2):65–66, 70.

Nelson, D. Information security: A holistic approach to network system security. *Journal of AHIMA.* 1997, May, 6 pg. Online. Available: http://www.ahima.org/publications/2f/focus.1.597.html

Sanchez-Swatman, L. Nurses, computers and confidentiality. *Canadian Nurse* 1997; August:47–48.

Vincze, L.S. Confidentiality and compliance: Political and public interests. *In Confidence.* 1997, Nov/Dec, 3 pg. Online. Available: http://www.ahima.org/publications/1a/inconf.nov.dec.1997.html

Zakoworotny, C., Rutz, C., and Zwingman-Babley, C. Information security: A team approach to managing an information security program. Journal of AHIMA. 1997, May, 7 pg. Online. Available: http://www.ahima.org/publications/2f/focus.597.html

American National Standards Institute Home Page
http://www.ansi.org

Canadian Institute for Health Information
http://www.cihi.ca

Canadian Information Highway Advisory Council
http://www.info.ic.gc.ca/info_highway/ih.html

Links to selected security standards
http://www.zeuros.co.uk/firewall/standard.htm

List of selected security websites and bulletin boards
http://www.carelink.ca/sites.html

Text of new European Data Protection Directive
http://www.echo.lu/legal/en/dataprot/datprot.html

United States Privacy Laws by State
http://www.epic.org

# 15
# Ergonomics

## Introduction

A major concern for nursing informatics is ergonomics. The word "ergonomics" comes from the Greek words "ergo," meaning work, and "nomos," meaning law. Ergonomics, a relatively new science, looks at the application of physiological, psychological, and engineering principles to the interaction between people and machines. Ergonomics attempts to define working conditions that will enhance individual health, safety, comfort, and productivity. This can be done by recognizing three things: the physiological, anatomical, and psychological capabilities and limitations of people, the tools they use, and the environments in which they function.

As the use of computerized nursing information systems increases, ergonomics is of increasing interest to nurses in their dual role as users of computers and as health care providers. Nurses are concerned with how computer workstations will affect the provision of patient care (see Chapters 7 and 8) and the nurse as an individual. These concerns include the physiological aspects (i.e., physical comfort), the cognitive aspects (i.e., comprehension of displayed information), and the practical aspects (i.e., infection control when using computers at the bedside). Ergonomics standards play a key role in improving the usability of systems and addressing many of the concerns identified here. They assist in the procurement of systems and systems components that can be used effectively, efficiently, safely, and comfortably. Ergonomics standards themselves do not guarantee good design but they do provide a means of identifying interface quality in design, procurement, and operational use. International standards for display screen equipment are being developed by the International Organisation for Standardisation (ISO). The ISO recommendations are developed by working groups whose members are representatives of the national standards bodies of member countries. There are 17 parts to the standard related to work with VDTs. Many of these parts are still works in progress. More information regarding ISO Standards can be obtained at http://www.iso.ch

The following is a list of the various parts of ISO 9241, *Ergonomics requirements for office work with visual display terminals (VDTs):*

- Part 1: General introduction
- Part 2: Guidance on task requirements
- Part 3: Visual display requirements
- Part 4: Keyboard requirements
- Part 5: Workstation layout and postural requirements
- Part 6: Environmental requirements
- Part 7: Display requirements with reflections
- Part 8: Requirements for displayed colors
- Part 9: Requirements for nonkeyboard input devices
- Part 10: Dialogue principles
- Part 11: Guidance on usability specification and measures
- Part 12: Presentation of information
- Part 13: User guidance
- Part 14: Menu dialogues
- Part 15: Command dialogues
- Part 16: Direct manipulation dialogues
- Part 17: Form-filling dialogues

Detailed discussion of ergonomics and the ISO standards is beyond the scope of this text, but this section addresses selected areas directly related to nurses. Chapter 16 provides a more in-depth examination of the principles of usability to be considered when evaluating software and hardware.

## The Nursing Computer Workstation

The nursing computer workstation has two components: hardware (the physical equipment) and software (the programs required to enter, retrieve, and process information). Both components affect the quality of patient care and the physical and psychological comfort of the nurse. The hardware normally has a way to enter data and commands and a way to display data and results. How this is accomplished primarily affects the physical comfort of the nurse. The quality of patient care is determined by how accurately data can be entered and how easily retrieved information can be interpreted and comprehended by the nurse. The effect of the presence of bedside terminals on the patient–nurse relationship has not been well documented.

Video display terminals (VDTs) are the usual point of contact between the nurse and most computerized nursing information systems. VDTs are the devices that show both input to, and output from, the central processing unit. Information is typed on the keyboard and presented on the display screen for verification by the operator before being transmitted to the computer. Output from the computer is presented to the operator in

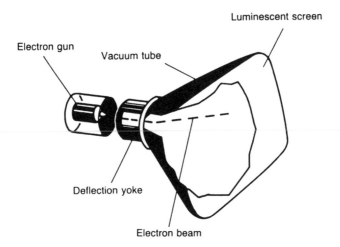

**FIGURE 15.1.** Cathode ray tube.

the same fashion, that is, as an image generated on the display screen (Figure 15.1).

## Physiological Concerns

Much research has been done regarding the physiological aspects of VDT workstations. The terms "video display terminal (VDT)," "video display unit (VDU)," "video matrix terminal (VMT)," "cathode ray terminal (CRT)," and "monitor" are synonymous. Users of VDTs complain of ergonomic shortcomings such as strained postures, poor photometric display characteristics, and inadequate lighting conditions. Others claim the complaints are symptoms of a health hazard requiring immediate measures to protect the health of operators. The National Institute for Safety and Health (NIOSH) in the United States has sponsored extensive research concerning a variety of ergonomics-related topics. These reports are available through the NIOSH website: http://www.cdc.gov/niosh/homepage.html. Additional reference articles, current journal listings, and related conferences can be accessed at the ERGOWEB site: http://www.ergoweb.com The following sections provide an overview of ergonomic concerns related to nursing informatics.

### *Eye Strain*

#### Size of Characters

The displayed size of the characters on the screen can contribute to eye strain. The character's image is generated on the display screen by a cathode ray tube. The cathode ray tube used in computer terminals is identical to those found in television sets. It is essentially a glass vacuum tube encased in a lead seal with an electron gun in opposition to a phosphor-coated screen. High-voltage electricity is used by the electron gun to generate a stream of electrons that can be directed to any display screen location. This electrical excitation of the phosphors eliminates the point on the screen at which the slender beam of electrons is being focused. A scanning mechanism generates letters and characters using a dot matrix pattern. The number of horizontal and vertical dots (usually $5 \times 7$ or $7 \times 9$ dots) in the matrix determines the resolution of the character. The best resolution, and therefore the clearest, easiest reading, at least for the reading of alphanumeric characters, is achieved using a $7 \times 9$ dot matrix (TFMS, 1996).

### Flicker

Flicker on the screen also causes eye strain. Two characteristics of the screen play a crucial role in reducing flicker: persistence, and refresh rate. *Persistence* is the length of time that the phosphors remain illuminated after being electrically excited. The *refresh rate* is the frequency with which each point on the surface of the screen is re-illuminated by electrical excitation. The refresh rate must be frequent enough so that the persistence of the phosphor is sustained; otherwise, the displayed characters will seem to fade away. Flicker occurs when the refresh rate is too low. The operator then notices the decay in the phosphor's illumination before it is reexcited. In this case, the operator can identify a pulsating luminescence in the display. The presence of flicker causes eye and mental fatigue for operators. Refresh rates of 70 Hz (cycles per second) are usually sufficient to prevent perceptible flicker on screens having light characters on a dark background, thus reducing eye strain (ISO, 9241, Part 3, 1996).

### Color

The color of the display does not seem to be a major physiological factor. The choice of the phosphor to be used in the screen is determined by the phosphor's grain, its luminescence, its color, and its persistence (rate of decay). There is considerable disagreement whether amber or green phosphors provide better legibility and color contrast. Generally, it is agreed that lighting conditions determine which is best in specific situations. Usually, green is preferred for highly illuminated rooms and amber for less well lit areas. Often the choice of color is more a matter of personal preference than of scientific determination considering the lighting conditions in most work environments.

### Glare

Glare also contributes to eye strain among users. Although lighting conditions do not appear to influence the choice of screen phosphor color, they are of considerable ergonomic significance in relation to glare. Glare occurs when the range of luminances in the visual field is too great; for example, when bright sources of luminares, windows, or their refracted images fall within the field of vision. Glare causes distractions, visual discomfort, reduced legibility, and reduced visual acuity. Engineers have attempted to reduce glare on display screens using three methods: etched glass and filters, optical coatings, and position of the screen. Etched glass and filters do reduce glare but also tend to simultaneously reduce legibility by defocusing the characters and reducing character brightness. In fact, some filters have been found to increase the operator's awareness of screen reflections! Optical coating of the screen glass has been found to be an effective but expensive solution concerning glare. The most effective, least expensive means of reducing glare is simply to make sure that the screen can be moved and positioned so that reflections are no longer visible. This can be accomplished by placing the screen at right angles to the source of light and by ensuring that the display screen is an independent, adjustable unit.

**Contrast**

Contrast examines how the use of color compatibility affects human performance under the effect of reflected glare. Performance may be improved by selecting proper color combinations. Most displays use light characters on a darker background (negative presentation). In general, white on black, white on blue, or amber on black is preferable to using black on white or white on yellow. Such displays appear to flicker less, but suffer from reduced contrast between characters and background as a result of high ambient light levels. The contrast between the brightness of the image and the brightness of the background is a key factor in determining the legibility of images on a VDT. It is recommended that the contrast ratio of characters and background on CRT screens be large, at least 3:1 and up to 15:1 (ISO, 9241, Part 3, 1996). As individual preferences for both brightness and contrast vary, the controls for these should be effective over the range of lighting and environmental conditions experienced at the workstation.

## *Posture*

The presence of rotating, tilt, and swivel mechanisms to allow adjustment of the screen is also important in helping the operator maintain proper posture. As illustrated in Figure 15.2, the National Institute for Occupation Safety and Health (NIOSH) in the United States recommends that the keyboard be 29 to 31 inches from the floor. The center of the display screen should be 10° to 20° below the user's vertical eye level. The angle between the upper and lower arm should be between 80° and 120°. The user's wrist angle in using the keyboard should be less than 10°, and ample leg room

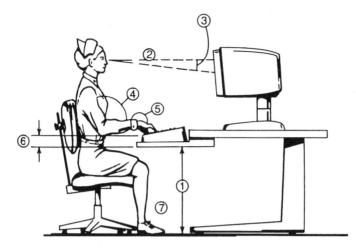

**Figure 15.2.** NIOSH specifications for VDT use show: (1) height of keys at 29–31 inches, (2) optimal viewing distance 17–25 inches, (3) screen center 10–20 degrees below plane of operator's eye height, (4) angle between upper and lower arm 80–120 degrees, (5) wrist angle under 10 degrees, (6) keyboard at or below elbow height, (7) ample leg room. (From *Computers and Medicine* 2, no. 5 (September 1982).)

must be available. It has also been found that swivel chairs with adjustable seat height and independent back support are helpful. Compliance with these criteria will reduce or prevent the pain or stiffness in the neck, shoulders, and lower back that results from poor posture at the workstation.

The user's workspace should be arranged so that the eye to display screen viewing distance is between 17 and 25 inches (see Figure 15.2), depending of course on the user's eyesight. To reduce eye strain induced by eye refocusing, the screen and keyboard, as well as any text that is being copied, should be at the same distance from the operator's eyes. Another factor, which has been shown to create itching, burning, and dry and irritated eyes, is the warm air flow created by floppy disk drives and terminal fans that often appears aimed at the user's face.

The previous postural concerns relate solely to workstations. Ergonomic concerns arising from bedside or notebook technology have not been explored.

## Other Health Concerns

The major debate surrounding cathode ray terminals is the question of potential radiation hazards. In North America, extensive testing was undertaken by NIOSH: measurements of ionizing and nonionizing radiation, analysis of workroom air for contaminants, administration of a questionnaire on health complaints to employees, and evaluation of ergonomic aspects in the workplaces. On the basis of this study, Murray et al. (1981) stated that "the results of these tests demonstrated that the VDT operators included in this investigation were not exposed to hazardous levels of radiation or chemical agents." NIOSH further concluded that routine monitoring of VDTs was unjustified. A similar position has been adopted by the Consumer and Clinical Radiation Hazards Division, Health and Welfare Canada (Charboneau, 1982).

In spite of these reassurances, other investigators, unions, employers, and the quasi-judicial bodies continue to have reservations. There has been a growing concern among CRT users that many health problems are associated with their machines. Currently, there is no valid research to indicate any direct cause-and-effect relationship between CRT radiation and user health hazard. However, more study is needed on the effects of ionizing radiation, non-ionizing radiation, and low frequency electromagnetic waves as well as possible synergistic interaction among these three.

Responsible nurses will monitor the literature and exercise a judicious use of caution and informed professional decision making to recognize media-generated hysteria and rebuttal by parties with vested interest.

## Psychological Concerns

The psychological aspects of computer ergonomics have been much less thoroughly researched and studied than the physiological aspects. To some extent, this situation is to be expected because physiological aspects are more easily measured and quantified than are the psychological aspects of computer use. However, as hardware costs decrease, as more software is developed, and as the physiological aspects of ergonomics are addressed, greater attention is being directed toward the psychological aspects of ergonomics. Unfortunately, the psychological aspects of the human–machine interface continue to be approached in a highly subjective, emotional, and personal fashion.

## *The Human–Machine Interface*

The latest techniques in computer program development consider the user's cognitive abilities including memory load, visual scanning, and formulation of mental models. These techniques make it easier for the user to enter data and comprehend information. These techniques address:

- Dialogue design: intelligent or adaptive interfaces
- Input methods: windows, icons, mouse, and pointer environments
- Screen design: graphical user interfaces
- Attention-getting techniques: use of color

- Consistency in appearance of screen information, error messages, and system usage

Also, these techniques meet the subjective criteria by which their advocates evaluate them. However, further research is required to determine if they meet the psychological ergonomic needs of other users. See Chapter 16 to identify a process for evaluating the usability of the interface when selecting software and hardware.

## *Variety of Input/Output Media*

There has been a move away from total reliance on the keyboard for input and the monochrome display for output. Individuals can use speech for both input and output, color graphics, physiological probes, and computer mice to facilitate keyboard use. There are also touch screens used for data entry. Pen-based notebook systems offer yet another form of a more naturalistic input device. Natural speech recognition programs also offer another naturalistic approach to input and output. Many users new to the computing environment find a greater degree of psychological comfort in using input devices not requiring keyboarding/typing skills (see Chapter 2 for a description of these input media).

## Research Needs/Opportunities

A psychological aspect of computing ergonomics that remains largely unstudied is the impact of a computerized workstation on individuals' behavior within an organization. We simply do not yet know the full effects on people when they work in a highly automated environment and, subsequently, have less need and opportunity for human contact. Interpersonal relations, group dynamics, personal stress levels, anxiety levels, and productivity among personnel in such organizations are unexplored. It is imperative that this kind of information be sought without delay.

The potential of bedside systems to affect the nurse–patient relationship must also be researched. As new technology is developed there is an ongoing need to evaluate not only the effectiveness of the technology, but also the ergonomic effects on both nurses and patients.

## *References*

Charbonneau, L. The VDT controversy. *The Canadian Nurse* 1982;October:30.

ISO 9241 Part 3. Online. Available: http://www.iso.ch

Murray, W.E., Cox, C., Moss, C., and Parr, W. *A Radiation and Industrial Hygiene Survey of Video Display Terminal Operation.* Cincinnati: National Institute of Occupational Safety and Health, 1981.

TFMS. "Understand display screen ergonomics." System Concepts Ltd. 1996. 18 pg. Online. Available: http://www.system-concepts.com/stds/hse4.html

## *Additional Resources*

Bragg, T.L. An ergonomics program for the health care setting. *Nursing Management* 1996;27(7):58–62.

Hasler, R.A. Human factors design: What is it and how it can affect you? *Journal of Intravenous Nursing* 1996;19(3S):S5–8.

TFMS. Using ergonomics standards for procurement and design. System Concepts Ltd. 15 pg. Online. Available: http://www.system-concepts.com/stds/hse5.html

Swanson, N.G., et al. NIOSH exploratory study on keyboard design finds no major differences in user comfort, fatigue. 2 pg. Online. Available: http://www.cdc.gov/niosh/keyboard.html

Stewart, T. Ergonomics standards concerning human-system interaction: Visual displays, controls and environmental requirements. *Applied Ergonomics* 1995; 26(4):271–274.

# 16
# Usability

KATHY MOMTAHAN

## Introduction

Usability is defined as "the extent to which a product can be used by specified users to achieve specified goals with effectiveness, efficiency and satisfaction in a specified context of use" (ISO, 1994, p. 2). There are 17 parts to the ISO usability standard, and many of these parts are still works in progress (see Chapter 15). This chapter presents an overview of usability testing methodologies. An example of the application of one type of usability testing method, called heuristic evaluation, in the hospital setting is presented. Related websites are listed where appropriate.

## Types of Usability Tests

There are various types of usability tests. An example of some of the types of usability testing procedures currently in use are user testing, objective evaluation methods, heuristic evaluation (sometimes classified as a usability inspection method) (Nielsen and Mack, 1994), and questionnaires.

### User Testing

The current "gold standard" of usability assessment is user testing (Landauer, 1995). User testing involves developing a set of tasks for users to try with a system while the tester watches, notes errors, and times the process. Users are usually asked to engage in a monologue as they think their way through the task. There are various ways of accomplishing user testing but most of them entail some form of observational methodology. For a detailed description of user testing and how to go about it, see Nielsen (1997).

### Objective Evaluation Methods

Although "objective" evaluation methods require the input of a human, this type of methodology formalizes the usability evaluation by guiding the evaluators through the evaluation of the software being tested, often in terms of its conformance to the ISO 9241 standards. The ISO 9241 evaluator developed by Oppermann and Reiterer (1997) is an example of this type of methodology.

## *Heuristic Evaluation*

Heuristic evaluation is referred to by Landauer (1995) as "a good second best" in terms of usability testing. Heuristic evaluation is a usability inspection method (Nielsen, 1992) that uses usability experts to perform an analysis of a computer interface. The usability experts use their knowledge and experience and a set of written usability guidelines, called heuristics, to guide them in their evaluation. The following is the set of usability principles that Nielsen (1994) identified as important to a well-designed user interface from a factor analysis of 249 usability problems (Nielsen, 1994).

*1. Visibility of system status:* The system should always keep users informed about what is going on, through appropriate feedback within reasonable time.

*2. Match between system and the real world:* The system should speak the users' language, with words, phrases, and concepts familiar to the user, rather than system-oriented terms. Follow real-world conventions, making information appear in a natural and logical order.

*3. User control and freedom:* Users often choose system functions by mistake and will need a clearly marked "emergency exit" to leave the unwanted state without having to go through an extended dialogue. Support undo and redo.

*4. Consistency and standards:* Users should not have to wonder whether different words, situations, or actions mean the same thing. Follow platform conventions. Platform conventions are guidelines to help software developers achieve consistent user interfaces across software products for a particular operating system (i.e., the Microsoft User Interface Style Guide) (Microsoft, 1995).

*5. Error prevention:* A careful design that prevents a problem from occurring in the first place is even better than good error messages.

*6. Recognition rather than recall:* Make objects, actions, and options visible. The user should not have to remember information from one part of the dialogue to another. Instructions for use of the system should be visible or easily retrievable whenever appropriate.

*7. Flexibility and efficiency of use:* Accelerators, unseen by the novice user, may often speed up the interaction for the expert user to such an extent that the system can cater to both inexperienced and experienced users. Allow users to tailor frequent actions.

*8. Aesthetic and minimalist design:* Dialogues should not contain information that is irrelevant or rarely needed. Every extra unit of information in a dialogue competes with the relevant units of information and diminishes their relative visibility.

*9. Help users recognize, diagnose, and recover from errors:* Error messages should be expressed in plain language (no codes), precisely indicate the problem, and constructively suggest a solution.

*10. Help and documentation:* Even though it is better if the system can be used without documentation, it may be necessary to provide help and documentation. Any such information should be easy to search, focused on the user's task, list concrete steps to be carried out, and be not too large.

The usability concepts just outlined are very similar to the concepts that have been highlighted by Lowery and Martin (1990) as being important to the evaluation of healthcare software. However, neither Nielsen (1992, 1994) nor Lowery and Martin rank these concepts by level of importance. Nielsen (1997) recommends combining other usability testing methods such as heuristic evaluation with user testing with real users. Other examples of heuristic criteria are the "ergonomic criteria" developed by Scapin and Bastien (1997). (See also http://www.cc.gatech.edu/classes/cs6751_97_winter/Topics/heur-eval and http://www.inria.fr/RRRT/RR-2326.html).

# Questionnaires

Questionnaires can be used to obtain the end-user's point of view. In the last few years, various questionnaires have been developed for this purpose. For example:

- The Questionnaire for User Interaction Satisfaction (QUIS 5.0) developed by Norman and Shneiderman (1989) http://www.lap.umd.edu/QUISFolder/quisHome.html
- The Purdue Usability Testing Questionnaire (PUTQ) developed by Lin, Choong and Salvendy (1997)
- The Software Usability Measurement Inventory (MUSiC, 1992) http://www.ua.ac.be/MAN/WP51/t38.html

# An Example of a Usability Test in a Hospital Environment

The heuristic evaluation method (Nielsen and Molich, 1990; Nielsen, 1992) was recently chosen to evaluate the computer interface of an automated pharmacy dispensing system (Momtahan, 1997). This usability method was chosen over user testing because it was practical; it involved about 4 months of the researcher's time and about 8 hours of each volunteer usability expert's time but involved very little of the pharmacy staff's time. Ten usability experts were recruited from university and industry to perform the evaluation. The automated pharmacy dispensing machine that was the focus of the evaluation was controlled by two computers. One computer (called the System 2 computer) directly controlled the dispensing machine and the other computer (called the System 1 computer) captured the patient and prescription information from the hospital mainframe and transcribed this information into a format that could be used by the System 2 computer.

As it was impossible to have usability experts manipulate the software that runs the equipment, a document was developed with screen pictures from the two computer interfaces and a description of how pharmacy staff navigate through the software to accomplish their daily automated dispensing of drugs. The document with screen pictures describing the navigation process was edited by the main technician running the machine and the pharmacy manager. This document is currently being used to train new staff in the pharmacy department. To have a quantitative as well as a qualitative assessment of the pharmacy software using the heuristic evaluation method, a questionnaire was developed. The following is a sample of the questions developed based on Nielsen's (1994) heuristics. For a complete list of the questions used in this survey, see Momtahan (1997).

### Visibility of system status:
The system does a(n)

| Bad | Poor | Reasonable | Good | Excellent |
|-----|------|------------|------|-----------|
| 1 | 2 | 3 | 4 | 5 |

job of keeping users informed about what is going on.

### Match between system and the real world:
Information is presented in a logical order.

| Strongly Disagree | Disagree | Neither Agree nor Disagree | Agree | Strongly Agree |
|-------------------|----------|----------------------------|-------|----------------|
| 1 | 2 | 3 | 4 | 5 |

### Recognition rather than recall:
Does the system make more use of users' recognition or recall?

| Recall | | | | Recognition |
|--------|---|---|---|-------------|
| 1 | 2 | 3 | 4 | 5 |

### Ease of learning versus ease of procedure once it's learned:
Taking the daily processing of file transfer orders only into account (pp. 1–12), how easy do you think it would be for new staff to learn this process?

| Very Difficult | Difficult | Neutral | Easy | Very Easy |
|----------------|-----------|---------|------|-----------|
| 1 | 2 | 3 | 4 | 5 |

Once a pharmacy worker has learned the process, how easy would you rate the process of running the file transfer procedure?

| Very Difficult | Difficult | Neutral | Easy | Very Easy |
|:---:|:---:|:---:|:---:|:---:|
| 1 | 2 | 3 | 4 | 5 |

## *The Results of the Usability Experts' Assessment*

The System 1 software was Windows based and ran on a PC. The System 2 software also ran on a PC computer but the software was DOS based. According to the usability experts, the main problems with the System 1 computer interface were these:

- The main menu names and icons were confusing
- The interface screen contained nonfunctional information
- There was no indication of how to complete tasks
- There were no error prevention tactics

The main problems with the System 2 computer interface were that it was considered:

- Too hierarchical
- Poorly organized
- To have poor labels for menus and function keys
- To lack error prevention opportunities

## Human–Computer Interaction: Usability Assessments and Other Ways to Improve Efficiency, Effectiveness, and Satisfaction

Using a questionnaire such as the one presented here is one way that a number of software products being considered can be evaluated for their usability. The best people to evaluate a computer interface are those known as "double experts," people who have training in human factors and who also have knowledge of the area for which the software was designed. However, double experts are difficult to find. One of the limitations of the heuristic evaluation reported here is that although the volunteers who performed the heuristic evaluation were experts in the area of human–computer interface evaluation, they were not familiar with the pharmacy tasks and environment and had to rely on the researcher to accurately describe the tasks and environment for them.

In addition to Nielsen's (1994) heuristic evaluation method, a number of other evaluation questionnaires, checklists, and guidelines have been developed, many of which were reviewed in a recent special issue on usability evaluation methods in the journal *Behaviour & Information Technology* (1997). There are also many style guides to help in the evaluation of a computer interface, e.g., the *Microsoft User Interface Style Guide* (Microsoft, 1995). Style guides can be helpful in the evaluation of healthcare software that is developed on particular platforms. Some software developers may do a better job than others of maintaining the conventions developed by Apple or Microsoft to help users transfer their skills from one software package to another. Someone who is familiar with *Word for Windows* should be able to feel as if they can transfer to other software developed for a Windows environment without having to relearn the software environment. Consistency among software interfaces in use in a hospital will go a long way to ensuring the efficient use of the hospital's computers.

Although usability in healthcare software interfaces is important, even more important is the usefulness of the software; i.e., does the software perform a function that is perceived as being useful to the people who are using it? Davis (1993) has developed a questionnaire designed to evaluate the perceived usefulness of information systems. He found that perceived usefulness was 50% more influential than ease of use in determining usage of information systems.

Some important areas concerning the study of human–computer interaction not covered here that may be of interest to healthcare professionals include research into mental models (Norman, 1983; Liu, 1997; Wickens and Carswell, 1997), task analysis (Gilbreth, 1914; Luczak, 1997), and allocation of functions (Fitts, 1951; Sharit, 1997). New technology, particularly computerization or recomputerization of entire hospitals, provides an opportunity to redesign how tasks are accomplished and by whom. It also provides an opportunity to reassess how information such as clinical records is organized.

## Conclusion

This chapter has reviewed the concept of usability and has provided an example of a usability assessment of the computer software interface of the two computer systems used to run a automated pharmacy dispensing machine. Usability evaluations conducted before purchase decisions are made can help avoid problems that users might encounter later, and may provide additional information to guide purchase decisions. Usability assessments can also aid in providing feedback to manufacturers or in-house software developers as well. A combination of a task analysis to determine the best method of performing a task and which parts of the task should ideally be performed by the healthcare worker and which are best performed by the computer, a knowledge of usability issues, and the purchase of software that is judged as useful by staff should help to avoid situations where software is purchased but never used or not used to its capacity.

## *References*

Davis, F.D. User acceptance of information technology: System characteristics, user perceptions and behavioral impacts. *International Journal of Man-Machine Studies* 1993;38:475–487.

Fitts, P.M. *Human engineering for an effective air-navigation and traffic-control system.* Report No. 593420. Washington, DC: National Research Council, 1951.

Gilbreth, L.E. *The Psychology of Management: The Function of the Mind in Determining, Teaching and Installing Methods of Least Waste.* New York: Sturgis, 1914.

International Standards Organization. *Ergonomic requirements for office work with visual display terminals (VDTs), Part 11: Guidance on usability (draft standard).* ISO/DIS 9241-11. Geneva: International Organization for Standardization, 1994.

Landauer, T.K. *The Trouble with Computers: Usefulness, Usability, and Productivity.* Cambridge: MIT Press, 1995.

Lin, H.X., Choong, Y., and Salvendy, G. A proposed index of usability: A method for comparing the relative usability of different software systems. *Behaviour & Information Technology* 1997;16(4/5):267–278.

Liu, Y. Software-user interface design. In: Salvendy G. (ed.) *Handbook of Human Factors and Ergonomics*, 2nd Ed. New York: Wiley, 1997:1689–1724.

Lowery, J.C., and Martin, J.B. Evaluation of healthcare software from a usability perspective. *Journal of Medical Systems* 1990;14(1/2):17–29.

Luczak, H. Task analysis. In: Salvendy G. (ed.) *Handbook of Human Factors and Ergonomics*, 2nd Ed. New York: Wiley, 1997:340–416.

Microsoft. *The Windows Interface Guidelines for Software Design.* Radmond, WA: Microsoft Press, 1995.

Momtahan, K.L. *Introducing new technology into hospitals—A case study of pharmacy automation during hospital restructuring.* Doctoral dissertation, Carleton University, Ottawa, 1997.

MuSiC. *Metrics for usability standards in computing* (ESPRIT II Project 5429). National Physical Laboratory, UK, 1992.

Nielsen, J. Finding usability problems through heuristic evaluation. *Proceedings ACM CHI '92 Conference* (Monterey, CA, May 3–7), 1992:373–380.

Nielson, J. Enhancing the explanatory power of usability heuristics. *Proceedings ACM CHI '94 Conference* (Boston, MA, April 24–28), 1994.

Nielson, J. Usability testing. In: Salvendy G. (ed.) *Handbook of Human Factors and Ergonomics*, 2nd Ed. New York: Wiley, 1997:1543–1568.

Nielson, J., and Mack, R.L. *Usability Inspection Methods.* New York: Wiley, 1994.

Nielson, J., and Molich, R. Heuristic evaluation of user interfaces. *Proceedings ACM CHI '90 Conference* (Seattle, WA, April 1–5), 1990:249–256.

Norman, D.A. Some observations on mental modes. In: Gentner, D., and Stevens, A.L. (eds.) *Mental Models.* Hillsdale, N.J.: Erlbaum, 1983.

Oppermann, R., and Reiterer, H. Software evaluation using the 9241 evaluator. *Behaviour & Information Technology* 1997;16(4/5):232–245.

Scapin, D.L., and Bastien, J.M.C. Ergonomic criteria for evaluating the ergonomic quality of interactive systems. *Behaviour & Information Technology* 1997;16(4/5):220–231.

Sharit, J. Allocation of functions. In: Salvendy G. (ed.) *Handbook of Human Factors and Ergonomics*, 2nd Ed. New York: Wiley, 1997:301–339.

Wickens, C.D., and Carswell, C.M. Information processing. In: Salvendy G. (ed.) *Handbook of Human Factors and Ergonomics*, 2nd Ed. New York: Wiley, 1997:89–129.

## *Additional Resources*

Carroll, J.M. Human-computer interaction: Psychology as a science of design. *Annual Review* of *Psychology* 1997;48:61–83.

Salvendy, G. (ed.) *Handbook of Human Factors and Ergonomics*, 2nd Ed. New York: Wiley, 1997.

Scapin, D.L., and Berns, T. (eds.) Usability evaluation methods. *Behaviour & Information Technology* 1997;16(4/5) (Special issue).

# 17
# Disaster Recovery Planning

## Introduction

Disaster recovery planning (DRP) is many things to many people. To some, it is planning how to recover or replace damaged computer systems. To others, it is planning how to maintain critical hospital/nursing functions during interruptions in computer service. To still others, it is planning how to avoid those interruptions, and to yet others, it is planning an organization's response to any emergency or crisis situation.

DRP is, of course, all these things and more. Disaster recovery planning, in its broadest sense, encompasses all measures taken to ensure organizational survival in the event of any natural or man-made calamity, and to minimize the impact of such an event on the organization's staff, patients, and bottom line. Disaster recovery planners are faced with an intimidating array of terms, techniques, and technologies: hot sites, cold sites, warm sites, mobile recovery, off-site storage, electronic vaulting, UPS, T1 links, Megastream, satellite transmission, . . . ! (see glossary). What does this have to do with nursing informatics?

Nursing has traditionally not been involved in disaster recovery planning. However, as nurses come to depend more and more on information technology, they must become involved in developing disaster recovery plans to safeguard patient care. The Disaster Recovery Plan is an extensive and inclusive statement of actions to be taken before, during, and after a disaster. The Plan must be regularly tested and updated to ensure the continuity of operations and the availability of critical data and processes in the event of a disaster. The goal of the planning process is to minimize the disruption of operations and ensure a measure of organizational stability and an orderly recovery after a disaster (Wold, 1997). In all but the smallest organizations or facilities, a formal planning method is needed to ensure quality, consistency, and comprehensiveness of disaster recovery contingency plans. Informal, ad hoc, or, worst of all, the "it will never happen to us" approaches must absolutely be avoided. It should also be noted that disaster recovery planning is not a one-time, finished product, but a process that must continually be used to update the contingency plans as elements in the organization change.

## Planning Process

The disaster recovery contingency planning process includes these steps:

- Risk identification: Which problems might occur?
- Risk analysis: What would be their impact?
- Risk prioritization: Which problems are the most critical?
- Risk reduction: How can I reduce the impact of the problems?
- Risk management planning: How will I apply this to the project?
- Risk monitoring and testing: How effective is our risk control?

The interaction of these activities is shown in the flowchart in Figure 17.1.

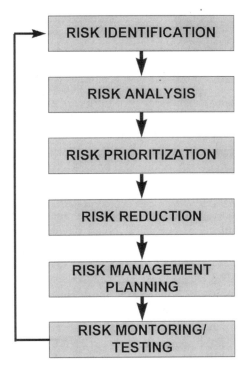

**FIGURE 17.1.** Disaster recovery contingency planning process.

# Planning Team

A fundamental premise of all types of planning applies to disaster recovery planning: plans are best developed by those who must actually implement them in the event of an actual disaster. A planning committee, including representatives from all functional areas of the organization, the operations manager, and the data processing manager should oversee the development and implementation of the plan. Many organization additionally appoint a Contingency Planner to work with a planning committee. Developing such a plan can be done completely in-house, with assistance from an external specialized disaster software or storage vendor, or by hiring an external disaster planning consultant. Often, a combination of these strategies provides the best value in the planning process. There are numerous software products available to guide a planning committee through the process. There are also national and regional professional organizations of Disaster Recovery consultants that will be able to provide guidance to novice planners. Access to a variety of disaster planning information, terminology, conference announcements, sample plans, and links to other related organizations is available at the website of the Disaster Recovery Journal at http://www.drj.com

# Risk Identification

Many risk assessments start with a group of project personnel gathering together to write down a list of potential risks. In general, this is not an effective starting point for risk identification. It constrains the identified risks to those which each individual thought was worth raising at the time. Many issues that are not considered as risks will not be raised, but such issues can combine in complex ways and develop into critical risks. The way to avoid this trap is to "brainstorm" the issues surrounding the project.

From the list of issues produced, obvious risks may be extracted. The remaining issues are kept for analysis. Further risks may be identified from analysis of project plans. Other techniques such as decision drivers exist. This method looks at the major decision points in the project and it is intended to identify when the decision may be driven by inappropriate influences. Application of these techniques should ensure that most of the risks surrounding the project are identified, including all the critical risks. The following hazard analysis checklist identifies some potential sources of risk that users of nursing information technology should consider (Government of Alberta, 1987; Wold and Shriver, 1997).

## *Possible Sources of Hazards*

### Natural Threats

1. Climate: Which materials in your collection are the most sensitive to extremes and fluctuations in temperature? Do you get heavy or prolonged snowfall, or rainfall or severe storms?
2. Topography: Is your building beside a lake or river? Is your basement below water table level? Is your area prone to avalanches, landslides or earthquakes?

### Technical Threats

1. Building structures: Has the roof a skylight, roof access, and drains? Are there water pipes running through the records area?
2. Dangerous goods: Are there any gas cylinders, solvents, or paints stored near the records? Are staff trained in the correct handling of dangerous goods?
3. Internal services: Are plumbing, electrical wiring, fire detectors, fire extinguishers, and security measures regularly inspected and maintained? Are there up-to-date plans and drawings of these? Are duplicates stored safely somewhere else?
4. Utility services: Which are you responsible for? How about sewers and telephones? Have you up-to-date plans of their locations, including master switches? Is there a backup? Is water pressure adequate for fighting fire?
5. Information systems: Are there alternate systems available if there is a malfunction or failure of the CPU? Failure of system software? Failure of application software?

### Human Threats

Is unauthorized access possible to either the physical site or information systems? What safeguards are in place related to bomb threats, extortion, burglary, work stoppage, or computer crime?

## Risk Analysis

### *Records*

When doing the risk analysis, consider the value of the records that need to be protected. Several factors affect the value of a record. Consider the following:

1. How much did it cost to create that record in the first place? What would it cost to recreate it now?

2. Does the information protect the rights of individuals, research, or the business interests of the agency?
3. Is the information complete, or would other documents be necessary if action had to be taken!
4. How available is it? If the information could be obtained from another source without too much delay, its value is reduced.

In assessing the value of your essential records for insurance purposes, there are two approaches:

- Recreating the information: Calculate the cost of gathering the information from scratch, e.g., by research, surveys, drafting, and then the cost of producing and reproducing it. This is estimated by the number of man-hours × $/hour for the project.
- Reproducing only: Calculate the cost of duplicating your essential records now for off-site storage, or the cost of reproducing your off-site records for use after a disaster. The most visible form of information is paper, closely followed by magnetic and film records.

One thing is certain, it would cost much less to duplicate now than to recreate later, after the information has been destroyed. For example, if you were to lose 100 cubic feet of records, it might cost $10,000 to recreate the information. But if you have off-site backup copies, the only additional cost is for transportation. It is necessary to keep reproduction to a minimum, and to use the cheapest means of reproduction consistent with the purpose or use of the information on the records. Remember, it is the information you are insuring, not the media. Before any reproduction is undertaken, consider the following questions:

1. Could the original record be stored at a safer location without causing great inconvenience?
2. Is the record available elsewhere, in a field office, in another department, or with the government, for example?
3. Would an extract or synopsis of the records meet the need, rather than a copy of the entire original record?
4. Does a summary type of record fulfill the need or is the original record necessary? For example, personal history cards instead of the personal file!
5. Are the records available now in printed or prepared form such as annual reports, machine run, or extra typed or printed copies?

## *Processing*

There is also a need to analyze the risk related to delivery of service in the event of a computer-related disaster. Computers are involved in the automatic delivery of intravenous medications, delivery of supplies throughout many hospitals, and even regulating everything from lights and heating to elevators. The risk exposure of all these systems must be considered in contingency planning. From a nursing perspective, there is extensive experience of the disruption caused when even one computerized IV delivery system malfunctions. Project the impact of a large-scale electrical or computer technology problem in an Intensive Care Unit if thorough contingency planning has not taken place.

## *Risk Prioritizing*

Risk prioritization is all about determining the "risk exposure" (Baxter, 1991):

Risk exposure = (Probability of unsatisfactory outcome) $\times$ (Loss, if outcome is unsatisfactory)

The components of "unsatisfactory outcome" may be cost, schedule, performance, or support, or may even relate to system evolution. The determination of the risk exposure will provide the disaster planning project manager with a prioritized list of risks. The ones near the top will require immediate action, whereas the bottom part of the list consists of risks that would be costly but unlikely to occur, or risks which will probably occur but would cause little loss. The type of risk reduction strategies used depend on the type of risk analysis performed. Where quantitative analysis has been used, a range of parameter values may be investigated so that the project manager can select an appropriate "level" of risk for a given likely outcome.

In all cases, the cost of reducing the risks must also be considered. A ratio may be calculated that is known as the "risk reduction leverage". This ratio assesses the risk exposure before and after the risk reduction processes have been carried out and compares them with the cost of those processes. A relative cost–benefit measure can then be achieved when this is applied to the prioritized risk list. This helps with planning risk reduction activities and may lead to a decision to "live with some risks."

## Risk Reduction

Sometimes simple steps can be taken that reduce the level of potential damage or risk to records. Here are a few "commonsense" suggestions (Government of Alberta, 1992).

## *Physical*

- Keep passages in storage areas unobstructed.
- Never store records on the floor.

- Do not leave original documents on desks overnight.
- Identify and store cellulose nitrate-base film safely apart from the rest of the collections and have it copied at the earliest opportunity. It is highly combustible, and it slowly decomposes under normal storage conditions, releasing gases harmful to paper and film.
- Do not pack files too tightly. This ensures that water will not cause them to swell to the point where they burst from their shelving.
- Shelve materials so that they are set back slightly from the edge; this prevents the vertical spread of fire from one shelf to another.
- Avoid basement storage. Water seeks the lowest level.
- Check areas where pipes and windows are subject to condensation.
- Install shelving at least 12 inches away from outside walls, 3 inches away from inside walls, and with the bottom shelves at least 4 inches above the floor.
- Store the more valuable material on upper shelves and upper floors.
- Do not install carpet in storage areas. It will retain water and prevent drainage, as well as interfering with temperature stabilization and relative humidity.
- Install and maintain fire detection and fire extinguishing systems.

## *Procedural*

Procedural prevention includes activities relating to security and recovery, performed on a day-to-day, month-to-month, or annual basis. Examples would include maintaining up-to-date backup copies of all computer files; annual verification of user IDs and passwords; maintaining a system for storing backup copies in a place discrete from the source computer; and scheduling inspections and testing of smoke detectors, sprinkler systems, and fire extinguishers. The goal of procedural prevention is to define activities necessary to preventing various types of disasters and ensure that these activities are performed as required.

## *Recovery Options*

Before a plan can be formalized, the planning committee must evaluate all the available recovery options. Such options include these:

- Off-site data storage at *hot sites, warm sites, or cold sites*
- Reciprocal agreements for data storage with other organizations
- Multiple data centers and multiple computers
- Consortium arrangements with many organizations sharing data storage

The key in evaluating recovery strategies is to identify the strategy that works best for your organization rather than opting for the newest and latest rage in recovery technology that does not provide a best match for your operations.

## The Disaster Recovery Plan

Document a written plan. Disaster Recovery Planning involves more than off-site storage or backup processing. Organizations must develop written, comprehensive disaster recovery plans that address all its critical operations and functions. It is essential that nurses are involved in this process to represent the data and processing needs related to patient care in whatever setting.

A disaster recovery plan should contain all the information necessary to maintain the plan as well as execute its action steps. Use of a standard format for all departmental planning allows for easy access of information and ongoing maintenance of the plan. A suggested format for the plan's document is outlined next (Government of Alberta, 1992; Wold, 1997; Wold and Shriver, 1997; Hussong, 1997).

- Part 1: Introduction and Statement of Purpose
  State why the plan has been written and what it is intended to achieve. You should say something about who developed it and how it is to be kept current.
- Part 2: Authority
  Document the authority for the preparation of the plan and subsequent action. In this part, you also designate who is to be responsible for the records during the emergency, that is, who will coordinate the execution of the plan, and the line of succession.
- Part 3: Scope of the Plan
  This part will generally have three sections.
  A. Events Planned For: Itemize each kind of emergency event dealt with in the plan. For each, indicate the circumstances under which the event might occur and indicate what its expected impact on the department could be. List the most serious or most likely events first.
  B. Locations Planned For: If the department's records are located only at one site this section may not be required. However, if more than one site or building is involved, indicate here which sites are covered by the plan and the circumstances under which the plan might or might not apply to each individual site. Alternatively, separate plans could be developed for each site or building if this would be more practical. The following equipment should be considered: mainframe computer system, personal computers, bedside systems, data communications, and voice communications.
  C. Relationship to Other Plans: If the organization has other action plans, such as a medical emergency plan or a fire reaction plan, it is usually a good idea to describe how all plans relate to and supplement

each other and to indicate the circumstances under which they may be executed individually or simultaneously.

- Part 4: Emergency Procedures

Business resumption planning theory usually suggests vital records should be backed up and stored off site. However, in practice, there are always documents too bulky or too valuable to be copied. There are also documents where only the original will do, and then there is always work in progress. To be realistic, contingency plans should address the probability of having to retrieve vital material from an evacuated site. Other contents of this section should include these points:

  - Who is to put the plan into action, under what circumstances the plan is to be fully or partially executed, and how all the actions will be carried out.
  - The location of the emergency operations center (EOC) should be specified. This will be a predetermined meeting site for the disaster action team.
  - A floor plan showing the locations of the essential records for all sites must be included.
  - Detailed procedures for contingency processing at an alternate site (i.e., fixed location hot site, mobile facility) must be in place and written down.
  - Detailed procedures for establishing voice and data communications with the alternate processing site must be in place.
  - Sample testing schedules and procedures, including types of tests, test participants, team test responsibilities, and test forms should be included.
  - Include maintenance procedures for keeping the plan current.

The following are some other questions your plans should address. You can probably think of others yourself (DRIE Digest, 1992).

- STORAGE

Are vital documents stored in a fireproof room/vault/cabinet? Is the fire rating sufficient? Is it rated for magnetic media? Is it waterproof?

- SECURITY

Will the room/vault/cabinet be closed in an emergency? How will you secure documents if they have been retrieved?

- ACCESS

How will you arrange access to a cordoned off building? Who would be assigned to retrieve the material?

- IDENTIFICATION

If you were allowed to retrieve only one box of material, how would you identify the most urgent or critical?

- RESTORATION
  If your documents are charred or soaked, do you know how to restore them?

## *Appendices*

Use as many appendices as may be needed to include information vital to the success of the plan, but which may change so often as to make its inclusion in Parts 1 to 4 impractical. Suggested subjects follow:

- A staffing chart of the department, an organization chart showing the department's relationship to other departments (such as city government or other outside governing authority), and a chart illustrating the disaster control organization within the department. Other organizational charts may illustrate the department's relationships to local civil preparedness authorities and to disaster and welfare agencies, including the Red Cross.
- Call-up lists of key personnel who will be valuable to the execution of the plan; include name, title, address, telephone numbers, and the duties assigned to each.
- Instructions for contacting outside organizations, such as the fire department, the police department, local electric, gas, water, and telephone companies, hospitals and ambulance services, plumbers, electricians, locksmiths and glass companies, guard and janitorial services, exterminators, attorneys, and any other key people or agencies that might be of assistance. State why each is to be called and what service each will be expected to render. It is critical to keep these lists current; review them at regular intervals, at least annually.
- An inventory of essential records and the priorities for their protection. The estimated cost of creating or reproducing valuable records for offsite storage.
- A summary of the arrangements that have been made for the relocation of records. This should include the names of persons to be contacted when temporary space is needed and information about alternative space in case the primary space also is suffering from the same disaster.
- Instructions for ensuring the emergency operation of the building's utilities and for service and operation of vital building support systems.
- Probably the most important appendix will be a list of resources that might be needed in an emergency. There should also be a list of local suppliers. Record the supplies and materials you will need, what they are to be used for, who is to buy them, who is to use them, and where they can be found. Record your arrangements for borrowing materials, equipment, and personnel from other departments, how to transport items, and whom to call. List specialists who can be called on for assistance in preserving damaged record materials.
- The final appendix should be a glossary of special terms that are used in the plan so that all its users will be speaking the same language.

## Plan Testing and Maintenance

After all the effort taken to develop a disaster recovery plan, many organizations make the mistake of thinking that the process is "finished"! The contingency plan must be audited and tested on a regular basis to know that proposed processes will actually serve the purpose of protecting the data and processes of the organization should a real disaster occur.

Because organizations change continually, disaster recovery plans must also be dynamic. A process must be included for regularly updating the plan. Most disaster recovery plans will require a complete review of all procedures every 5 years. This review should focus on refining the requirements, exploiting new technology, and using a fresh approach to consider new solutions to old problems. With regular testing and an annual audit, the plan should be effective in processing critical data after a catastrophe occurs.

## Summary

Disasters such as fires, earthquakes, hurricanes, power blackouts, and floods will continue to occur. Less dramatic disasters such as power "bumps" or broken water pipes also claim data vital to patient care. To minimize losses, hospitals must establish and maintain effective computer contingency plans. Health care agencies should identify the most suitable plan for their organization, obtain management's commitment to the plan, and then implement the plan. Nursing must ensure that information vital to patient care is considered in disaster recovery planning.

## *References*

Baxter, K. Avoiding the inevitable. The British Journal of Health Care Computing 1991;8(2):33–34.

Government of Alberta. Disaster planning for Government of Alberta records. Unpublished document, 1992.

Hussong, W.A. So you're the company's new contingency planner! Disaster Recovery Journal 1997, 8 pg. Online. Available: http://www.drj.com/new2dr/w3_001.htm.

Points to Ponder. DRIE Digest 1992;1(2):2.

Wold, G.H. Disaster recovery planning process: Parts I, II, & III. Disaster Recovery Journal. 1997, 19 pg. Online. Available: http://www.drj.com/new2dr/w2_002.htm.

Wold, G.H., and Shriver, R.F. Risk analysis techniques. Disaster Recovery Journal 1997, 7(3) 8 pg. Online: Available: http://www.drj.com/new2dr/w3_030.htm.

# 18
# Implementation Concerns

WITH CONTRIBUTIONS BY CHERYL PLUMMER

## Introduction

Successful implementation of a Nursing Information System (NIS) depends on promoting nursing user acceptance of the system. In this chapter, the focus is on identifying and responding to sources of resistance to information systems and computers in health care and the management of change.

## Sources of Resistance to Information Systems and Computers in Health Care

To address the reason why health care professionals, nurses, physicians, and technologists, among others, have been slow in using computers and information technology, extensive research was conducted and countless discussions held, which resulted in the identification of seven major sources of resistance (Ball and Snelbecker, 1982). The results of this classic study continue to be applicable (Adderly et al., 1997; Doyle and Kowba, 1997; FitzHenry and Snyder, 1996; Marasovic et al., 1997).

### Oversell by Vendors

The first reason is the tendency for some vendors to overstate or to oversell their product. Of course, not every vendor or salesman oversells every time. Nonetheless, if you had to come up with a general statement describing the way many vendors have conducted themselves when dealing with clients in the health care field, it would be fair to say that the vendor would promise the moon to health professionals if only they would buy Brand X machines. All too often the computer has been presented as a panacea for all health care's organizational and overall management problems.

Until recently, health care professionals were unschooled in computer use and tended to believe that the vendor had the solution to their problems. Often the health professional turned the decision power over to the information systems personnel, who knew little of the nurses' or other health professionals' information needs. This practice typically has led to serious communication problems for the users and those who assume responsibility for the design and initial implementation of the computer system. This breakdown in communication thus impairs the quality of the system initially designed and by continued poor communication handicaps progress in the basic use of computers in hospitals.

## Unrealistic Expectations

A second source of resistance stems from unrealistic expectations regarding the actual contributions of computer systems in nursing. This attitude is unfortunate because it may lead to inappropriate concepts about what computer systems can do. At other times, it tends to mask otherwise desirable and feasible contributions.

Numerous illustrations of this theme have accompanied some of the inroads made by computerization in health care. Often the computer was looked upon as a panacea for administrative or political problems in the nursing practice. When the promises and expectations did not materialize, the health care professionals soon found that many of the promised applications offered were not forthcoming. In some cases, however, a 40% to 60% solution to the problem was achieved, which in itself should have been viewed as a monumental advance. However, health care professionals had been promised an unrealistic 100% solution, blinding them to the help they were indeed receiving. As a consequence, the entire program was disregarded, with hope for a much more general solution in the future.

A specific example of this phenomenon is the use of computers for EKG analysis. At present, a high degree of certainty with regard to normal EKG interpretation can be attained using the computer as a diagnostic tool. Less success, however, is possible in specific diagnosis of abnormalities. Quite often, health care practitioners wait for a perfect system to be developed to solve 100% of the problem, not wanting to acknowledge that an available system providing 60% assistance with a routine task is a giant step forward.

Users' unrealistic expectations typically lead to mixed feelings and resistance concerning computer technology. Only a small minority of nurses and hospital administrators presently can identify the ways in which computers and information technology can be used. Thus, this sense of diffidence results either in giving information systems specialists full authority regarding computers and information systems or in puzzling and inconsistent resistances to any use of computers and information technology.

## Changes in Traditional Procedures

Computers and information technology can pose threats to long-established, sound procedures in nursing. Nursing has a traditional set of rules, laws, ethics, and codes of confidentiality. Computerization has an impact on all of this, just as all types of technological innovations appear to pose a major threat when first introduced.

For nurses, skepticism is, to a very large degree, a most desirable professional trait. Nurses are entrusted with the welfare of their patients, and in that context skepticism about new fads and resistance to change in one's mode of practice are well placed. Potential danger to a patient's welfare can be perceived if the nurse does not feel confident about how successful or reliable computers and information technology might be in the care of the patients. Particularly threatening is the possibility that the nurse may not sufficiently understand the new technology so that the patients' welfare, entrusted to the nurse, may be in danger. Some health computer experts think it is unrealistic to expect the current generation of nurses, who have not become acquainted with computers as a natural part of their training and education, to accept a wide range of computer systems applications in their actual practice of nursing.

It is important to note here the variation in the extent to which information technology has been applied in different potential areas (Ball and Snelbecker, 1982). For example, information technology is quite frequently used in financial management matters but less frequently for patient care and for educational purposes.

## *Insufficient Involvement of Nurses*

Administrators and nurses are often not adequately and consistently involved in critical decisions about the use of information technology. Naiveté of health and hospital top management concerning the new information technology has often proved detrimental to the success of computer installations in health centers. In addition, there seems to be a lack of top management involvement when developing short and long range planning in the selection and installation of hospital and medical information systems.

Management sometimes treats the installation of a medical health care or patient information as though it were a new telephone system or a new air conditioning system. There seems to be a gap in perceiving that installation of an information system will have a major impact on all aspects of the institution, from financial management, to patient management, right down to a total reorganization of ancillary services and staffing practices in general. It is urgent that key hospital decision makers realize that they have the major responsibility in deciding how this "new tool" is to be used. Without the use of competent consultants, good vendor contracts, responsible systems analysis, and involved administration, fully the vast potential of computers and information systems cannot be utilized fully in such areas as administration, patient care, research and education.

## *System Improvement Versus New Approaches*

In many cases resistance occurs when nursing personnel hold on to existing systems rather than exploring new technologies. While "new" is not necessarily better, such resistance can preclude becoming aware of advances in nursing and patient care. A common tendency is to view a particular function solely in terms of existing systems characteristics rather than to recognize alternative ways of conceptualizing how patient care may be improved. It is not adequate to use new technologies simply to complete old tasks faster (see Chapter 12). Change management approaches such as TQM/CQI and Business Process Redesign can assist nursing staff in optimizing the role of information technology in the performance of their patient care and other duties.

The problem of medical records provides a typical illustration. Basically, the medical records mission is one of data storage and access—a major communications problem. It cannot be resolved simply through extending the ancient, inaccurate manual code, which has grown to monstrous dimension and exorbitant cost. The computer as a communications controller and file manager could provide greater flexibility in the functions and use of medical record systems. However, computer technology should also aid us in finding the best means for maintaining and gaining access to needed information.

The general objective of the medical record is to make information about the ongoing care of patients accessible so that subsequent diagnosis and treatment will constitute high-quality patient care. To do this requires data storage and retrieval by means that will facilitate communication among health professionals. Unfortunately, the way medical records systems operate is sometimes dictated by existing systems. For example, existing manual systems have certain characteristics that determine how information can be stored and retrieved. Weed (1991) has addressed this subject by formulating his concepts of the problem-oriented medical record (POMR) and Knowledge Coupling. In Weed's approach, medical records in their new form, utilizing computerized methods, can bring invaluable patient data to the physician and nurse at the point where the best benefits from the data result in better care. New technology could not have been applied to this major advance of integrating computers in the medical records as early as it has if Weed had not devised a new way of conceptualizing goals and problems. Through this paradigm, it is now possible for computer technology to provide health care providers with information about patients when and where it is needed.

## *Fear of Leaving the "Gutenberg Culture"*

Another form of resistance is linked to the tremendous impact of the printing press and the way information is maintained through printed records. We sometimes fail to recognize that the printed word has certain limitations in addition to providing certain opportunities. Computer-based information systems not only provide storage and retrieval of information but also afford new opportunities for increasing our knowledge. This interactive characteristic can have important implications for the ways we use information. However, it necessitates changes in our present "printed word" views about information. Gabrieli (1981) maintained:

Knowledge is a formalized and organized representation of scientific facts. Computers can store and retrieve such facts much easier, more efficiently and far more economically than the human. We can now construct a synergistic man-machine system for clinical medicine where many facts are stored in a readily retrievable form by a computer so that the machine is fully under the control of the human user. In this system, the machine is merely an electronic extension of the human memory. Such an electronic information system will overcome the major restriction of the Gutenberg culture, the limitation of the human memory.

## *Fear of the Unknown*

This last point concerns fear and change. Seldom has an individual given a more concise analysis of the acceptance or acknowledgment of change within a traditional system or discipline than did Machiavelli (1513). His analysis on the establishment of new systems is as follows:

It must be remembered that there is nothing more difficult to plan, more doubtful of success, nor more dangerous to manage, than the creation of a new system. For the initiator has the enmity of all who would profit by the preservation of the old institutions and merely lukewarm defenders in those who would gain by the new ones.

## Management of Change

A major potential source of resistance involves the confidential and personal aspects inherent in the nurse–patient relationship. Nurses are greatly concerned that unauthorized persons may gain access to information about patients if computer-based records are used. Stories occasionally reported in the mass media about breakdowns in the security of computer systems lend support to such fears. The fears become more personally and professionally relevant if the nurse feels that some "machine" is intruding on their relationships with patients. In reality, with proper procedures, the nurse can enhance confidentiality rather than jeopardize it (see Chapter 14). The information system also can serve as an extremely helpful tool in aiding the nurse to spend more professional time in fostering personal-professional relationships with patients.

The key to resolving the problems lies in fostering collaboration among nurses, physicians, other health professionals, and computer technologists in designing and maintaining systems that enhance cost-efficient, quality patient care. In anticipating the broad scale implementation of computerized information systems in health care institutions and agencies, it is fast becoming clear that such transformation is frequently complex and always accompanied by a shift in values and priorities that can conflict with vested interests. Machiavelli's ancient advice still holds true.

It is unfortunate that tasks related to implementation of a computerized information system frequently become the focus rather than the process. The emphasis must be process oriented rather than task oriented. Priority must be given to the acceptance of and familiarization with a change of this magnitude. A substantial body of empirically based knowledge related to change theory can provide the basis for implementation of any system, as has been discussed in preceding chapters. A detailed discussion of change theory, however, is beyond the scope of this text.

Lewin's (1969) classic work suggested that behavior in an institutional setting is not a static habit or pattern, but a dynamic balance of forces working in opposite directions within the social-psychological space of the institution (see Figure 18.1). Lewin goes on to identify three stages in accomplishing changes in behavior: unfreezing the existing equilibrium, movement toward a new equilibrium, and refreezing the new equilibrium. To initiate the unfreezing of the equilibrium, there are three strategies:

- Increase the number of driving forces
- Decrease the number of resisting forces
- A combination of these

The nursing profession is beginning to experience the profound impact computers and information systems ultimately will have on nursing practice and patient care. Previously, nurses were faced with the choice of whether to act traditionally and have change thrust on them from outside the ranks of the profession through an increase in the driving force. This approach of

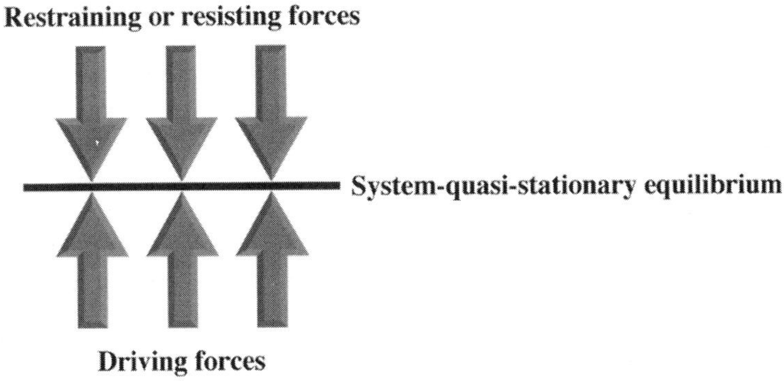

**Restraining or resisting forces**

**System-quasi-stationary equilibrium**

**Driving forces**

FIGURE 18.1. Lewin's dynamic balance of forces.

resistance to this change (i.e., introduction of health care information systems) merely results in increasing the resisting forces that produce consequential increase in the driving forces (e.g., societal trends, government, and administration). Ultimately, because the driving forces in this case also have the power and authority, the change would be instituted but probably be accompanied by increased tension, instability, and unpredictability in nursing practice and patient care. This option is totally unacceptable to nurses who, as patient advocates, are committed to using every means at their disposal to ensure the highest quality care for patients. Computers and information systems are only one tool to be used in achieving this goal. No longer is the question "Should the nursing profession resist automation?" Given present societal, governmental, and technical trends, the change to and expansion of computerized information systems in health care agencies is inevitable. The question now becomes one of coping with the resisting forces within and among the profession so that the result is a stable, predictable, rational approach to improving the quality of nursing practice and thus the quality of patient care.

In another classic reference, Benne and Chin (1969) identified several models for accomplishing change. We believe that their normative-educative approach provides a comprehensive framework for the implementation of concepts discussed in this and preceding chapters. Benne and Chin perceive the normative-educative process of change as follows:

Change in a pattern of practice or action, according to this view, will occur only as the persons involved are brought to change their normative orientations to old patterns and develop commitments to new ones. And changes in normative orientations involve changes in attitudes, values, skills and significant relationships, not just changes in knowledge, information or intellectual rationales for action and practice.

This approach to change emphasizes both cognitive and affective components when determining an individual's behavior. That is, it recognizes that what a person believes (i.e., values, attitudes, and social norms) is just as important as what a person knows in terms of influencing that person's actions. Thus, successful change can only be accomplished by addressing both cognitive and affective aspects of individual behavior. Obviously, concepts related to adult education are essential to promoting change in the cognitive (knowledge) domain and concepts related to values clarification will be used in promoting change in the affective (attitude) domain.

In addition, all the factors that determine the impact of the group on individual behavior must be taken into account—for example, group norms and values, role theory, power, and formal and informal leadership structure. Thorough understanding of change theory and its application is vital to the successful implementation of the technological applications discussed in this book.

Nursing is without question the single largest group of care providers in any health care organization. The ability to positively influence the nursing population regarding the implementation of computer-based systems is a major factor in determining the success of the implementation. Nursing is, by tradition, a militaristic profession. Its roots were in the military with the crusaders, in the religious nursing orders, which were very hierarchical, and then with Nightingale in the Crimea. Nursing's traditions were very much militaristic, and change was by command rather than cooperation. Modern nurses with better academic credentials and better education no longer accept change simply on the basis of position authority. They now expect to have input into the change. Also they expect that changes will be based on knowledge, logic, and research rather than on whim and emotion. Nurses also expect greater sophistication from their leaders in the use of skills and strategies for introducing changes that will affect the practice of nursing. To this end, numerous nursing authors have reported their strategies and experiences in implementing such change. Repeatedly, the importance of the following factors is identified (Adderly et al., 1997; Doyle and Kowba, 1997; FitzHenry and Snyder, 1996; Marasovic et al., 1997):

- Involve nursing early in the preplanning that includes all departments.
- Involve the user actively in planning.
- Designate a person in the nursing department at the senior management level to coordinate the implementation process within the nursing department.
- Designate the nursing implementation coordinator as liaison between nursing department and other departments.
- Establish a user's committee within the nursing department chaired by the nursing implementation coordinator; include the enthusiastic, the uncommitted, and the mildly negative on the committee.
- Make resource people available as consultants to the nursing implementation coordinator and their departmental committee.
- Develop a training program that includes explanation of rationale for the computerization, nurses' responsibilities related to the new system, expected effect of the system on nurses, and nursing care in the organization as well as actual use of the system.
- Use professional colleagues and peers to train other nurses (i.e., a core group of trained nursing users train other nursing staff to use the system).
- Time training to occur just before the new system goes "on-line"; allow sufficient learning time; provide training time to all shifts.

## Summary

Computers and information systems are as much a part of nursing practice today as the stethoscope. Resistance can be overcome if a collaborative effort is launched by health personnel and information technology specialists. Through cooperation and free exchange of ideas, information systems technology can facilitate major advances in improving patient care.

## *References*

Adderly, D., Hyde, C., and Mauseth, P. The computer age impacts nurses. *Computers in Nursing* 1997;15(1):43–46.

Ball, M.J., and Snelbecker, G.E. Overcoming resistances to telecommunications innovations in medicine and continuing medical education. *Computers in Hospitals* 1982;3(4):40–45.

Benne, K.D., and Chin, R. General strategies for effecting changes in human systems." In: *The Planning of Change: Readings in Applied Behavioural Sciences*, 2nd Ed. New York: Holt, Reinhart, & Winston, 1969.

Doyle, K., and Kowba, M. Managing the human side of change to automation. *Computers in Nursing* 1997;15(2):67–68.

FitzHenry, F., and Snyder, J. Improving organizational processes for gains during implementation. *Computers in Nursing* 1996;14(3):171–180.

Gabrielli, E.R. 1981. Memorized versus computerized medical knowledge. Annual Harry Goldblatt Lecture, Mt. Sinai Hospital, Cleveland, Ohio.

Lewin, K. Quasi-stationary social equilibria and the problem of permanent change. In: Bennis, W.G., Benne, K.D., and Chin, R. (eds.) *The Planning of Change*. New York: Holt, Reinhart, & Winston, 1969:235–238.

Machiavelli, N. *The Prince* (1513). Translated by George Bull. New York: Penguin Books, 1961.

Marasovic, C., Kenney, C., Elliott, D., and Sindhusake, D. Attitudes of Australian nurses toward the implementation of a clinical information system. *Computers in Nursing* 1997;15(2):91–98.

Weed, Lawrence L. *Knowledge Coupling*. New York: Springer-Verlag, 1991.

# Part V
# Professional Nursing Informatics

# 19
# Nursing Informatics Education: Past, Present, and Future

WITH CONTRIBUTIONS BY JO ANN KLEIN AND JUDITH V. DOUGLAS

## Introduction

Today's health care environment continually places increasing demands on nurses to communicate, share, and synthesize information and data through the use of information systems, with or without the assistance of computers (Chapman et al., 1994; Ngin and Simms, 1996). Nurses who are computer literate, in addition to having knowledge of information systems, have the opportunity to use the power and efficiency of computer systems to play an important role in enhancing patient care delivery and shaping nursing practice.

Computer-literate nurses are defined as licensed nurses who demonstrate competency in the understanding and use of computer hardware, software, terminology, and operating systems (Saba and McCormick, 1996). In today's information age, nurses are expected to keep pace with rapidly advancing technology. Appropriate utilization of computers and information systems can help nurses make well-informed decisions regarding management and patient care issues. It is, therefore, critical that education in the use of computerized health care knowledge systems be included as an important component of basic, as well as advanced, nursing curricula.

Nurse educators are expected to teach how to develop, retrieve, and implement electronically stored data to optimize information-dependent clinical decisions. Also, the nurse educator is expected to provide guidelines concerning newly emerging nursing knowledge and ways that this knowledge can be accessed. This need requires the nurse educator to keep abreast of the advancing technology on a theoretical as well as practical basis.

The intent of this chapter is to explore the development of graduate-level nursing informatics education from its inception to the present, with an emphasis on the importance of computer literacy as an integral part of the educational program. After discussing the evolution of nursing informatics education and incorporating an existing nursing informatics model, goals and objectives for future nursing informatics education are suggested.

A review of the literature provides a historical overview of nursing informatics education, including a discussion of the recognition of nursing informatics as a formal specialty by the American Nurses Association (ANA) with certification through the American Nurses Credentialing Center. Through this recognition, the specialty of nursing informatics has assumed standards of practice that should be integrated into the graduate-level nursing informatics educational curriculum. Studies that have been conducted to determine the educational needs of nursing informatics students were also examined.

## Review of the Literature

### *Historical Overview of Nursing Informatics Education*

During the 1980s, nurses who were involved in informatics were primarily self-educated because of the small number of graduate programs available to formally prepare nurses to work in this specialty. During that time, the number of faculty involved in these graduate programs was small enough so that they could independently network in an effort to exchange course content. Education focused on teaching the use of computers as a tool for word processing, spreadsheet analysis, graphics production, and statistical applications (Arnold, 1996). These early programs addressed only the nature of information systems and their selections for nursing practice (Graves et al., 1995; McGonigle, 1991).

In 1988, Dr. Barbara Heller was instrumental in establishing the first graduate program in nursing informatics at the University of Maryland School of Nursing in Baltimore. The focus of this formalized program included an understanding of nursing informatics science and systems theory in a clinical and management context, with particular emphasis on its impact on nursing practice (Romano and Heller, 1990).

The Maryland program was developed in close collaboration with the university's information services division, headed by Dr. Marion J. Ball, who worked with the School of Nursing to launch their technology assisted learning centers, develop an outside advisory board for the program, and initiate innovations in the curriculum. Together with Dr. Kathryn Hannah, she contributed the major initial texts for the program (Ball and Hannah, 1984; Ball et al., 1988; Ball et al., 1995; Hannah et al., 1994).

A second graduate school program followed in 1990 when the University of Utah initiated a nursing informatics program that focused on the transformation of nursing data into information to support clinical decision making. Students learned about nursing informatics theory, design and analysis of clinical nursing systems, clinical nursing database design, decision support, and administration of clinical nursing information systems (Arnold, 1996). This program followed on the heels of a discontinued grant-funded summer postdoctoral seminar for nursing informatics that began at Utah during the summer of 1988 and ended before the opening of that university's graduate program in nursing informatics.

Since the inception of Utah's graduate-level nursing informatics program, a lack of federal funding has limited the development of other similar programs. Funding resources are critical to provide adequate computer hardware, software, support services, faculty, and individual implementation strategies for these programs. Only recently has any organization been awarded grant funding to implement a pilot nursing informatics graduate program. In September 1998, New York University School of Nursing, under the direction of Dr. Barbara Carty, anticipates offering the newest nursing informatics graduate track. This program is expected to include theory and clinical applications with multiple preceptorship experiences encompassing all aspects of nursing informatics.

Despite a lack of funding for new programs, the need for nursing informatics courses has been recognized by other nursing schools. These educational institutions have integrated nursing informatics courses within their undergraduate, as well as graduate, curricula in the form of required courses, electives, conferences, and continuing education workshops. Furthermore, the traditional classroom has expanded beyond its walls to include distance education, telemedicine, and continuing education offerings. An example of an accredited nursing education distance learning program is the one offered by Regents College, based in New York, which has utilized the U.S. postal service and the Internet to teach courses leading to baccalaureate degrees in nursing.

## *Recognition as a Nursing Specialty*

In 1992, nursing informatics was formally recognized as a nursing specialty by the American Nurses Association. This recognition of nursing informatics as its own specialty was followed by the development of nursing informatics standards of practice, which were published by the American Nurses Association in 1995. These standards require that informatics nurses acquire and maintain current knowledge in nursing informatics practice (American Nurses Association, 1995). To achieve this, the informatics nurse is required to seek additional knowledge and skills appropriate to the practice setting by participating in educational programs and activities, conferences, workshops, interdisciplinary professional meetings, and self-directed learning. Thus, nursing informatics educators are needed to provide appropriate learning opportunities. The standards also suggest that each informatics nurse keep a record of his or her own learning activities and seek certification when eligible.

Nursing Informatics certification became available in 1995 through the American Nurses Credentialing Center (ANCC). Topics on the certification exam include: (1) system analysis and design, (2) system implementation and support, (3) system testing and evaluation, (4) human factors, (5) computer technology, (6) information/database management, (7) professional practice/trends and issues, and (8) theories (American Nurses Credentialing Center, 1995).

To be eligible to take the nursing informatics certification examination, applicants are required to have a baccalaureate or higher degree in nursing, maintain licensure, and have 2 years of active experience as a registered nurse. In addition, each candidate must have a minimum of 2000 hours of experience in the field of nursing informatics in the 5 years before taking the examination. In lieu of this experience, 12 semester hours of academic credit in informatics in a nursing graduate program and a minimum of 1000 hours in informatics nursing may be substituted (American Nurses Credentialing Center, 1995). Since 1997, the certification exam has been available by computer at 55 testing facilities throughout the United States. It was the first computerized ANCC certification exam.

## *Nursing Informatics Graduate-Level Education Today*

Many educational and practice institutions have initiated programs to prepare nurse clinicians simply as users of automated systems, while others are preparing health care information systems specialists. Despite the increased use of computer systems in nursing informatics, the management component of informatics presented by Graves and Corcoran (1989) remains essential. The nursing informatics student is still taught to have the "functional ability to collect, aggregate, organize, move, and represent information in an economical, efficient way that is useful to users of the system" (Graves and Corcoran, 1989).

Today, nurses can take advantage of the virtual classroom where the educational process occurs outside the formal classroom setting. In this environment, use of telecommunication technologies through computer-based intranets, extranets, and the Internet make innovative multimedia teaching possible. This teaching methodology is ideal for students who require flexible class schedules secondary to work and family obligations. The virtual classroom, as an interactive process, enables nursing students and their teachers to utilize telecommunication software applications such as interactive video instruction, electronic mail, bulletin boards or newsgroups, and chat conferencing as a learning milieu. To supplement virtual classroom activities, students are guided to utilize the Internet, where databases of nursing and health care information and other applicable learning resources can be accessed from school and home computers. It is, therefore, the responsibility of nurse educators to actively train students to access, retrieve, and implement this growing base of virtual learning tools and to provide feedback to students regarding their success in implementing these tools.

## Studies Examining Nursing Informatics Educational Needs

As early as 1990, when no formal nursing informatics program existed in their school, recommendations were made by the Computing Advisory Council (CAC) at The University of Texas Health Science Center School of Nursing at San Antonio for integration of nursing informatics within graduate research coursework (Noll and Murphy, 1993). At that time, it was recommended that students achieve the following competencies upon completion of the graduate program, regardless of their major: (1) analyze and select relevant information sources; (2) access existing Internet resources for nursing and related disciplines; (3) extract, manage, and organize data; (4) analyze the nurse's role in data security and integrity; (5) analyze the impact of nursing information systems; (6) evaluate and use appropriate software for advanced practice; and (7) demonstrate information transfer between computer systems (Noll and Murphy, 1993).

These programs, which incorporate nursing informatics coursework in their graduate-level curricula, confirm that achieving computer competency is not easy for all the participants. Magnus et al., (1994) participated in a graduate course titled "Nursing Informatics" at the Hunter-Bellevue School of Nursing that emphasized the integration and use of computer and information technology as it related to the management and process of data, information, and knowledge to support nursing practice and the delivery of care. At that time, there was noted resistance to using computers, because of fear of the unknown. Magnus and her classmates suggested that participating in the course helped to diffuse the 'mystery' surrounding the material (Magnus et al., 1994). Noll and Murphy (1993) reported that integration of nursing informatics material with hands-on application facilitated learning. In addition, students noted that information about software packages, particularly bibliographic databases, was very helpful and would be useful in the development of their graduating theses.

A study conducted by Saranto and Leino-Kilpi (1997) identified and described computer skills required in nursing and what should be taught about information technology in nursing education. A three-round Delphi survey was conducted with a panel of experts representing nursing practice, nursing education, nursing students, and consumers. The experts agreed that nurses must know how to use the computer for word processing purpose as well as for accessing and using hospital information systems and electronic mail (e-mail). Nurses must also be aware of system security and show a positive attitude toward computers. Conclusively, the study determined that hospital information systems and nursing informatics should be integrated into laboratory and hospital training (Saranto and Leino-Kilpi, 1997).

In 1996, Dr. Jean Arnold of the College of Nursing, Rutgers, the State University of New Jersey, conducted a survey among 497 respondents in a northeastern metropolitan area to determine the informatics needs of professional nurses. The subjects primarily represented informatics specialists, nurse educators, and nurse managers, many with masters or doctoral degrees. Respondents were asked to indicate their current knowledge and desired knowledge of nursing informatics in 23 content areas that are included in the ANCC Nursing Informatics Certification Exam.

The survey revealed that 73% of the respondents were interested in returning to school to earn certification in nursing informatics while 59% of the respondents were interested in a graduate degree (Arnold, 1996). Decision support, integration of nursing informatics, advanced nursing informatics, decision analysis, and graphics presentations were the content areas most highly ranked by informatics nurses. In addition, informatics trends and issues information were the foremost educational needs identified by informatics nurses in the survey. The results reported by informatics nurses in both areas differed from the responses by nurse educators and nurse managers, suggesting that position titles and responsibilities have an impact on a subject's interest in advanced education in addition to the subject's use of computer applications (Arnold, 1996).

As a result of her survey, Arnold recommended that informatics nursing curricula content include "graphic presentation of data, decision support, electronic communications, integration of nursing informatics within basic and other specialty programs, critique of computer-assisted clinical data analysis, and expert knowledge acquisition" (Arnold, 1996). She also recommended including review courses for the informatics certification examination and emphasized the need for more graduate and continuing education programs to meet the increased demand for informatics knowledge.

# The Future of Nursing Informatics Education

Clearly, there is a need for standardization of graduate nursing informatics curricula based upon the standards of nursing informatics practice defined by the ANA, nursing informatics certification requirements defined by the ANCC, and utilization of a nursing informatics model such as that developed by Riley and Saba incorporating the suggested adaptations.

For the nurse educator to effectively teach and reinforce this newly acquired nursing informatics knowledge, computer systems should be readily available at all sites where nursing education occurs or clinical decisions are made, and in any place where nursing is practiced. Students must be allowed to experience situations where computer applications related to nursing informatics can be used, which includes utilization of the virtual classroom.

One of the primary barriers to utilization of the virtual classroom in nursing informatics education has been the speed with which telecommunication and computer technology has been developing, resulting in frequently changing software and hardware requirements and a financial investment that many schools are not able to sustain. It is hoped that as the cost of computer hardware and accompanying software systems continues to decline, computerized educational modalities and clinical information banks will become more readily accessible.

The development of nursing informatics curricula for graduate-level nursing students demands that the minimum standards be based on an understanding of the ANA's nursing informatics standards or practice. Optimally, the curricula should be based upon the understanding as well as the application of the ANA's nursing informatics standards of practice in addition to the requirements for achieving certification in nursing informatics through the ANCC.

To achieve these goals, there must be practical application of the presented information systems theory. This should include not only additional educational experiences but also substantial hands-on experience through preceptorship arrangements. First-hand experience will ensure that all master's level nursing informatics graduates will display a high level of competency in both theory and practice. Because this is such a crucial goal, coursework should continue to focus on computer applications and related issues in nursing practice, nursing administration, nursing education, and nursing research.

# Defining an Educational Model for Graduate-Level Nursing Informatics

Not only is there a need for more nursing informatics programs, but a need also exists for an educational framework to promote standardization and structure within the nursing informatics curricula. Because the specialty is so new, there has been limited research regarding development of models specifically designed for nursing informatics education. Utilization of educational models would provide the needed framework not only for theoretical education but also for practical applications.

Riley and Saba's Nursing Informatics Education Model (NIEM) is an educational application aimed at undergraduate students that can be adapted for graduate students. Riley and Saba's model can fulfill the need for a theoretical can practical framework in addition to meeting the desired requirements of informatics nurses cited in Arnold's survey (Saba and McCormick, 1995).

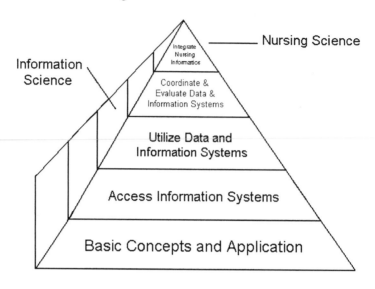

Nursing Science

Information
Science

Computer Science

**FIGURE 19.1.** Riley and Saba's Nursing Informatics Education Model (NIEM). (From Saba, V., and McCormick, K. *Essentials of Computers for Nurses.* New York: McGraw-Hill, 1995:558, with permission.)

Riley and Saba's Nursing Informatics Education Model emerged and evolved with the development of computer technology in the health care industry. As illustrated in Figure 19.1, NIEM identifies three dimensions of content that comprise nursing informatics computer science, information science, and nursing science. NIEM further identifies the educational outcomes that must be addressed in the three domains of learning: cognitive, affective, and psychomotor. Once the objectives are achieved in each domain of learning, students can integrate nursing informatics into their nursing roles. This integration of knowledge and competence in nursing education requires that a program include content, hand-on application, and attitude: The model supports the integration of computer technology into nursing education to enhance critical thinking skills and provide an active learning experience. Confidence, psychomotor skill level, and knowledge attainment are enhanced in the process. An advantage of using this model is the ability for the student nurse to make decisions in simulated case studies without risk to the patient (Saba and McCormick, 1995).

As detailed in Appendix E and summarized here, NIEM's objectives occur in four steps. Because basic computer skills are germane to fundamental nursing education, the first step gives students the knowledge and technical skills to function effectively (Lawless, 1993; Saba and McCormick, 1995). Computer application content at this level includes concepts of computer hardware and software as well as computer system components. Students are required to use a word processing program for assignments and to format documents in American Psychological Association (APA) format. System content includes the use of computerized databases and search engines for reference material (Saba and McCormick, 1995). While it is hoped that all students entering a graduate-level program would be proficient in basic computer skills and applications, this step provides the needed content and practical experience for those students entering graduate-level programs with little or no computer knowledge.

As noted in Appendix F, this author recommends student application of word processing, database, presentation, and spreadsheet software programs; this is in addition to bibliographic retrieval using CD-ROM software as well as Internet searches. This hands-on computer experience is augmented by the assignment of e-mail addresses and required subscription to a class e-mail discussion group, which can be utilized for discussion and assignments. Nursing literature supports the use of e-mail, as an informal exchange of communication, in helping new computer users cope with the stress of using new technology and to enhance critical thinking skills (Magnus et al., 1994; Todd, 1998).

The second step of Riley and Saba's model involves application of computer technology to document and access health information for the purposes of patient assessment. On an undergraduate level, Riley and Saba introduce the Saba Home Health Care Classification of Nursing Diagnosis and Intervention in the classroom to develop patient care plans and in the hospital patient information system for recording care (Saba and McCormick, 1995).

This author suggests that, on the graduate level, step 2 can be adapted to include organizational theory and associated computer applications such as utilization of Microsoft Project for project management simulation. In addition, students can apply computer applications to health care financial management coursework in determining staffing needs, cost–benefit ratios, and budgets. It is during step 2 that this author suggests the computerized patient record (CPR) be introduced, particularly in regard to classification systems and taxonomies, managed care, and the social, legal, and ethical issues associated with the CPR.

The third step of the Riley and Saba model introduces undergraduate students to advanced concepts utilizing existing information systems in clinical agencies to plan and implement patient care (Saba and McCormick, 1995). This author proposes that, on a graduate level, this step can be adapted to include telecommunications in health care with an emphasis on understanding the policy development that led to the current trend toward telemedicine and telenursing applications in addition to its utilization. Also, knowledge about system requirements and design and development applications should be imparted through actual student experience working in venues such as outpatient agencies, vendors, hospital information system departments, and consulting firms.

Riley and Saba's fourth and final step requires students to integrate computer technology into nursing care and includes evaluation, quality improvement, multidisciplinary collaboration, and utilization of available resources with the technology. In addition, students are required to examine the social, legal, and ethical issues they encounter through the use of computer technology (Saba and McCormick, 1995).

This final step has been integrated into earlier steps of the graduate-level adapted model. Therefore, this author suggests revising the fourth step to include implementation of a full systems analysis. To achieve this, the student would need to have the opportunity to work on a systems development life cycle in a preceptor-based practicum real-life experience during the course of a 1-year internship. This plan would allow the student to benefit from long-term hands-on experience under the guidance of an experienced practitioner. In turn, this experience, coupled with earlier short-term practical experience, would enable students to claim credible nursing informatics experience when searching for employment after graduation.

Clearly, Riley and Saba's model is adaptable and can be applied to all levels of nursing informatics education. Because the practice of nursing informatics can occur in any area where nurses practice, this model is applicable in all practice settings (Lange, 1997). It is, therefore, a realistic model for standardizing nursing informatics education methodology.

## Conclusion

Informatics knowledge, in this age of information, is necessary for the growth of the nursing profession. Increasing the number of available of nursing informatics graduate-level programs is critical if the nursing profession is to meet the challenges presented by the integration of this rapidly advancing technology into health care. Therefore, the graduate-level nursing informatics educational environment must continue to strive to become a forum where educator and student meet in an expanded capacity made possible by an increase in the integration of computer competencies within the nursing informatics curricula.

This practice does not undermine the importance of noncomputerized systems in the field of nursing informatics, but responds to the challenge of keeping pace with the changing regimen. By creating a pilot nursing informatics program utilizing the suggested adaptations of Riley and Saba's Nursing Informatics Education Model, increased computer literacy and competency can be achieved in a graduate-level nursing informatics program. Therefore, it is suggested that research be conducted to determine the effectiveness of such a program to (1) measure the effectiveness of the proposed program in relation to improving computer literacy and, therefore, increasing competency, (2) determine the feasibility of developing an actual program, and (3) add to the current knowledge base about nursing education curriculum requirements for nursing informatics graduate-level programs.

Once validated through research, this proposed model can serve as a guideline for schools of nursing that are in the process of considering, planning, developing, or implementing graduate-level nursing informatics curricula.

## *References*

American Nurses Association. *Standard of Practice for Nursing Informatics.* Washington, D.C.: American Nurses Publishing, 1995.

American Nurses Credentialing Center. *Informatics Certification Catalog.* Washington, D.C.: American Nurses Credentialing Center, 1995.

Arnold, J. Nursing informatics educational needs. *Computers in Nursing* 1996;14(6):333–339.

Ball, M.J., and Hannah, K.J. *Using Computers in Nursing.* Reston, Va: Reston Publishing, 1984.

Ball, M.J., Hannah, K.J., Gerdin Jelger, U., and Peterson, H. *Nursing Informatics: Where Caring and Technology Meet.* New York: Springer-Verlag, 1988.

Ball, M.J., Hannah, K.J., Newbold, S.K., and Douglas, J.V. *Nursing Informatics: Where Caring and Technology Meet,* 2nd Ed. New York: Springer-Verlag, 1995.

Chapman, R., Reiley, P., McKinney, J., Welch, K., Toomey, B., and McCauslan, M., Implementing a local area network for nursing in a large teaching hospital. *Computers in Nursing* 1994;12(2):82–87.

Graves, J., and Corcoran, S. The study of nursing informatics. *Image: Journal of Nursing Scholarship* 1989;21(4):227–231.

Graves, J., Amos, L., Hueber, S., Lange, L., and Thompson, C. Description of a graduate program in clinical nursing informatics. *Computers in Nursing* 1995;13(2):60–69.

Hannah, K.J., Ball, M.J., and Edwards, M.J.A. *Introduction to Nursing Informatics.* New York: Springer-Verlag, 1994.

Lange, L. Informatics nurse specialist: Roles in health care organizations. *Nursing Administration Quarterly* 1997;21(3):1–10.

Lawless, K. Nursing informatics as a needed emphasis in graduate nursing administration education: The student perspective. *Computers in Nursing* 1993;11(6):263–268.

Magnus, M., Co, M., Jr., and Cerkach, C. A first-level graduate studies experience in nursing informatics. *Computers in Nursing* 1994;12(4):189–192.

McGonigle, D. Establishing a nursing informatics program. *Computers in Nursing* 1991;9(5):184–189.

Ngin, P., and Simms, L. Computer use for work accomplishment. *Journal of Nursing Administration* 1996;26(3):47–53.

Noll, M., and Murphy, M. Integrating nursing informatics into a graduate research course. *Journal of Nursing Education* 1993;32(7):332–334.

Romano, C., and Heller, B. Nursing informatics: A model curriculum for an emerging role. *Journal of Nursing Education* 1990;15(2):16–19.

Saba, V., and McCormick, K. *Essentials of Computers for Nurses.* New York: Mc-Graw-Hill, 1996.

Saranto, K., and Leino-Kilpi, H. Computer literacy in nursing: Developing the information technology syllabus in nursing education. *Journal of Advanced Nursing* 1997;25(2):377–385.

Todd, N. Using e-mail in an undergraduate nursing course to increase critical thinking skills. *Computers in Nursing* 1998;16(2):115–118.

# 20
# The Future for Nurses in Health Informatics

## Introduction

As a new millennium approaches the emphasis in health informatics is increasingly changing. The initial focus was on hardware and moved to an emphasis on software. As understanding of health informatics evolves, increasingly that hardware and software are recognized as merely means of capturing, transporting, and transforming data into information that enables caregivers to provide people with the best possible health services. There is an information rich environment with new and powerful tools to assist caregivers and care recipients alike to seek and use information to make health-affecting decisions and to generate new health knowledge. Expanded understanding of how people seek and use information by drawing on cognitive science and organizational development (Tang and Patel, 1992; Lorenzi et al., 1995) is essential.

## A Vision of the Future

Haux (1998) has described a vision of medical informatics. Ball et al. (1997) have explored the implications of these aims for nursing.

- Aim 1. Diagnostics: the visible human body. Remote access to high-quality digital images supports new modes of care delivery (Dayhoff and Siegel, 1998; Zimmerman, 1995). These images can be minimized, ensure access to specialists, and create new requirements for coordinating and managing care. Other developments include the incorporation of images of various types into electronic patient records. These advances will enhance the information available to caregivers, including nurses, and impact the ways in which they deliver care. The National Library of Medicine's (NLM's) Visible Man and Visible Woman are now accessible via the Internet or CD-ROM; the availability of such images can increase the knowledge of the human body and ultimately contribute to nursing assessment and intervention.

- Aim 2. Therapy: medical intervention with as little strain on the patient as possible. Noninvasive diagnostics and minimally invasive surgery are growing significantly, thanks to laparoscopic procedures and computer-aided visualization. Clearly these advances affect nurses involved in the procedure itself: they also affect nurses involved throughout the care process, joining with other forces limiting the number of hospital days and changing the role of the hospital-based nurses.
- Aim 3. Therapy simulation. Nurse educators have been leaders in using simulation-based training for their students, offering simulation labs for basic skills. Further development of simulation technologies will allow nurses to refine advanced skills. Multimedia computer based training will supplement hands-on lab experiences.
- Aim 4. Early recognition and prevention. Today increasing numbers of nurse practitioners are providing primary care, and nurse-managed clinics are becoming the mechanism for delivering affordable primary care. Both trends suggest that nursing will become responsible for patient education, working with patients to develop health behaviors that prevent illness and promote wellness.
- Aim 5. Compensating physical handicaps. A device used on an ongoing basis by the patient tends ultimately to involve nursing in its support, as a daily living skill. These skills have long been the concern of nursing. New informatics applications in this area will require a new level of knowledge and sophistication among nursing staff.
- Aim 6. Health consulting: the informed patient. Patient education is receiving new attention. Multimedia programs guide patients in deciding on interventions for prostate cancer and videotapes are available for purchase in pharmacies addressing titles ranging from alcoholism to gastrointestinal ulcers. As more health-related information becomes available to consumers via the Internet, patients will definitely need guidance in evaluating and using information, guidance which nursing has often provided in the past and will do so increasingly as counselors and teachers of patients and clients.
- Aim 7. Health reporting. To date, public health has relied on retrospective reports to control disease. Today the information infrastructure offers the capability to intervene in a more timely manner through ongoing surveillance of certain conditions and through programs such as the NLM'S clinical alerts. The National Institute of Health is extending the boundaries through its Human Genome Project and Gene Bank. We have yet to realize the benefits that can result from large-scale data repositories providing population-based health statistics. Nursing will play a role in using and understanding outcome information to improve the management and quality of care.
- Aim 8. Enterprise information systems. Nurses have long been the frontline users of information systems in health care. Many such systems have, regrettably, come between the nurse and the patient. Clinical informatics

must focus on making information tools an integral component of the care process, noticeable only by their absence. Technology should free up the caregiver, eliminating cumbersome and repetitive data entry. Increasingly, technology will need to support health professionals including nurses in a wide variety of settings within large-scale integrated health service networks. As members of the health care team, nurses will continue to be at the hub, or center of patient care—even when they are functioning within a telehealth/telemedicine setting.

- Aim 9. Medical documentation. Movement toward the computer based patient record (CPR) and electronic health record (EHR) continues, albeit less rapidly than hoped. The major obstacles are nontechnical: questions remain regarding medical knowledge representation and structure of the record. Work is underway to integrate the Unified Nursing Language System (UNLS) into the NLM'S Unified Medical Language System (UMLS); the Telenurse project in the European Community; the International Classification of Nursing Practice initiative of the International Council of Nurses along with other initiatives both national and international. All of these hold promise for improved nursing documentation. Of course, data protection and patient confidentiality remain key critical issues, as do standards for access.

- Aim 10. Comprehensive documentation of medical knowledge and knowledge-based decisions for case management. These efforts are closely linked to outcomes and quality assurance. Self-learning systems like APACHE continuously construct their own databases from data gathered in the caregiving process and revise the probabilities that guide their users. New ethical considerations arise. How will these systems affect issues of clinical judgment and responsibility? Clearly the nursing profession will have to address these questions, both in concept and in practice.

## New Roles for Nurses in Nursing and Health Care Informatics

As the discipline known as nursing informatics (see Chapter 1) evolves in the context of the vision of health informatics, what must nurses contribute to the use of informational technologies in the delivery of health care? Nurses can and should contribute in the areas of research, education, and practice.

In the area of research, nurses with appropriate preparation have participated in developmental projects. All the major developers and vendors of computerized hospital information systems employ nurses as consultants, advisors, systems engineers, systems analysts, or programmers. Major research initiatives, led by nurse researchers, are underway to study the use of the Internet and World Wide Web for delivery of patient care or education.

Nurses have also participated in government funded investigations studying the effects of the implementation of such systems on health care delivery and nursing practice. In addition, nurses have been extensively involved in research related to the development of international data and information standards for health data and information as well as nursing data and information.

Most recently, nurses are developing information management methods and tools for use in transforming health and nursing data into information. Similarly, nurses have been in the forefront of projects exploring the educational and instructional uses of large mainframe computers, personal computers, multimedia, and the Internet. These nurses are actively involved in developing and evaluating computer hardware, software, and multimedia materials used by organizations providing patient care and in educational institutions. In the future, nurse researchers should be initiating studies of the ergonomic effects associated with the use of information technologies in nursing practice and nursing education.

In the area of practice, nurses have traditionally been the interface between the client and the health care system. In the application of nursing informatics, nurses with masters or baccalaureate preparation can and should participate in the selection and implementation of systems. Parker and Gassert (1996) have concluded that Informatics Nurse Specialists (INS) are eminently qualified to assist the health care industry in implementing the Joint Commission on the Accreditation of Healthcare Organizations (JCAHO) standards (Joint Commission on the Accreditation of Healthcare Organizations, 1994) in the clinical environment. In fact, Parker and Gassert (1996) assert that INSs will function more effectively and appropriately as systems analysts in patient care settings than will the nonclinical systems analyst, who may have a background in computer science, engineering, or another discipline. Nurses must articulate for the computer program designers and systems engineers the automated systems needs of health care professionals and clients. A related role is that of change agent, who facilitates the business process design (or redesign) related to delivery of patient care. This role enables organizations and the people within them (including nurses) to use information and information systems with the maximum degree of effectiveness and efficiency. The development and wide dissemination of Telehealth applications ultimately may provide an expanded scope of practice for nurses as the delivery of health services is transformed.

In the area of education, INSs should be teaching and interpreting the jargon and basic tenets of modern nursing for the information specialists. They should also be preparing their professional colleagues for the inevitable widespread implementation of automated information systems. This preparation can be accomplished through basic and ongoing education programs. In facilities where information systems are being installed or upgraded, nurses are and should continue to be the trainers for nurses using new or upgraded applications software. The American Nurses Association (ANA) officially recognized and defined the Informatics Nurse specialist in 1992 and has put in place a process for certifying Informatics Nurse Specialists (Newbold, 1996).

The goal of these new roles for nurses is to create patient-centered, enterprise health information systems for use in health care agencies and institutions that will meet the needs of the users. Health care professionals should not be required to change their patterns of practice to conform to a computer system. Thus, for information systems to best assist in the process of patient care decision making by nurses, nursing informatics must receive and respond to input from nursing. Nurses and information specialists must cooperate in the development of information systems that produce the types of information needed by nurses in their practice. Information specialists and nurses must establish a dialogue that results in each group understanding the needs and constraints under which the other functions.

As early as 1971, Singer warned that the more complex the system, the higher the cost of change and, therefore, the more rigid and inflexible the system becomes. Thus, caution in the designing and implementation of any information system is essential. Future nursing needs must be anticipated and provision made for flexibility in the design of programs in the information system selected for use. Again, a general understanding is needed between nurses and information specialists regarding the functions and limitations of computers and the dynamic nature of nursing so as to select flexible hardware and design satisfactory computer programs. Only nurses can provide the input necessary to ensure nursing needs are met by health care information systems.

Because of the widespread integration of nursing informatics into health care agencies and institutions, the role of the nurse will intensify and diversify. Redefinition, refinement, and modification of the practice of nursing will intensify the nurse's role in the delivery of patient care. At the same time, nurses will have greater diversity by virtue of employment opportunities in the nursing informatics field. Nursing's contributions can and will influence the evolution of health care computing. The contributions of nurses are essential to the expansion and development of health care computing. By providing leadership and direction nurses can ensure that health care computing and nursing informatics evolve to benefit the patient. That expected benefit is to expand and improve the quality of health care received by patients.

## Role of Professional Associations

Nurses interested in having a positive impact on the development of the information management aspects of their profession are faced with the formidable task of keeping up with a body of knowledge that becomes quickly outdated. "State-of-the-art" technology changes with meteoric haste. The slightest lapse in an individual's monitoring of new technological developments can result in one's knowledge becoming historical.

How does an individual maintain currency of information? Obviously, the professional journals and trade magazines provide an important service. Unfortunately, the people on the frontiers of developing new technology and its applications are often too busy developing, with no time left for writing about their activities. Thus, a curious dichotomy is occurring. People are reverting to more informal means of communication to disseminate information about the newest developments in high-technology information processing.

The professional associations fulfill the vital function of facilitating the exchange of the current information on informatics developments. Individuals involved in the health informatics field are more than willing to welcome "new blood" with fresh ideas. They are also more than eager to expound on their ideas to new listeners. Often contact initiated on a face-to-face basis at professional associations annual meetings results in the establishment of an informal network of colleagues. These informal networks maintain contact between conferences for the purpose of sharing information and ideas. In addition, the professional associations provide a forum for the communication and exchange of ideas. Formal addresses by leaders in the field and informal discussions in the corridors and at social events during conferences facilitate this exchange of ideas. The professional associations also publish newsletters, journals, and conference proceedings. These media are aimed at accelerating wide dissemination of information about new information management methods, technology, or software and their use or application.

Nurses with interest and expertise in health informatics should seek membership in three types of organizations:

- The first direction is affiliation with multidisciplinary associations whose focus is health informatics. The purpose of membership in this type of an organization is for nurses to maintain and expand their expertise in health informatics.
- The second type of organizational membership is maintenance of affiliations with nursing professional organizations. This membership should be maintained for the dual purpose of providing leadership and sharing ideas and information about health informatics within the nursing community.
- The third type of affiliation is membership in vendor-sponsored user groups.

## Multidisciplinary Professional Associations

In addressing the first type of professional affiliation, it is readily apparent that, although very few nurses have achieved a high level of preparation in nursing informatics and health informatics, there is a growing cadre of nursing colleagues with a shared interest in health informatics. The value of affiliating with a multidisciplinary association is in the scope and depth of expertise, information, and perspectives available from contact with experts in the health informatics. In the United States, the American Medical Informatics Association (AMIA) offers a variety of activities:

- Conducting scientific, technical and educational meetings, one of which is the annual meeting of the association Fall Symposium (formerly known as SCAMC, Symposium on Computer Applications in Medical Care)
- Publishing and disseminating digests, reports, proceedings, and other pertinent documents, independently and in professional literature
- Advising and coordinating functions and matters of interest to the membership
- Stimulating, sponsoring, and conducting research into the application and evaluation of technological systems as they apply to health care and medical science
- Representing the United States in the international arena of medical systems and informatics

In 1982, the nurse members of this association formed a Nursing Professional Specialty Group (PSG) within the organization that later became AMIA. This subgroup meets at the same time as the AMIA annual meeting and the spring congress. It is also active in promoting and facilitating communication among its members between meetings. The objectives of the AMIA Nursing PSG are as follows:

- Obtain basic knowledge about computers and systems
- Share information about computer applications in nursing
- Integrate knowledge about the nursing process into health care systems
- Develop new knowledge through the use of computer support for nursing research
- Use computer systems for both professional and patient/health education
- Communicate with other practitioners regarding nursing systems

In Canada, COACH, Canada's Health Informatics Association, is a multidisciplinary group of health care and information-processing professionals who are active in the area of medical informatics and health care computing. The purpose of COACH is to create a forum for the exchange of ideas, concepts, and developments in the information-processing field within the Canadian health care environment.

Within this framework, COACH's objectives are these:

1. To further continuing dialogue among health care institutions, associations, and governments relative to all health information processing applications, and
2. To disseminate information on applications or approaches through media such as seminars, workshops, conferences, or newsletters, thereby

providing various sectors of the health care system with a source of information and expertise.

There is a growing cadre of nurses active in COACH. The Nursing Informatics Special Interest Group has developed the following goals and objectives:

- Establish and maintain communication at the national level
- Provide leadership in the establishment of provincial Nursing Informatics interest groups
- Promote nursing informatics education
- Act as a resource to agencies and professionals interested in nursing informatics
- Establish liaison with the provincial Nursing Informatics Groups
- Maintain communication with the Canadian Nurses' Association
- Network with nursing informatics professionals at the national and international levels by providing a forum for exchanging experiences and ideas
- Contribute to the advancement of the Nursing Informatics discipline

The two preceding national organizations provide membership opportunities for individuals. These organizations also have counterparts in 38 other countries. Internationally, these various national health (medical) informatics societies constitute the membership of the International Medical Informatics Association (IMIA). IMIA is a nonpolitical, international, scientific organization, whose mandate is the open exchange of scientific information and assistance in health informatics between member countries. IMIA defines itself as an international and world representative federation of national societies of Health Informatics and affiliated organizations. IMIA does not have individual members although there may be several delegates from each country as observers; each country has only one designated representative with one vote.

IMIA has long held the position that "the term 'medical informatics' is a compromise between several relevant adjectives and is considered synonymous with 'health informatics.'" IMIA's prime function is educational with dissemination of knowledge regarding health information processing. To accomplish this IMIA organizes these:

1. Triennial MEDINFO series, which were held in Stockholm (1974), Toronto (1977), Tokyo (1980), Amsterdam (1983), Washington, D.C (1986), China and Singapore (1989), Geneva (1992), Canada (1995), and Seoul, Korea (1998). These large conferences form an excellent review of the state of the art of Medical Informatics. Information forthcoming MEDINFO conferences can be found at their web site (http://www.hon.ch/medinfo).

2. Working groups on special topics such as nursing, education, EKG processing, and confidentiality, security, and privacy.

3. Working conferences, of which more than 30 have been held in the past 15 years.

IMIA also represents International Federation of Information Processing (IFIP) in the Health Informatics field to such organizations as World Health Organization (WHO) and World Medical Association and at world conferences such as the Alma Ata WHO/UNICEF conferences on primary health care. Finally, IMIA disseminates knowledge by means of publication and distribution of MEDINFO and working conference proceedings. Additional information is available from the IMIA web site (http://www.imia.org).

In the fall of 1982, following an IMIA-sponsored working conference on the Impact of Computers on Nursing, the IMIA General Assembly accepted the proposal that an international working group on nursing be formed (see Chapter 3). Working Group 8 provides an international focus for activity in nursing informatics and an international core of interested and committed people who work toward implementing IMIA objectives regarding nursing. In 1985, the first meeting of this group was held in Calgary, Canada. The working group organizes an international symposium at 3-year intervals. Each symposium produces a volume of proceedings to provide the widest possible distribution of the information presented at the meeting. Information on the Working Group and its Nursing Informatics symposia can be found on their web site (http://www.gl.umbc.edu/~abbott/nurseinfo.html).

Nursing educators will find the Association for the Development of Computer Based Instructional Systems (ADCIS) a useful resource. ADCIS defines itself as an "international, not for profit, organization with members throughout the United States, Canada, and various other countries. These members represent elementary and secondary school systems, colleges and universities, business and industry, as well as military and government agencies." The published purposes of ADCIS are as follows:

- Advance the investigation and utilization of computer-based instruction (CAI) and/or management (CMI).
- Promote and facilitate the interchange of information, programs, and materials in the best professional and scientific tradition.
- Reduce redundant effort among developers.
- Specify requirements and priorities for hardware and software development and encourage and facilitate their realization.

The Health Education Special Interest Group (HESIG) within ADCIS is the subgroup with which most nurse educators are aligned.

## Nursing Professional Organizations

The second type of membership that nurses interested in health care computing should maintain is their affiliation with the nursing professional associations. The importance of this type of membership is in the obligation of professionals to share their expertise and knowledge with colleagues. The banding together of nurses having expertise in nursing informatics within national nursing organizations raises other members' awareness of this aspect of nursing. It also provides a contact point for nurses desiring to expand their knowledge in this area.

## *Vendor-Sponsored User Groups*

Practically all major vendors of software applications for health encourage and support the establishment of formal organizations for users of their products. This type of affiliation facilitates the exchange of ideas and approaches among users of similar software applications. This practice prevents the duplication of effort related to experience with use of a software application. It also provides a forum for users to communicate with the vendor about changes or upgrades to the software.

## Summary

Nurses will find professional organizations valuable for having a positive impact on the information-processing aspects of their profession. Participation in three types of organizations (multidisciplinary, nursing, and vendor sponsored) is recommended.

This chapter also considered the trend toward new roles for nurses as a result of the widespread use of computer-based enterprise health information systems. Without question, new roles for nurses will continue to develop. At the same time, the current role of the nurse is changing. The survival and advancement of the profession, however, depend on nurses abandoning their previous professional stance of passive reaction and adopting a new anticipatory, proactive stance. Nursing must be prepared to exploit information technology fully and to participate actively in information management so as to advance the practice of nursing.

## *References*

Ball, M.J., Douglas, J.V., and Hoehn, B.J. New challenges for nursing informatics. In: Gerdin, U., Tallberg, M., and Wainwright, P. (eds.) *Nursing Informatics: The Impact of Nursing Knowledge on Health Care Informatics.* Amsterdam: IOS Press, 1997:39–43.

Dayhoff, R.E., and Siegel, E.L. Digital imaging within and among medical facilities. In: Kolodner, R.M. (ed.) *Computerizing Large Integrated Health Networks: The V.A. Experience.* New York: Springer-Verlag, 1998.

Haux, R. Aims and tasks of medical informatics. *International Journal of Biomedical Computing,* 1998. Joint Commission on the Accreditation of Healthcare

Organizations. *Accreditation Manual for Hospitals*. Oakbrook Terrace, Ill.: JCAHO, 1994.

Lorenzi N.M., Riley, R.T., Ball, M.J., and Douglas, J.V. *Transforming Health Care Through Information: Case Studies*. New York: Springer-Verlag, 1995.

Newbold, S.K. The informatics nurse and the certification process. *Computers in Nursing* 1996;14(2):84–88.

Parker, C.D., and Gassert, C. JCAHO's Management of information standards: The role of the Informatics Nurse Specialist. *Journal of Nursing Administration* 1996;26(6):13–15.

Singer, J.P. Hospital computer systems: Myths and realities. *Hospital Topics* 1971;4:9 (January).

Tang, P.C., and Patel, V.L. Major issues in user interface design for health professional workstations: Summary and recommendations. *International Journal of Biomedical Computing* 1992;34:139–148.

Zimmerman, K.L. Clinical imaging: Applications and implications for nursing. In: Ball, M.J., Hannah, K.J., Newbold, S.K., and Douglas, J.V. (eds.) *Nursing Informatics: Where Caring and Technology Meet*, 2nd Ed. New York: Springer-Verlag, 1995:320–330.

# Appendices

# Appendix A
## Generic Request for Proposal*

The request for proposal (RFP) is the culmination of the planning phase of the systems process. The purpose of the RFP is to report the planning phase findings and make recommendations regarding (1) changing the existing information system, (2) instituting a new information system, or (3) incorporating a proposed system into an existing larger system. The RFP recommends systems and components that will help resolve the organizational problem for which the system is being developed. It is the method by which an organization seeking to build a system spells out its objectives, functional requirements, budget limitations, and available resources to internal management as well as outside vendors.

The RFP should be approved by the organization's information systems planning committee before it is disseminated to outside vendors for solicitation bids among prospective bidders. Outside vendors view the RFP as a standard document that outlines system objectives and design requirements. The RFP provides the basis for judging the vendor's ability to meet system requirements.

While requirements and objectives differ based on the needed system, all RFPs should include the following:

- Background information about the organization including its mission, goals, objectives, and critical success factors
- Identification of the Information Systems Planning Committee who will be responsible for the installation and maintenance of the system
- Financial situation of the organization including the method of financing
- Benefit–cost analysis to determine the feasibility of the project
- Clear identification of the organizational problem for which the system is being developed
- Clear identification of the scope of the systems project

---

* Contributed by Jo Ann Klein, who wishes to acknowledge Victor Casamento, Don Taber, and Terry Walsh for their input in the development of this Request for Proposal.

- Description of the existing system, if applicable
- Framework and model on which the proposed system is based
- Clear identification of the general requirements of the system
- Proposed information architecture developed during the planning phase of the systems process
- Statement of specific hardware and software requirements
- Proposal instructions and schedule
- Criteria for evaluation proposals
- Site visit requirements

Activity Log

Maintaining a log of information systems planning committee activities from week to week serves as a project management tool. It enables the committee leader to ascertain the work activities of individuals as well as the group in meeting the goals of the committee. While this is not a formal part of the RFP document, it is recommended that the committee utilize this methodology during the course of preparing and evaluating the RFP. Details of the recommended sections of the RFP are included in the following example:

Background Information
- Introduction
  Includes organization's mission, vision, and values
  Includes organization's business goals and objectives
  Includes organization's critical success factors
  Includes profit status of the organization
  Includes demographics of the population addressed by the system
- Financial Background
  Includes the operating budget
  Includes funding status of the organization
  Includes project funding status
  Includes benefit–cost ratio to determine feasibility of the project
- Problem Statement
  Clearly depicts issues requiring system development
  States organizational problem that system addresses
- Scope of the Project
  Defines organizational parameters from which the system will be developed
- Description of the Current System
  Description of the existing system, if applicable
  Includes a functional decomposition diagram that illustrates the system processes
  Includes a location decomposition diagram defining the system in relation to its users utilizing a hierarchical model
  Includes a detailed data flow diagram depicting system inputs, processes, and outputs

Include a system location connectivity diagram to illustrate geographic distance between sites if the system is networked

- Framework and Model
  System should be developed based upon an established model such as a communications model or information systems model that has been researched and validated; this provides a framework from which the system is built
  Relationship of proposed system to the framework and model should be addressed
- Information Systems Planning Committee
  Exists to be made knowledgeable of the information needs of the organization
  Should include representatives from all levels of the organization affected by the system as well as members of the community affected by the system, including funding sponsors
  Include a Systems Administrator who has knowledge important for planning and project design
- Recommended Hardware
  Recommendations should be based upon budget restrictions, existing and proposed system processes, software considerations, and the geographic architecture of the organization
  Completed system should provide a system life cycle of at least 5 years
  Include advantages and disadvantages of recommended hardware for the system
- Recommended Software
  Recommendations should be based upon budget restrictions, existing and proposed system processes, hardware considerations, and the geographic architecture of the organization
  Include advantages and disadvantages of recommended software for the system
  Include source code procurement as part of the requirement; this will not only provide intellectual property security, but may enable in-house programmers to change the system as needed
- Objectives of the New System
  Clearly identify the objectives of the new system in regard to the organization, its personnel, and the community it will serve
  Indicate functions the system will address as well as applications that it will provide; these functional requirements indicate what is needed by the organization to provide the support and services necessary to accomplish business goals and objectives
- Benefit–Cost Analysis
  Examined to indicate the feasibility of the project
  Includes cost of construction and installation of the system in addition to training of staff
  Usually determined for no less than a 5-year period

Identify results of the analysis and include the detailed analysis in the RFP Appendix

Example: Proposal Instructions and Schedule
General Instructions. The procedures set forth in this RFP must be followed to ensure consideration of your proposal.

Proposal Submission. All proposals must be received by ⟨name of organization⟩ no later than ⟨specific time and date⟩. Proposals received after the deadline may not be considered. The ⟨name of the organization⟩ reserves the right to reject all bids. The ⟨name of the organization⟩ reserves the right to reject any vendor not responding in the manner specified in this document. The ⟨name of the organization⟩ also reserves the right to invite other vendors to submit proposals at a later date.

Submit 12 copies of your proposal and one complete set of user and technical documentation to the address shown below:

Systems Analyst
Name of Organization
Address
City, State, Zip Code
Telephone Number

We recognize the proprietary nature of your documentation. We will sign a nondisclosure agreement to protect your materials if you require.

Inquiries. Questions regarding the RFP and/or this process should be directed to:

Systems Analyst
Name of Organization
Address
City, State, Zip Code
Telephone Number

A written summary of questions and answers of general interest will be provided to all vendors who have received this RFP. The identity of the company asking the question will not be disclosed.

Supplements to the RFP. In the event changes or revisions must be made to this RFP, a written supplement will be prepared and issued to all vendors who received it. The proposal due date may be altered at the discretion of the ⟨name of organization⟩ if a supplement is issued.

Evaluation Process. Proposals will be evaluated based on the vendor's acknowledgment of meeting the ⟨name of organization⟩ information system requirements, the cost-effectiveness of the proposed system, the vendor's commitment of resources and proven ability to meet an implementation schedule, the vendor's experience and reputation, the quality of the vendor's training and customer service, and the vendor's responsiveness to the RFP process.

The vendors that most closely meet the requirements outlined in the RFP will be invited to present a live presentation of their product during the week of ⟨date⟩. At that time, a thorough review will be made of your ability to meet RFP requirements through a formal presentation of your product.

Site Visits. Two finalists will be selected after the on-site presentations. Site visits to one of your client sites must be scheduled for the week of ⟨date usually 1–2 weeks after the presentation⟩. The site should be an organization similar to ours, utilizing a ⟨type of system⟩. The site must be an established user of your system with an installation of system features and options that illustrate the real-world use of your product.

Intention to Propose. Vendors receiving this RFP must respond in writing to ⟨name of the organization⟩ by ⟨time and date⟩, stating your intention to bid. In your letter of intent, include the name and address of a company contact person responsible for our account.

Use of Vendor Proposal and Documentation. All materials submitted become the property of ⟨name of organization⟩, but user and technical documentation will be returned if requested. If you intend to submit confidential or proprietary information as part of the proposal, any limits on the use of, or distribution of, material must be clearly stated in writing. The proposals will be evaluated by the ⟨organization⟩ Information Systems Planning Committee, and, at its discretion, external experts may be consulted.

## Proposal Requirements: General Information

Proposal Format and Content. Your response to the RFP must be submitted in the format outlined below. The information required in each section of your response is described below:

I.  Introduction
    A.  Introductory Letter: Provide standard letter, on company letterhead, introducing the company and its representatives with whom the ⟨name of organization⟩ Information Systems Planning Committee will be meeting.
    B.  Executive Summary of Proposal: In the introductory letter, provide a brief summary of what is being proposed for ⟨name of organization⟩.
II. Vendor Company Backgroud
    A.  Company Overview: Provide a brief statement of your company's background, approach to information systems, evolution of your product line, and scope of services.
    B.  Financial Profile: Give a brief description of your company's financial structure, including ownership and general financial strength. Include copies of the two most recent annual reports and financial statements.

C. <u>Organization</u>: Provide a brief description of the company's organization. Include organizational charts that relate to pertinent departments and functions. Indicate the number of personnel in these departments.

III. <u>System Description: Overview</u>
   A. <u>System Summary</u>: Present a brief summary of the systems and various product lines you offer. Summarize the applications available on these product lines. Outline methods used to update and enhance your system once it is installed in the ⟨organization⟩.
   B. <u>Current Development Efforts</u>: Describe efforts to improve or change current system functions. If necessary, indicate the impact of these efforts in the proposal. Provide time estimates for the availability of any products described that are under development.
   C. <u>Hardware and Software</u>: Discuss which hardware and software are currently operational. Distinguish between that which is installed and that which is in the testing phase.

IV. <u>System Description: Software</u>
   A. <u>Proposed Application</u>: Describe in detail the system you are proposing.
   B. <u>Application Software</u>: Describe the programming environment used to support the application and its characteristics including:
      1. Ability to modify delivered system on-site
      2. User interface design strategy
      3. Required languages
   C. <u>Database Architecture</u>: Describe the database supporting the application, including:
      1. Database architecture
      2. Required database software
      3. Capability to add data elements to the database
      4. Limitation to the use of those data elements
      5. Ad hoc reporting capabilities (e.g., data extraction)
   D. <u>Operating System</u>: Describe the system software capabilities, including, but not limited to:
      1. Communications protocols
      2. Interface capabilities
      3. File maintenance
      4. Range of hardware that will support the proposed system
      5. Requirements for scheduled system downtime
      6. Describe file recovery procedures required in the event of a system failure during
         a. on-line update
         b. batch update
      7. Estimate time required for recovery from system failures described in (f) based upon statistics provided in this document

E. <u>System Security</u>: Describe how the following security concerns are met:
   1. Access to overall application functions and databases
   2. Access to specified functions by responsibility
   3. Access to specified functions by location
   4. Access to files and database using tools
   5. Ability to track security violations
F. <u>Other Software Characteristics</u>: Describe other software characteristics, including, but not limited to:
   1. User interface design strategy
   2. Data input validation and controls
   3. Retention of all detail transactions
   4. Remote or terminal printer capabilities
   5. Ability to 'hot-key' between terminal sessions
   6. Regular batch-processing requirements
   7. Messaging and/or e-mail capabilities
G. <u>Ownership of Programs</u>: Specify the arrangements normally included in a standard contract regarding ownership of programs customized for client, restrictions on client modification of software, and program changes.
H. <u>Conversion Assistance and Acceptance Testing</u>
   1. Describe procedures used to install the system
   2. Describe procedures for system testing modifications
   3. Describe the period during which software changes can be implemented without incurring cost
   4. Functions that cannot be changed
   5. Assistance provided to user departments during system installation and acceptance testing
   6. Proposed system acceptance criteria
I. <u>Interfaces</u>
   1. Describe communication protocols you have worked with and which protocols you can demonstrate with the current release of your software
   2. Identify likely modifications required by your software so that you can interface to systems identified in this RFP
   3. The scheduling and billing systems will likely be required to interface with ⟨name of system⟩. Indicate existing interfaces and outline your general interface strategy.
   4. Describe your experience in providing modem access for PCs and the capability to support cooperative processing because this system will most likely interface with ⟨name of system⟩.
   5. Describe your experience in interfacing within a complex environment
V. <u>System Description: Hardware</u>

A. <u>Proposed Configuration</u>:
   1. Describe the proposed hardware configuration based upon information provided regarding the model and framework, organizational process diagrams, organizational context data flow diagram, organizational location decomposition diagram, the geographic architecture of the organization, and the proposed organizational system topology.
   2. Complete a proposed configuration table to summarize the hardware configuration.
B. <u>CPU and Peripherals</u>: Address the following based on your software and recommended system configuration, including an estimate of system response times.
   1. CPU sizing
   2. Disk storage
   3. Tape drives
   4. Optical storage
C. <u>Terminals</u>: Estimate the numbers and type of each device the system should include, being sure to indicate specific requirements for proprietary devices.
   1. CRTs
   2. Bar code readers
   3. Bar code printers
   4. Printers
   5. Scanners
D. <u>Expandability</u>: Describe the expansion capabilities of the proposed system. Indicate the system upgrades available. Provide the following technical information for the proposed configuration and for upgraded systems.
   1. Maximum number of devices on proposed configuration
   2. Maximum memory expansion
   3. Number of systems in upgrade line
E. <u>Reliability</u>: Describe the hardware reliability of all equipment in the proposed configuration including the following information:
   1. Mean time between failures
   2. Scheduled preventive maintenance intervals
   3. Number and type of redundant devices
   4. Remote diagnostic capabilities
F. <u>User Interface</u>: Describe the hardware configuration in terms of user ease in working with the equipment including the following information:
   1. Light pen support
   2. Bar code support
   3. Mouse input
   4. Voice input
   5. Text editors

VI. <u>Vendor Support</u>
  A. <u>Software and Hardware</u>
    1. Location of the appropriate corporate and field offices
    2. Describe warranties on the software and hardware including time frame and provided support services
  B. <u>Implementation Support</u>: Specify the implementation support provided. This support should include, but not be limited to, the following products and services:
    1. Necessary modifications as specified ⟨name of organization⟩
    2. Acceptance testing
    3. Implementation planning with the provision of a copy of the actual implementation plan developed by your company for a ⟨type of system⟩ serving ⟨actual population numbers and type being served by the system on a monthly basis⟩
    4. Implementation support
      a. Assist in application modification
      b. Assist in application installation
      c. On-site support during final stages of implementation
      d. On-site project management
Provide any costs associated with these implementation services in the cost tables of this RFP.
  C. <u>Training and Customer Service</u>
    1. Describe the training program you provide in the use of the proposed system
    2. Describe the percent of training provided by vendor staff
    3. List all formal training courses provided by your company
    4. Specify the scope of in-house training
    5. Describe available additional customer services
Provide any costs for training services in the cost tables found in the RFP appendix.
  D. <u>Documentation</u>: Describe the documentation and number of sets provided to the organization on the use of the system. Complete documentation for the application software should be available immediately and should include:
    1. User documentation
    2. Training manuals
    3. Operator manuals, including control procedures
    4. Overall system flowcharts
    5. Program descriptions
    6. File descriptions
    7. Source code
  E. <u>Continuing Support</u>: The following support is required:
    1. Software: vendor should provide 7-day, 24-hour phone service for problem consultation and resolution

2. Hardware: vendor should provide 7-day, 24-hour phone service for problem consultation and resolution
3. System enhancements
   a. New releases should be distributed electronically or on magnetic type
   b. System should provide a mechanism to automatically apply enhanced code
4. System performance: vendor will participate in the review of system performance on an ongoing basis to determine if the system is performing within acceptable parameters
5. User groups: vendor should sponsor a user group that meets on a regular basis
6. Consulting: vendor should have analysts available to consult and support ⟨name of organization⟩ personnel with modifications/enhancements that may be required to support the ⟨name of organization⟩ evolving information system needs

Provide any costs for training services in the cost tables found in the RFP appendix.

F. Assigned Personnel: Identify personnel that will be assigned to the project.

The ⟨name of organization⟩ reserves the right of refusal of any vendor project team members. Cite language in your support agreement that facilitates the removal of staff from the project.

G. Experience and References: Provide the following information:
   1. List applications features requested by the ⟨name of organization⟩ that have been installed in at least one similar area of practice serving the same population and number as ⟨name of organization⟩
   2. List similar organizations now served by your company, the date of service commencement, and a contact name and telephone number for each of these organizations
   3. Provide the total number of organizations nationwide that use the system
   4. Identify a minimum of three organizations with installed configurations similar to the one you have proposed that may be contacted as references. List the features installed and the stage of implementation of the application. Provide the name of contacts in the Information Systems Departments of these organizations.

H. Disaster Services: Provide the following information:
   1. Services provided when a client experiences a disaster
   2. Equipment delivery time commitments
   3. Off-site arrangements

VII. Site Preparation Requirements: Describe all necessary site preparation requirements for the recommended configuration.

VIII. Implementation Time Frame
   A. Provide a copy of the proposed implementation timetable.
   B. Indicate the sequence of features to be installed.
   C. Estimate the elapsed time and proposed vendor support in days for each application.

IX. Standard Contract
   A. Provide a copy of your standard contract.
   B. Indicate the sequence of features to be installed.

X. Costs
   A. Costs should be itemized following the format of the cost tables provided in the RFP appendix.
   B. One-time costs (licensing fees) must cover a minimum of 5 years.
   C. If our parent company should decided to use your system at affiliate organizations, how may this affect your pricing?

XI. Response to Systems Capabilities Questionnaire
   The last section of the RFP addresses the functional capabilities of the ⟨type of system⟩. This section is divided into various functional requirements. These sections have the ⟨name of organization⟩ requirements listed under them. Respond to the requirements as follows:
   A. Indicate whether or not the requirement is being met by the system:
      1. Answer "Yes" if the current release meets the requirement
      2. Answer "Custom" if the software can be modified to meet the requirement
      3. Answer "No" if the software cannot be modified to meet the requirement
   B. Respond to each item contained within the functional requirement.
   C. If you answer "Custom", provide rough cost and time estimates in the timetable.
   D. Where necessary, comments concerning how the system meets a requirement should be provided. Make certain that your proposal provides adequate detail where the RFP specifically asks for vendor comment and information about a particular requirement.
   E. When responding to the requirements, use the format as presented. When a requirement requires a narrative response, place your response on a separate page following the appropriate section.
   F. An officer of your company must sign a statement similar to the sample found on the next page. Use your letterhead.

Vendor Please Note:

## YOUR RESPONSES TO THE FUNCTIONAL SPECIFICATIONS
## WILL BE INCORPORATED INTO THE CONTRACT

The responses provided in this proposal are accurate. Responses are based on features found in

_____,  _____.

        Version                        Application

_____,  _____

        Signature                        Date

_____

        Title

**Cost Tables**

One-Time Costs

| Procedure | Quantity | Costs |
|---|---|---|
| Software Modules | | |
| Hardware Equipment (itemize) | | |
| Communications Equipment (itemize) | | |
| Supplies Descriptions | | |
| Training Description | | |
| Documentation Description | | |
| Shipping | | |
| Installation/Conversion | | |
| Interface Description | | |
| Travel and Lodging | | |
| Custom Modifications | | |
| Other (itemize) | | |

Monthly Costs

| Procedure | Quantity | Cost/Month |
|---|---|---|
| Hardware Maintenance | | |
| Software Maintenance | | |
| Communications | | |
| Supplies | | |
| Other (itemize) | | |

Note: Use these categories in your presentation. If there are items that are priced separately within one category, show the cost of each in detail.

**Sample Case Management System Capabilities Questionnaire**

| Ref # | Functional Requirement | Yes | No | Custom |
|---|---|---|---|---|
| 1.1 | Patient assessment module, including history and physical, for the initial interview, each patient encounter, and QA evaluation to include case notes. | | | |
| 1.2 | Patient assessment module to include standard and custom questionnaires with ability to score answers and get numeric totals of assessment. | | | |
| 1.3 | Patient assessment module to include all questions are reportable data elements capable of being extracted for reporting purposes. | | | |
| 1.4 | Patient assessment module to include provides memo scroll screens with multilingual capabilities. | | | |
| 1.5 | Patient assessment module to include storage of the completed assessment questionnaire as part of the case record. | | | |
| 2.1 | Scheduler module for appointments and events per individual client and per nurse practitioner to include listings of messages, appointments, and tasks. | | | |
| 2.2 | Scheduler module to include the ability to forward schedule to other Nurse Practitioners within the organization. | | | |
| 2.3 | Scheduler module to include the ability to assign priority. | | | |

| Ref # | Functional Requirement | Yes | No | Custom |
|-------|------------------------|-----|-----|--------|
| 2.4 | Scheduler module to include the ability to link notes or events to a schedule item. | | | |
| 2.5 | Scheduler module to include the ability to view by case. | | | |
| 2.6 | Scheduler to include ability to view by Nurse Practitioner. | | | |
| 2.7 | Scheduler module to include the ability to view by day, week, or month. | | | |
| 2.8 | Scheduler module to include the ability to view by screen. | | | |
| 2.9 | Scheduler module to include the ability to view by report. | | | |
| 2.10 | Scheduler module to include the ability to configure series of schedule entries with implementation by a button click (e.g., 6 weeks of weekly reports). | | | |
| 3.1 | Patient profiles module to include custom case coding messages, appointments, and tasks. | | | |
| 3.2 | Patient profiles module to include the ability to forward scheduler information to other NPs on the local system and extract to the parent company system. | | | |
| 4.1 | Provider profiles module to provide an independent repository of referral resources. | | | |
| 5.1 | Timesheets/billing module must be flexible and comprehensive. | | | |

| Ref # | Functional Requirement | Yes | No | Custom |
|-------|------------------------|-----|-----|--------|
| 5.2 | Timesheets/billing module must provide complete accounts receivable system or ability to interface with parent company network. | | | |
| 5.3 | Timesheets/billing module must have the ability to track time for reporting. | | | |
| 5.4 | Timesheets/billing module must have the ability to store and retrieve fee schedules for insurers and managed care providers. | | | |
| 5.5 | Timesheets/billing module must have the ability to generate automate time slips that note time and activity per user authentication. | | | |
| 5.6 | Timesheets/billing module must have the ability to bill on percent of savings. | | | |
| 5.7 | Timesheets/billing module must have the ability to bill by rate schedules. | | | |
| 5.8 | Timesheets/billing module must have the ability to bill per hour or per activity or by flat rate charges. | | | |
| 5.9 | Timesheets/billing module must have the ability to customize invoices. | | | |
| 5.10 | Timesheets/billing module must have the ability to export data to a general ledger within the system or extract for reporting to the parent company | | | |
| 6.1 | Care plan module must have the ability to generate and store generic care plans with customizing capabilities and rate tracking. | | | |

| Ref # | Functional Requirement | Yes | No | Custom |
|-------|------------------------|-----|----|--------|
| 6.2 | Care plan module must provide authorization for precertification purposes (critical for managed care contracts). | | | |
| 6.3 | Care plan module must have the ability to create new care plans. | | | |
| 6.4 | Care plan module must have the ability to build in cost savings data (treatment types, number of treatments, date of treatments, billing rates). | | | |
| 6.5 | Care plan module must have the ability to compare and contrast rates for instant cost reports. | | | |
| 6.6 | Care plan module must allow for billing by percentage of savings. | | | |
| 7.1 | Document management module to create standard form letters launched within the case for referrals and insurance. | | | |
| 7.2 | Document management module must have the ability to merge case information directly into the document. | | | |
| 7.3 | Document management module must have the ability to print all documents. | | | |
| 7.4 | Document management module must have the ability to log dates and name of created documents and maintain addressed in a separate document log. | | | |

| Ref # | Functional Requirement | Yes | No | Custom |
|-------|------------------------|-----|-----|--------|
| 7.5 | Document management module must have the ability to produce heavily formatted documents using Word, Word Perfect, or any other word processing program compatible with the network. | | | |
| 7.6 | Document management module must have the ability to import multimedia files to a case history (e.g., graphics, sounds). | | | |
| 7.7 | Document management module must have the ability to launch multimedia embedded files within the program for review. | | | |
| 8.1 | Reports module must have ability to create reports from memo notes. | | | |
| 8.2 | Reports module must have ability to create reports from the scheduler. | | | |
| 8.3 | Reports module must have ability to create financial reports. | | | |
| 8.4 | Reports module must have ability to create case summary reports. | | | |
| 8.5 | Reports module must have ability to create custom reports. | | | |
| 8.6 | Reports module must have ability to create outcome reports through data extraction determined by preconfigured templates. | | | |

Appendices to Include:
- Organization Mission Statement
- Organization Goals and Objectives Statement
- Organization Critical Success Factors

## Organization Systems Project Plan Worksheet

| Task/Objective | Person(s) Responsible | Complete Date |
|---|---|---|
| I. Assessment | | |
| Site Survey | | |
| Assess written documentation | | |
| Evaluate current computer system<br>1. Age<br>2. Availability<br>3. Degree of amortization<br>4. Need for upgrades (include hardware/ software) | | |
| Rough estimate of resources (cost/benefit)<br>1. People<br>2. Time<br>3. Space<br>4. Equipment | | |
| Deliverables<br>a. Needs assessment | | |
| II. Planning | | |
| Selection of development team<br>1. Project manager<br>2. Nurse representative<br>3. Staff physician<br>4. Computer consultant<br>5. Other appointed members | | |

| Task/Objective | Person(s) Responsible | Complete Date |
|---|---|---|
| Team meeting to review organization structure, responsibilities, assignments, plan | | |
| Define specific responsibilities of development team members | | |
| Establish schedule for team meetings | | |
| Define and establish sign-off process | | |
| Define the project | | |
| Define problems | | |
| Define goals and objectives | | |
| Determine scope | | |
| Determine information needs | | |
| Deliverables<br>1. Written overview of project, problems, goals and objectives, and scope<br>2. Develop task time line | | |
| III. Analysis | | |
| Define user specifications<br>1. Inputs<br>2. Outputs<br>3. Edits | | |

| Task/Objective | Person(s) Responsible | Complete Date |
|---|---|---|
| Identify system benefits | | |
| Deliverables<br>1. Model and framework<br>1. Process diagram<br>2. Data flow diagram<br>3. Location decomposition diagram<br>4. Geographic architecture diagram<br>5. Proposed system topology | | |
| Written program specifications<br>1. Personnel<br>2. Time frame<br>3. Cost and budget<br>4. Facilities and equipment<br>5. Data manipulation and output<br>6. Operational considerations<br>7. Human–computer interactions<br>8. System validation plan | | |
| IV. Implementation design | | |
| Design inputs | | |
| Preliminary procedures for use of the system | | |
| Design outputs | | |

| Task/Objective | Person(s) Responsible | Complete Date |
|---|---|---|
| Design controls | | |
| User documentation | | |
| Functional flow chart | | |
| Deliverables<br>1. Data element definitions<br>2. Screen definitions<br>3. File definitions<br>4. Selection of file structure and programming language | | |
| V. Development Phase | | |
| Create RFP | | |
| Evaluate RFP responses | | |
| Negotiate contract | | |
| User test data developed | | |
| User test scheduled | | |
| Perform complete user cycle | | |
| Deliverables<br>1. RFP<br>2. Contract<br>3. User testing plan<br>4. User testing evaluation forms | | |

**Organizational Site Survey**

| Questions and Observations | D<br>Date | N<br>N/A | Comments |
|---|---|---|---|
| General Observations | | | |
| 1. Observe work flow processes that are automated and those that are manual. Determine the reason for the manual process. | | | |
| 2. Observe a wide variety of transactions being entered on the system. What percentage of transactions are being entered via:<br>a. Light pen _____<br>b. Keyboard _____<br>c. Mouse _____<br>d. Trackball _____<br>e. Glidepoint _____<br>f. Trackpoint _____<br>g. Bar code reader _____<br>h. Touch screen _____<br>i. Portable hand-held device _____<br>f. Voice activation _____ | | | |
| 3. Perform user assessment (See User Assessment Survey) | | | |
| 4. Ask how long the database is maintained on-line? What information is kept on the database? | | | |
| 5. Determine who from the facility comprised the project team for system selection and implementation? | | | |
| 6. Ask for details about implementation strategies and organizational structures? | | | |
| 7. How did the facility select the installed vendor? What went into make this decision? | | | |

| Questions and Observations | D<br>Date | N<br>N/A | Comments |
|---|---|---|---|
| 8. What were the goals for the facility and each of its departments in implementing the system? Have the goals been realized? | | | |
| 9. Ask about the knowledge and experience of the vendor's implementation personnel. Were health care professionals involved on the team? | | | |
| 10. Ask about current and planned projects for computerization in the area being visited. Do plans include interfacing or integrating products? | | | |
| 11. Review all computer-generated reports, documents, and forms. How flexible is design and content? How easy are changes to implement? What additional reports would be facility like generated? | | | |
| 12. Closely examine the look of the screens, content, layout, depth and breadth of available information, and ease of use. | | | |
| 13. What is the response time between entering data on one screen and being able to enter data on a new screen? | | | |
| 14. What hardware is used to run the system? What is the average downtime—scheduled/unscheduled? | | | |
| 15. What is the total number of operational terminals on the system? | | | |

| Questions and Observations | D Date | N N/A | Comments |
|---|---|---|---|
| 16. Does the system offer help and wizard screens for basic use of the system? for system reports? | | | |
| 17. Does the vendor have an active and productive user group? How would they rate the responsiveness of the vendor to request for changes? | | | |
| Nursing Information Systems | | | |
| 1. Observe the user working with a:<br>a. Care plan<br>b. Nursing worksheet<br>c. Assessment document<br>d. Discharge planning guide for specific patient<br>e. Quality assurance record<br>f. Nursing charting record | | | |
| 2. Is the charting method flexible enough to support a variety of methodologies (e.g., ABC, SOAP, exception)? | | | |
| 3. Is the care planning system flexible enough to support a variety of methodologies (e.g., diagnosis-oriented, problem-oriented, etc.)? | | | |
| 4. Observe the following activities:<br>a. End-user charting<br>b. Updating care plan<br>c. Entering nurse treatment order<br>d. Confirming nurse treatment order and physician-ordered treatment<br>e. Entering/updating patient assessment | | | |

| Questions and Observations | D<br>Date | N<br>N/A | Comments |
|---|---|---|---|
| 5. Are physician orders automatically loaded into the system and available, without redundancy, in the:<br>  a. Careplan?<br>  b. Nursing worksheet?<br>  c. Assessment report?<br>  d. Discharge planning record? | | | |
| 6. Ask to see system-generated research and QA reports. | | | |
| 7. Speak to the head nursing administrator to gain an administrative-level perspective of the system. | | | |
| Personnel Systems | | | |
| 1. Determine if this exists in the current system? | | | |
| Staffing and Scheduling Systems | | | |
| 1. Determine if this exists in the current system? | | | |
| If a system exists: | | | |
| 2. Verify that staff's preferred hours are considered in scheduling. | | | |
| 3. Verify the time frame for advanced scheduling. | | | |
| 4. If applicable, determine if an interface exists between the personnel system and scheduling system. | | | |
| Interfacing Systems | | | |

| Questions and Observations | D Date | N N/A | Comments |
|---|---|---|---|
| General observations | | | |
| 1. To what if any systems outside of the network, is the facility system interfaced with? | | | |
| 2. Determine facility use of interfaced systems. | | | |

User Assessment Survey to be given to all users being interviewed for system requirements:

Name: _____

Job Title: _____

Job Description: _____

1. Do you own your own computer: _____ Yes _____ No
   If yes, describe your computer: _____
2. Have you used DOS applications? _____ Yes _____ No
3. Have you used Windows applications? _____ Yes _____ No
4. Are you familiar with networks and network applications? _____ Yes _____ No
5. Have you used electronic mail? _____ Yes _____ No
6. What kinds of pointing devices have you used (mouse, trackball, glidepoint, trackpoint)? _____
7. For what purposes have you used computers at work? _____
8. For what purposes have you used computers at home? _____
9. Which of the following applications software do you use? Please describe the frequency of use per day, purpose, and brand of software (e.g., word processing, 3×/day, Word 7.0)

| Application | Freq/Day | Purpose | Name of Software |
|---|---|---|---|
| Word Processing | | | |
| Database Management | | | |
| Spreadsheet | | | |
| Internet | | | |
| Graphics | | | |

10. How would you rate your level of "know-how" in using computer applications?
Beginner _____ Intermediate _____ Above-Avg _____ Superior _____
11. How would you rate your level of comfort in using the computer for basic applications?
Petrified _____ Uncertain _____ Neutral _____ Content _____
Comfortable _____
12. What would help you overcome your fear of using a computer system to perform your job duties? _____
13. What do you like most about the current system being used? _____ _____
14. What do you like least about the current system being used? _____ _____
15. Do you believe the current system provides flexibility in design and content? _____
16. If you could design this system to meet your personal needs, what would it include? _____
Observation of Screens:
17. What are your suggestions for types of screens? _____
18. What changes would you suggest for layout of the screens? _____ _____
19. What changes would you suggest for depth and breadth of available information? _____
20. What would help make these screens easier to use? _____

- Model upon which system is based
- Process diagram
- Context data flow diagram
- Location decomposition diagram
- Geographic architecture of the organization
- Proposed system topology
- List of recommended hardware
- List of recommended software
- Detailed benefit–cost analysis

*Acknowledgments.* The author wishes to acknowledge Victor Casamento, M.S., R.N., Don Taber, B.S.N., R.N., and Terry Walsh, M.S., R.N., for their assistance in developing the RFP example.

# *References*

Ball, M., Hannah, K., Newbold, S., and Douglas, J. *Nursing Informatics: Where Caring and Technology Meet*, 2nd Ed. New York: Springer-Verlag, 1995.
Ball, M., Simborg, D., Albright, J., and Douglas, J. *Healthcare Information Management Information systems*, 2nd Ed. New York: Springer-Verlag, 1995.

Casper, M. A non-traditional request for proposals. *Healthcare Informatics* 1993; January:22, 24.

Mills, M., Romano, C., and Heller, B. *Information Management in Nursing and Health Care*. Springhouse, Pa.: Springhouse, 1996.

Nelson, R., and Anton, B. A format for surveying computer-related learning needs in health care settings. *Computers in Nursing* 1996;14(3):150–155.

Saba, V., and McCormick, K. *Essentials of Computers for Nurses*, 2nd Ed. New York: McGraw-Hill, 1996.

Staggers, N., and Repko, K. Strategies for successful clinical information system selection. *Computers in Nursing* 1996;14(3):146–147.

Ward, W. *Health Care Budgeting & Financial Management for Non-financial Managers*. Westport, Conn.: Auburn House, 1994.

# Appendix B
## Addresses for Professional Societies

American Academy of Nursing
600 Maryland Avenue, SW, Suite
100 West
Washington, DC 20024-2571
(202) 651-7238
*http://www.nursingworld.org/aan/
index.htm*

American Association of Colleges
of Nursing
One Dupont Circle, NW
Suite 530
Washington, DC 20036
(202) 463-6930
*www.aacn.nche.edu*

American Nurses Association
Council on Nursing Services and
Informatics
America Nurses Association
600 Maryland Avenue
Suite 100 West, SW
Washington, DC 20024-2571
(202) 651-7000
*www.ana.org*

American Medical Informatics
Association (AMIA)
Nursing Informatics Working
Group
4915 St. Elmo's Avenue, Suite 302
Bethesda, MD 20814

(301) 657-1291
*www.amia2.amia.org*

Canadian Organization for the
Advancement of Computers in
Health (COACH)
16460 Afield Road
Edmonton, Alberta
Suite 1200
TSP 4P4 Canada
(403) 489-4553

Healthcare Information and
Management Systems Society
(HIMSS)
230 East Ohio Street, Suite 600
Chicago, IL 60611-3201
(312) 664-44677
*www.himss.org*

IEEE Computer Society
1730 Massachusetts Avenue, NW
Washington, DC 20036
(202) 371-0101
*www.iccad.com/ieee.html*

International Medical Informatics
Association (IMIA)
Nursing Informatics Special
Interest Group
Ulla Gerdin, RN, Chair

Swedish Institute for Health
  Services Development (SPRI)
Box 70487
Stockholm, Sweden
(011) 46 8 702 4600
ulla.gerdin@spri.se
*www.imia.org*

Medical Group Management
  Association
104 Inverness Terrace, East 112
Englewood, CO 80112
(303) 799-1111
*www.mgma.com*

Midwest Nursing Research Society
  (MNRS)
4700 W. Lake Avenue
Glenview, IL 60025
(847) 375-4711
*http://www.mnrs.org/*

National League for Nursing
  Council on Nursing Informatics
National League for Nursing
350 Hudson Street
New York, NY 10014
(800) 669-1656

*www.nln.org*
*nlninform@nln.org*

National Institute of Nursing
  Research
31 Center Drive, Room 5B09,
  MSC 2178
Bethesda, MD 20892-2178
*http://www.nih.gov/ninr/*

Sigma Theta Tau International
Honor Society of Nursing
550 West North Street
Indianapolis, IN 46202
(317) 634-8171
*www.stti.iupui.edu*

Society for Medical Decision
  Making
c/o The George Washington
  University
Office of Continuing Education in
  the Health Professions
2300 K Street, NW
Washington, DC 20037
(202) 994-8929
www.gwu.edu/*h*/~*smdm*

# Appendix C
## Sources of Additional Informatics and Health Care Information

AAOHN Journal
6900 Grove Road
Thorofare, NJ 08086-9447
609-848-1000

Administrative Radiology Journal
1305 West Glenoaks Boulevard
Glendale, CA 91201-2203
818-500-1872

Advance for Nurse Practitioners
650 Park Avenue West
King Of Prussia, PA 19406-1434
610-265-7812

Advance for Physician Assistants
650 Park Avenue West
King Of Prussia, PA 19406-1434
610-265-7812

Advances in Nursing Science
200 Orchard Ridge Drive Suite
    2000
Gaithersburg, MD 20878-1978
301-417-7500

AHA News
737 North Michigan Avenue
Chicago, IL 60611-2615
312-440-6800

American Journal of Nursing
555 West 57th Street

New York, NY 10019-2925
212-582-8820

American Journal of Public Health
1015 15th Street, NW
Washington, DC 20005-2605
202-789-5600

The American Nurse
600 Maryland Avenue, SW, Suite
    100W
Washington, DC 20024-2520
202-651-7000

ANNA Journal
East Holly Avenue
Pitman, NJ 08071
609-256-2300

AOHA Progress
5301 Wisconsin Avenue, NW, Suite
    630
Washington, DE 20015-2015
202-686-1700

AORN Journal
2170 South Parker Road
Denver, CO 80231-5711
303-755-6300

The APCO Bulletin
2040 South Ridgewood Avenue

Daytona Beach, FL 32119-2257
904-322-2500

Archives of Environmental Health
1319 18th Street, NW
Washington, DC 20036-1802
202-296-6267

ARN News
5700 Old Orchard Road, First
    Floor
Skokie, IL 60077-1036
708-966-3433

AWHONN Voice Newsletter
700 14th Street, NW, Suite 600
Washington, DC 20005-2010
202-662-1600

Biomedical Safety & Standards
1351 Titan Way
Brea, CA 92621-3708
714-738-6400

BNA's Health Care Policy Report
1231 25th Street, NW
Washington, DC 20037-1157
202-452-6526

Bulletin of the Pan American
    Health Organization
525 23rd Street, NW
Washington, DC 20037-2847
202-293-8130

Boletin de la Oficina Sanitaria
    Panamericana
525 23rd Street, NW
Washington, DC 20037-2847
202-293-8130

Catholic Health World
4455 Woodson Road
Saint Louis, MO 63134-3701
314-427-2500

CCH Pulse: The Health Care
    Reform Newsletter
2700 Lake Cook Road
Deerfield, IL 60015-3867
708-267-7000

California Hospitals
4471 D Street
Sacramento, CA 95819
916-452-6200

California Nurse
1145 Market Street, Suite 11000
San Francisco, CA 94103-1545
415-864-4141

The Case Manager
10809 Executive Center Drive,
    Suite 105
Little Rock, AR 72211-6020
501-954-7444

Chicago Healthcare
800 Roosevelt Road, Suite A-14
Glen Ellyn, IL 60137-5814
708-858-1980

Competitive Healthcare Market
    Report
3100 Highway 138
Wall Township, NJ 07719
908-681-1133

Computers in Nursing
University of Southern Maine
96 Falmouth Street
Portland, ME 04103-4899
207-780-4568

Connecticut Nursing News
377 Research Parkway Suite 2-D
Meriden, CT 06450-7155
203-238-1207

Economic Trends
840 North Lake Shore Drive

Chicago, IL 60611-2431
312-422-3000

Educacion Medica y Salud
525 23rd Street, NW
Washington, DC 20037-2847
202-293-8130

E M A News
4350 Dipaolo Center, Suite C
Glenview, IL 60025-5212
708-699-6362

Emergency Preparedness News
951 Pershing Drive
Silver Spring, MD 20910-4432
301-587-6300

Harvard Public Health Review
116 Huntington Avenue
Boston, MA 02115-592
617-351-0150

Healthcare System Reform Alert
3100 Highway 138
Wall Township, NJ 07710
908-681-1133

Health Care Authority
89 Main Street Drawer 20
Montpelier, VT 05601-0020
802-828-2900

Health Care Innovations
One Bridge Plaza Suite 350
Fort Lee, NJ 07024-7502
201-947-5545

Health Care Professional Magazine
110 Main Street
East Greenwich, RI 02818-3827
401-984-9330

Health Styles
1115 Clifton Avenue

Clifton, NJ 07013-3641
201-777-5888

Health Funds Development Letter
3100 Highway 138
Wall Township, NJ 07719
908-681-1133

Healthcare Advertising Review
1866 Colonial Village Lane
Lancaster, PA 17601-6704
717-393-1000

Healthcare Fund Raising
  Newsletter
3100 Highway 138
Wall Township, NJ 07719
908-681-1133

Healthcare Community Relations
  and Marketing Letter
3100 Highway 138
Wall Township, NJ 07719
908-681-1133

Health Care Management Review
200 Orchard Ridge Drive Suite 200
Gaithersburg, MD 20878-1978
301-417-7500

Healthcare Management Team
  Letter
3100 Highway 138
Wall Township, NJ 07719
908-681-1133

Health Care Risk Management
3525 Piedmont Road
North East 6
Piedmont Center, Suite 4000
Atlanta, GA 30305-1515
404-262-7436

Health Law Week
590 Dutch Valley Road N.E.

Atlanta, GA 30324-5330
404-881-1141

Health Care Community News
233 Commerce Building
Sioux City, IA 51101
712-255-0012

Healthcare Executive
One North Franklin Street, Suite
 1700
Chicago, IL 60606-3421
312-424-2800

Health Care Facility Management
2700 Lake Cook Road
Deerfield, IL 60015-3867
708-267-7000

Healthcare Financial Management
2 Westbrook Corporate Center,
 Suite 700
Westchester, IL 60154-5723
708-531-9600

The Healthcare Forum Journal
425 Market Street, 16th Floor
San Francisco, CA 94105-2406
415-356-4300

Healthcare Informatics
4530 West 77th Street, Suite 300
Minneapolis, MN 55435
612-835-3222

Healthcare Marketing Abstracts
P.O. Box 40959
Santa Barbara, CA 93140-0959
805-564-2177

Healthcare Marketing Report
P.O. Box 76002
Atlanta, GA 30358-1002
770-457-6106

HealthCare New Jersey
760 Alexander Road CN 1
Princeton, NJ 08540-6305
609-275-4071

Healthcare New Orleans
111 Veterans Boulevard, Suite
 1810
Metairie, LA 70005
504-834-9292

Health Care Reform Week
11300 Rockville Pike, Suite 1100
Rockville, MD 20852-3003
301-816-8950

Healthcare Supervisor
1121 Spring Lake Drive
Itascam, IL 60143-3200
708-285-1121

The Health Care Supervisor
200 Orchard Ridge Drive, Suite
 200
Gaithersburg, MD 20878-1978
301-417-7500

Health Care Strategic Management
5350 South Roslyn Street, Suite
 400 South
Englewood, CO 80111-2125
303-290-8500

Health Care Systems Strategy
 Report
1101 King Street, Suite 4440
Alexandria, VA 22314-2944
703-683-4100

Healthcare Trends & Transition
808 Priscilla Street, Second Floor
Salisbury, MD 21801-384
410-749-3200

Health Data Management
118 South Clinton Street, Suite 700

Chicago, IL 60661-3628
312-648-0261

Health Education Reports
4401-A Connecticut Avenue, NW,
    Suite 212
Washington, DC 20008-2322
202-362-3444

Health Facilities Management
737 North Michigan Avenue, Suite
    700
Chicago, IL 60611-2615
312-440-6800

Health Management Technology
6300 South Syracuse Way, Suite
    650
Englewood, CO 80111-6726
303-220-0600

Health Marketing Quarterly
10 Alice Street
Binghamton, NY 13904-1503
510-524-6144

Health Progress
4455 Woodson Road
Saint Louis, MO 63134-3701
314-427-2500

Health Scene
Polyclinic Medical Center
2601 North 3rd Street
Harrisburg, PA 17110-2098
717-782-4141

Health System Leader
P.O. Box 2106
Rockville, MD 20847-2106
301-468-1610

Health Systems Review
1405 North Pierce, Suite 308

Little Rock, AR 72207-5357
501-661-9555

Health Texas
6225 U.S. Highway 290 East
Austin, TX 78723
512-465-1000

Health Values: The Journal of
    Health, Behavior, Education &
    Promotion
P.O. Box 4593
Star City, WV 26504-4593
304-293-4699

HMO Magazine
1129 20th Street, NW, Suite 600
Washington, DC 20036-3403
202-778-3250

HMO Practice
900 Guaranty Building
Buffalo, NY 14202
716-857-6361

Holistic Nursing Practice
200 Orchard Ridge Drive, Suite
    2000
Gaithersburg, MD 20878-1978
301-417-7500

Homecare
23815 Stuart Ranch Road
Malibu, CA 90265-4897
310-317-4522

Hospice Forum
519 C Street, NW
Washington, DC 20001-2103
202-547-7424

Hospice Letter
3100 Highway 138
Wall Township, NJ 07719
908-681-1133

Hospital Admitting Monthly
3525 Piedmont Road
North East 6
Piedmont Center, Suite 4000
Atlanta, GA 30305-1515
404-262-7436

Hospitals & Health Networks
737 North Michigan Avenue
Chicago, IL 60611-2615
312-440-6800

Hospital & Health Services
  Administration
1021 East Huron
Ann Arbor, MI 48104-1628
313-764-1380

Hospital Employee Health
P.O. Box 740056
Atlanta, GA 30374-0056
404-262-7436

Hospital Infection Control
P.O. Box 740056
Atlanta, GA 30374-0056
404-262-7436

Hospital Litigation Report
4590 Dutch Valley Road N.E.
Atlanta, GA 30324-5330
404-881-1141

Hospital News & Healthcare
  Review
604 Broad Street
Nashua, NH 03063-3314
603-880-0223

Hospital News and Health-Care
  Review
P.O. Box 10180
Westborough, MA 01581-6018
508-366-2225

Hospital News–Greater
  Philadelphia Edition
2022 East Allegheny Avenue
Philadelphia, PA 19134-3817
215-739-2033

Hospital News–Southern New
  Jersey Edition
2022 East Allegheny Avenue
Philadelphia, PA 19134-3817
215-739-2033

Hospital Physician
125 Strafford Avenue, Suite 220
Wayne, PA 19087-3318
610-975-4541

Hospital Peer Review
3525 Piedmont Road Northeast
Atlanta, GA 30305
404-262-7436

Hospital Topics
1319 18th Street, NW
Washington, DC 20036-1802
202-296-62678

Imprint
555 West 57th Street, Suite 1327
New York, NY 10019-2925
212-581-2211

Infocare
2902 Evergreen Parkway, Suite 100
Evergreen, CO 80439-7958
303-674-2774

JOGNN: Journal of Obstetric,
  Gynecologic & Neonatal
  Nursing
227 East Washington Square
Philadelphia, PA 19106
215-238-4200

Journal for Healthcare Quality
5700 Old Orchard Road, 1st Floor
Skokie, IL 60077-1036
708-966-9392

Journal of Child and Adolescent
  Psychiatric Nursing
1211 Locust Street
Philadelphia, PA 19107-5409
215-545-7222

Journal of Community Health
  Nursing
10 Industrial Avenue
Mahwah, NJ 07430-2205
201-236-9500

Journal of Continuing Education in
  Nursing
6900 Grove Road
Thorofare, NJ 08086-9447
609-848-1000

Journal of Gerontological Nursing
6900 Grove Road
Thorofare, NJ 08086-9447
609-848-1000

Journal of Health, Politics, Policy
  and Law
P.O. Box 9066
Durham, NC 27708-0660
919-687-3636

Journal of Hospital Marketing
10 Alice Street
Binghamton, NY 13904-1503
510-524-6144

Journal of Perinatal and Neonatal
  Nursing
200 Orchard Ridge Drive, Suite
  2000
Gaithersburg, MD 20878-1978
301-417-7500

Journal of Nursing Care Quality
200 Orchard Ridge Drive, Suite
  2000
Gaithersburg, MD 20878-1978
301-417-7500

Journal of the New York State
  Nurses Association
2113 Western Avenue
Guilderland, NY 12084-9559
518-456-5371

Journal of Nursing Education
6900 Grove Road
Thorofare, NJ 08086-9447
609-848-1000

Journal of Nurse-Midwifery
655 Avenue of the Americas
New York, NY 10010-5017
212-633-3876

Journal of Psychosocial Nursing
  and Mental Health
6900 Grove Road
Thorofare, NJ 08086-9447
609-848-1000

Journal of School Nursing
92 South Highland Avenue
Ossining, NY 10562-5615
914-762-6498

Journal of Trauma Nursing
1211 Locust Street
Philadelphia, PA 19107-5409
215-545-7222

Journal On Quality Improvement
One Renaissance Boulevard
Villa Park, IL 60181-4294
708-916-5453

Kansas City Nursing News
7373 West 107th Street

Overland Park, KS 66212-2547
913-381-4949

Legislative Network for Nurses
951 Pershing Drive
Silver Spring, MD 20910-4432
301-587-6300

Managed Care Executive
11300 Rockville Pike, Suite 1100
Rockville, MD 20852-3003
301-816-8950

Managed Care Outlook
1101 King Street, Suite 4440
Alexandria, VA 22314-2944
703-683-4100

Managed Healthcare
859 Williamette Street
Eugene, OR 97401-2918
503-343-1200

Managed Care Law Outlook
1101 King Street, Suite 4440
Alexandria, VA 22314-2944
703-683-4100

Managing Senior Care
4951 Pershing Drive
Silver Spring, MD 20910-4432
301-587-6300

Massachusetts Association of
  Health Boards Quarterly
56 Taunton Street
Plainville, MA 02762-2144
508-643-0234

The Massachusetts Nurse
340 Turnpike Street
Canton, MA 02021-2700
617-821-4625

Medical Staff Leader
737 North Michigan Avenue, Suite
  700
Chicago, IL 60611-2615
312-440-6800

The Missouri Nurse
1904 Bubba Lane
Jefferson City, MO 65109-56344
314-636-4623

Modern Healthcare
740 North Rush Street
Chicago, IL 60611-2525
312-649-5342

Morbidity and Mortality Weekly
  Report
1600 Clifton Road NE
Mailstop C-08
Atlanta, GA 30329-4018
404-332-4555

National Report on Computers &
  Health
P.O. Box 10525
Burke, VA 22009-0525
703-451-7324

The Nation's Health
1015 15th Street, NW
Washington, DC 20005-2605
202-789-5600

NASN Newsletter
092 South Highland Avenue
Ossining, NY 10562-5615
914-762-6498

Neonatal Network
1304 Southpoint Boulevard, Suite
  2800
Petaluma, CA 94954-6861
707-762-2646

New Jersey Nurse
320 West State Street
Trenton, NJ 08618-5704
609-392-4884

New York State Medical News
208 Townsend Street
Syracuse, NY 13203-2339
315-472-6948

NMCN-American Journal of
   Maternal Child Nursing
555 West 57th Street
New York, NY 10019-2925
212-582-8820

Northern California Medfax
1611 Telegraph Avenue Suite 1201
Oakland, CA 94612-2146
510-832-3364

NP News
655 Avenue of the Americas
New York, NY 10010-5017
212-989-5800

NRN Magazine
5 Paragon Drive
Montvale, NJ 07645-1725
201-358-7314

Nurse Educator
227 East Washington Square
Philadelphia, PA 19106
215-238-4200

The Nurse Practitioner
655 Avenue of the Americas
New York, NY 10010-5017
212-989-5800

Nurseweek-Texas Edition
3001 LBJ Freeway, Suite 211
South Dallas, TX 75234-2715
214-488-8200

Nurseweek-California Edition
1156 Aster Avenue, Suite CO
Sunnyvale, CA 94086-6810
408-249-5877

Nursing
1111 Bethlehem Pike
Spring House, PA 19477-1114
215-646-8700

Nursing Administration Quarterly
200 Orchard Ridge Drive, Suite
   2000
Gaithersburg, MD 20878-1978
301-417-7500

Nursing & Health Care
350 Hudson Street
New York, NY 10014-4504
212-989-9393

Nursing Diagnosis
1211 Locust Street
Philadelphia, PA 19107-5409
215-545-7222

Nursing Economics
East Holly Avenue
Pitman, NJ 08071
609-256-2300

Nursing Forum
1211 Locust Street
Philadelphia, PA 19107-5409
215-545-7222

Nursing Management
8672 Neeb Road
Cincinnati, OH 45233-4614
513-347-7000

Nursing News
48 West Street
Concord, NH 03301-3553
603-225-3783

Nursing Research
555 West 57th Street
New York, NY 10019-2925
212-582-8820

Nursing World Journal
470 Boston Post Road
Weston, MA 02193-1529
617-899-27024

OACCH Advocate
7910 Woodmont Avenue, Suite 300
Bethesda, MD 20814-3015
301-654-6549

Orthopaedic Nursing Journal
East Holly Avenue
Pitman, NJ 08071
609-256-2300

Pediatric Nursing
East Holly Avenue
Pitman, NJ 08071
609-256-2300

Pennsylvania Nurse
P.O. Box 68525
Harrisburg, PA 17106-8525
717-657-1222

Physician Assistant
105 Raider Boulevard
Belle Mead, NJ 08502-1510
908-874-8550

Physician Manager
1050 17th Street, NW, Suite 480
Washington, DC 20036-5503
202-775-9008

Pittsburgh Hospital News
Mount Lebanon Boulevard, Suite
   201A
Pittsburgh, PA 15234-1507
412-341-1775

Plymouth County Health Update
P.O. Box 9180
Dennis, MA 02638-0918
508-790-2761

The PMAO
20 North Wacker Drive, Suite 1575
Chicago, IL 60606-2903
312-899-1500

The PPO Report
1101 King Street, Suite 4440
Alexandria, VA 22314-2944
703-739-6444

Progress in Cardiovascular Nursing
227 East Washington Square
Philadelphia, PA 19106
215-238-4200

Public Health Nursing
238 Main Street
Cambridge, MA 02142-1016
617-876-7000

Public Risk Magazine
1815 North Fort Myer Drive, Suite
   1020
Arlington, VA 22209-1805
703-528-7701

Re: American Journal of Practical
   Nursing
1418 Aversboro Road
Garner, NC 27529-4547
919-779-0046

Rehabilitation Nursing
5700 Old Orchard Road, First
   Floor
Skokie, IL 60077-1036
708-966-3433

Report on Healthcare Information
   Management

1101 King Street, Suite 4440
Alexandria, VA 22314-2944
703-739-6444

Report on Health Care Solutions
4951 Pershing Drive
Silver Spring, MD 20910-4432
301-587-6300

Report: The Official Newsletter of
  New York State Nurses
  Association
2113 Western Avenue
Guilderland NY 12084-9559
518-456-5371

The Schiff Report
1129 Bloomfield Avenue
West Caldwell, NJ 07006-7123
201-227-1830

Sharings
Shore Memorial Hospital
Somers Point, NJ 08244
609-653-3670

Southern California Medfax
1611 Telegraph Avenue Suite 1201

Oakland, CA 94612-2146
510-832-3364

Today's O. R. Nurse
6900 Grove Road
Thorofare, NJ 08086-9447
609-848-1000

TJFR Health News Report
545 North Maple Avenue
Ridgewood, NJ 07450-1612
201-444-6061

Topics in Health Care Financing
200 Orchard Ridge Drive, Suite
  200
Gaithersburg, MD 20878-1978
301-417-7500

Trustee
737 North Michigan Boulevard
Chicago, IL 60611-2615
312-440-6800

Women & Infants Quarterly
  Newsletter
101 Dudley Street
Providence, RI 02905-2401
401-274-1100

# Appendix D
## Research Databases of Interest to Nurses

**AgeLine** 1978–present

Produced by the American Association of Retired Persons, AgeLine provides bibliographic references and original abstracts for materials related to aging and middle age from an interdisciplinary perspective. Works from the fields of psychology, economics, sociology, gerontology, public policy, business, health and health care services, and consumer issues are covered. Documents on health care and policy comprise about half the database. (OVID, Dialog)

**AIDSLINE** 1980–present

AIDSLINE (AIDS Information Online), produced by the U.S. National Library of Medicine, is a collection of bibliographic citations focusing on research, clinical aspects, and health policy issues related to AIDS (acquired immune deficiency syndrome). This database includes articles from more than 3000 journals published worldwide, as well as government reports, letters, technical reports, meeting abstracts and papers, monographs, special publications, theses, books, and audiovisual materials. Information in the AIDSLINE database is derived from the following sources: MEDLINE, CancerLit, Health Planning and Administration, CATLINE, AVLINE, meeting abstracts from the International Conferences on AIDS, the Symposia on Non-human Primate Models of AIDS, and AIDS-related abstracts from the Annual Meetings of the American Society of Microbiology. (OVID, Dialog, MEDLARS)

**Alcohol and Alcohol Problems Science Database** 1972–present

The Alcohol and Alcohol Problems Science Database (ETOH) contains more than 92,000 bibliographic records with abstracts to alcohol-related scientific documents from U.S. and international sources. It is produced by

*Acknowledgment.* This table was prepared with the assistance of John Cole, Head, Medical Library; Lorraine Toews, Head, Public Services; and Denise Genereux, Reference Library Assistant; at the Medical Library, The University of Calgary, Alberta, Canada.

the U.S. National Institutes of Health and the U.S. National Institute on Alcohol Abuse and Alcoholism. The database covers all aspects of alcoholism research, including psychology, psychiatry, physiology, biochemistry, epidemiology, sociology, animal studies, treatment and prevention, employee assistance programs, drinking and driving, and public policy. (OVID)

**Allied and Alternative Medicine** 1985–present

Covers the fields of complementary or alternative medicine and allied health. Descriptors used in indexing the records are based on MeSH (Medical Subject Headings). The information in this database will be of interest to anyone who needs to know more about alternatives to conventional medicine, such as doctors, nurses, podiatrists, and other medical practitioners, therapists, and members of health care libraries, specialist colleges, self-help groups and the pharmaceutical industry, as well as allied health professionals such as physiotherapists and occupational therapists whose practice is conventional. Approximately 350 biomedical journals are indexed regularly, and relevant articles are taken from other journals. The database includes English-language and European sources; newspapers and books are also indexed. (Dialog)

**BioethicsLine** 1976–present

Produced jointly by the Kennedy Institute of Ethics and the U.S. National Library of Medicine, the BioethicsLine database includes more than 47,000 records of English-language materials on bioethics. Documents are selected from the disciplines of medicine, nursing, biology, philosophy, religion, law, and the behavioral sciences. Selections from popular literature are also included. Covered document types include journal and newspaper articles, monographs, court decisions, bills, laws, and audiovisual materials. Approximately 100 primary sources and 40 indexes and databases are scanned for citations. (OVID, MEDLARS)

**BIOSIS Previews®** 1969–present

Produced by BIOSIS, BIOSIS Previews is the world's most comprehensive reference detabase in the life sciences. It covers original research reports and reviews in biological and biomedical areas. Coverage includes traditional areas of biology, such as botany, zoology and microbiology, as well as related fields such as plant and animal science, agriculture, pharmacology and ecology. Interdisciplinary fields such as biochemistry, biophysics, and bioengineering are also included. Nearly 7,000 serials are monitored for inclusion. In addition, the database covers content summaries, books (including software from 1992 to present), and information from meetings. Content summaries include notes and letters, technical data reports, reviews, U.S. patents from 1986 to 1989, translation journals, meeting reports from 1980 to present, bibliographies, nomenclature rules, and taxonomic keys. (OVID, Dialog)

**CancerLit** 1983–present.

Produced by the U.S. National Cancer Institute, CancerLit is an important source of bibliographic information pertaining to all aspects of cancer therapy, including experimental and clinical cancer therapy; chemical, viral and other cancer-causing agents; mechanisms of carcinogenesis; biochemistry, immunology, and physiology of cancer; and mutagens and growth factor studies. Some of the information in CancerLit is derived from the MEDLINE database. Approximately 200 core journals contribute a large percentage of the 750,000+ records in this database. In addition, other information is drawn from proceedings of meetings, government reports, symposia reports, theses, and selected monographs. (OVID, Dialog, MEDLARS)

**CA Search/CA Condensates**

Produced by Chemical Abstracts Service, the CA Search (CHEM) and CA Condensates (CHEB) databases provide comprehensive international coverage of literature published in all fields of chemistry. In addition to standard access points, chemical literature is searchable by CAS Registry Number, patent assignee and patent number. The extensive coverage of these two databases make them valuable resources not only for research and bench chemists, but also for professionals and students in technology and life sciences disciplines. (OVID, Dialog)

**Cumulative Index to Nursing and Allied Health Literature (CINAHL)** 1982–present

Produced by CINAHL Information Systems, The Nursing & Allied Health (CINAHL) database provides comprehensive coverage of the English-language journal literature for nursing and allied health disciplines. Material from more than 950 journals are included in CINAHL, covering fields such as cardiopulmonary technology, emergency services, health education, med/lab technology, medical assistance, medical records, occupational therapy, physical therapy, radiologic technology, respiratory therapy, social sciences, surgical technology, and the physician's assistant. Also included are health care books, nursing dissertations, selected conference proceedings, standards of professional practice, and educational software. There is selective coverage of journals in biomedicine, the behavioral sciences, management, and education. The database currently contains more than 250,000 records. (OVID)

**Drug Information Full Text**–Current Edition

Produced by the American Society of Health-System Pharmacists, Drug Information Full Text contains the complete text of evaluative monographs from AHFS Drug Information and the Handbook on Injectable Drugs. DIFT contains detailed information on virtually every single drug entity available in the United States, including some drugs and intravenous infusion solutions under investigation, as well as commercial drugs. Data on concentration, usage, stability, pH, dosage, administration, compatibility, chemistry, pharmacology, interactions, and toxicity are included. Users are advised that decisions regarding drug therapy are the responsibility of the clinician, and that this file is provided for informational purposes only. The entire monograph for a drug should be reviewed for a thorough understanding of the drug's actions, uses, and side effects. (OVID, Dialog)

### Educational Resources Information Centre (ERIC) 1966–present

Produced by the U.S. Department of Education, ERIC is a national bibliographic database that indexes more than 775 periodicals dealing with the subject of education. It is the premier resource for references to these materials. Targeted to teachers, administrators and other education professionals, ERIC combines information from two printed sources: Resources in Education (RIE) and the Current Index to Journals in Education (CIJE). The database currently contains more than 879,000 records. (OVID, Dialog)

### EMBASE 1974–present

EMBASE, the Excerpta Medica database, produced by Elsevier Science, is a major biomedical and pharmaceutical database indexing more than 3500 international journals in the following fields: drug research, pharmacology, pharmaceutics, toxicology, clinical and experimental human medicine, health policy and management, public health, occupational health, environmental health, drug dependence and abuse, psychiatry, forensic medicine, and biomedical engineering/instrumentation. There is selective coverage for nursing, dentistry, veterinary medicine, psychology, and alternative medicine. EMBASE is one of the most widely used biomedical and pharmaceutical databases because of its currency and in-depth indexing. Frequent updates allow access to the latest medical and pharmacological trends. The database currently contains more than 6 million records, with more than 375,000 citations and abstracts added yearly. The EMBASE Psychiatry and EMBASE Drugs and Pharmacology subset databases are also available from Ovid Technologies, Inc. (OVID, Dialog)

### HealthSTAR 1975–present

HealthSTAR contains citations to the published literature on health services, technology, administration, and research. It focuses on both the clinical and nonclinical aspects of health care delivery. The following topics are included: evaluation of patient outcomes; effectiveness of procedures, programs, products, services and processes; administration and planning of health facilities, services and manpower; health insurance; health policy; health services research; health economics and financial management; laws and regulation; personnel administration; quality assurance; licensing; and accreditation. HealthSTAR is produced cooperatively by the U.S. National Library of Medicine and the American Hospital Association. The database contains citations and abstracts (when available) to journal articles, monographs, technical reports, meeting abstracts and papers, book chapters, government documents, and newspaper articles from 1975 to the present. Citations are indexed with the National Library of Medicine's Medical Subject Headings to ensure compatibility with other NLM databases. Information in HealthSTAR is derived from MEDLINE, CATLINE, the Hospital Literature Index, and selected journals. Additional records specially indexed for this database do not appear in any other NLM database. HealthSTAR replaces the former Health Planning and Administration database (HEALTH). (OVID, HealthSTAR)

**International Pharmaceutical Abstracts** 1970–present

Produced by the American Society of Health-System Pharmacists, International Pharmaceutical Abstracts (IPAB) provides worldwide coverage of pharmaceutical science and health-related literature. Its comprehensive bibliographic citations are valuable to researchers, librarians and medical professionals. Coverage includes drug therapy, toxicity, and pharmacy practice, as well as legislation, regulation, technology, utilization, biopharmaceutics, information processing, education, economics, and ethics as related to pharmaceutical science and practice. The database currently contains more than 246,000 records. (OVID, Dialog)

**Life Sciences Collection** 1982–present

Contains abstracts and bibliographic citations from recent worldwide research literature in major areas of biology, medicine, biochemistry, biotechnology, ecology, and microbiology, and some aspects of agriculture and veterinary science. LIFE SCIENCES COLLECTION is produced by Cambridge Scientific Abstracts and corresponds to print series of more than 20 abstracting journals. Informative abstracts are included for about 90% of the records.

Print counterparts:

Animal Behaviour Abstracts
Biochemistry Abstracts
Biotechnology Research Abstracts
Calcified Tissue Abstracts
Chemoreception Abstracts
Ecology Abstracts
Entomology Abstracts
Genetics Abstracts
Virology and AIDS Abstracts
Human Genome Abstracts
Immunology Abstracts
Marine Biotechnology Abstracts
Microbiology Abstracts
CSA Neurosciences Abstracts
Oncology Abstracts
Toxicology Abstracts

**MEDLINE** 1966–present

Produced by the U.S. National Library of Medicine, the MEDLINE database is widely recognized as the premier source for bibliographic coverage of biomedical literature. MEDLINE encompasses information from Index Medicus, Index to Dental Literature, and International Nursing, as well as other sources of coverage in the areas of communication disorders, population biology, and reproductive biology. More than 8.5 million records from more than 3,600 journals are indexed. (OVID, Dialog, MEDLARS)

**Mental Health Abstracts** 1967–present

Cites worldwide information relating to the general topic area of mental health. Sources include 1200 journals from 41 different countries, in 21 different languages, books, monographs, technical reports, workshop and conference proceedings, and symposia. Also included are Far Eastern literature and nonprint media. There is no equivalent print version of the database. There are, however, publications that contain some of the records available online. They are Psychopharmacology Abstracts and the one-time publications, Abstracts of the Standard Edition of Freud, Abstracts of the Psychoanalytic Study of the Child, Woman and Mental Health, and Bibliography on Racism. Material included in Mental Health Abstracts is drawn from approximately 1500 primary sources, both domestic and international, including periodicals, technical reports, monographs, dissertations, conference proceedings, grant reports, and nonprint materials. Print counterparts: None (Dialog)

**Occupational Safety and Health (NIOSH)** 1973–present

A product of the Clearinghouse for Occupational Safety and Health, a division of the National Institute for Occupational Safety and Health. It includes citations to more than 400 journal titles as well as more than 70,000 monographs and technical reports. NIOSH covers all aspects of occupational safety and health, and includes such topics as hazardous agents, unsafe workplace environment, and toxicology. The ongoing sources for the database are about 159 core English-language technical journals, which provide the majority of records. Supplementing these are abstracts of all NIOSH publications and selected articles from journals of special importance to the occupational health and safety field. Print counterparts: None (Dialog)

**POPLINE (POPulation information onLINE)** 1970–present

POPLINE provides worldwide coverage of population, family planning, and related health issues, including family planning technology and programs, fertility, and population law and policy. In addition, POPLINE focuses on particular developing country issues including demography, AIDS and other sexually transmitted diseases, maternal and child health, primary health care communication, and population and environment. The file is produced by the Population Information Program at the Johns Hopkins School of Public Health. The database is funded primarily by the United States Agency of International Development. Primarily English-language items but international in scope; publications from 1970 to the present with selected citations dating back to 1886. (MEDLARS)

**PsycINFO** 1967–present

Produced by the American Psychological Association, PsycINFO covers the professional and academic literature in psychology and related disciplines, including medicine, psychiatry, nursing, sociology, education, pharmacology, physiology, linguistics, and other areas. PsycINFO's coverage is worldwide, and includes references and abstracts to over 1300 journals in more than 20 languages, and to book chapters and books in the English language. The database includes information from empirical studies, case studies, surveys, bibliographies, literature reviews, discussion articles, conference reports, and dissertations. PsycINFO currently contains more than 1 million references, with over 57,000 references added annually. PsycINFO is the world's most comprehensive source for bibliographic coverage of psychology and behavioral sciences literature. The PsycLIT and ClinPSYC subsets of PsycINFO are also available from Ovid. (OVID, Dialog)

**Social SciSearch** 1972–present

International, multidisciplinary index to the literature of the social, behavioral, and related sciences, produced by the Institute for Scientific Information (ISI®). SOCIAL SCISEARCH contains all the records published in the Social Sciences Citation Index. SOCIAL SCISEARCH indexes all significant items (articles, reports of meetings, letters, editorials, correction notices, etc.) from the more than 1500 most important worldwide social sciences journals. Additional articles relevant to the social sciences are selected from over 2400 journals in the natural, physical, and biomedical sciences. Print counterparts: Social Sciences Citation Index (Dialog)

**Sociological Abstracts** 1963–present

Sociological Abstracts is the premier online resource for researchers, professionals, and students in sociology and related disciplines. Three subfiles are included within the single database label SOCA. The first subfile includes citations and abstracts from more than 2000 journals indexed by Sociological Abstracts, plus relevant dissertation listings and abstracts of conference papers. The second subfile covers citations to book reviews from the International Review of Publications in Sociology. The third subfile includes citations and abstracts from Social Planning/Policy & Development Abstracts. The following subjects are covered in SOCA: activism and action research, gerontology, case work, community organization, demographics, family studies, feminist studies, media, policy sciences, political science, social security programs, and sociology. The subset version of this database is sociofile, also available from Ovid. (OVID, Dialog)

# Appendix E
## Riley and Saba's Nursing Informatics Education Model: Basic Computer Content for Undergraduate Students*

First Step
- Computer overview
- Computer components
  Hardware
  Software
- Word processing software
  Computer-based papers
- Bibliographic retrieval systems
  Conduct literature searches

Second Step
- Overview of information systems
- Patient care documentation
- Social/legal/ethical issues
  Computer-based patient record (CPR)
- Educational applications
  Computer-assisted instruction (CAI)
  Interactive videodisk instruction (IAV)

Third Step
- Use advanced software programs
- Implement nursing care documentation
  Drug administration systems
  Physiological monitoring
- Care planning documentation
- Patient instruction
- Evaluation of instruction

Fourth Step
- Coordinate patient care data
- Analyze databases
- Quality assurance program
- Utilize computer networks
- Evaluate computer hardware
- Evaluate computer software
- Assure ethical standards

---

* *Source:* Saba, V., and McCormick, K. *Essentials of Computers for Nurses.* New York: McGraw-Hill, 1995: 561 (with permission).

# Appendix F
## Proposed Nursing Informatics Education Model for Graduate Nursing Informatics Students

First Step
- Computer overview
- Computer components
  Hardware
  Software
- Word processing software (e.g., Microsoft Work, WordPerfect)
  Computer-based papers using APA format
- Database software (e.g., Microsoft Access, Paradox)
  Design and develop a database for health care delivery
- Project presentation software (e.g., Microsoft PowerPoint)
  Design, develop, and present presentation related to topic within nursing informatics
- Spreadsheet software (e.g., Microsoft Excel, Lotus 1-2-3)
  Develop spreadsheet to be included in word-processed paper or project presentation
- Bibliographic retrieval systems
  Conduct literature searches using CD-ROM software (e.g., CINAHL)
  Conduct literature searches using the Internet
- Email and Listserv Discussion groups
  Assign e-mail address to every student
  Utilization of Listserv for class discussion and assignments

Second Step
- Organizational Theory
  Project management: introduction to project management software (e.g., Microsoft Project)
  Health care financial management: e.g., benefit–cost ratio, budgeting using spreadsheet
  Resource utilization
  Basic organizational theory: e.g., critical thinking, conflict, change theory, management
- Overview of nursing informatics
  Nursing information models: application to computerized systems
  Introduction to nursing and health care information systems
    Communication networks
    Data capturing and sharing
    Decision support
    Patient classification/staffing
    Patient documentation
    Quality assurance

- Computerized patient record
  Introduction to classification systems and taxonomies
  Managed care
  Social, legal, and ethical issues
- Educational applications
  Computer-assisted instruction (CAI): analyze and/or develop CAI
  Interactive videodisk instruction (IAV)

Thrid Step
- Telecommunications in health care
  Telemedicine policy development
  Telenursing applications
- Advanced computerized patient record
  Requirements
  Systems design and development applications
- Implement nursing care documentation
  Clinical pathways (careplan documentation)
  Patient instruction
  Outcomes development
- Development of a Request for Proposal in response to a simulated case study
- Use advanced software programs
  Decision support system development (e.g., create DSS to address nursing problem)
  Internet software development (e.g., create website related to nursing and health care)
  Integrate software programs to develop system to meet needs of an organization
    Recommend weekly practical application to real-life situation (e.g., practicum experience)

Fourth Step (to be implemented in a preceptor-based practicum real-life experience requiring a system to be developed or modified)
- Systems analysis: full systems development life cycle analysis including executive summary, background information, information architecture (ERD, FDD, LDD), models (DFD, LCD), structure chart, program design, database design, screen design, and recommendations for training, implementation, and evaluation
  Involves evaluation of computer hardware
  Involves evaluation of computer software
- Utilization of CASE tool to assist in systems analysis

# Glossary

**Acoustic coupler**: A specific type of modem which uses the standard telephone set.

**A/D**: Analog-to-digital converter.

**Analog**: A computer that compares and measures one quantity with another.

**ANSI**: American National Standards Institute

**Application program**: A computer program written to solve a specific problem or perform a specific task.

**Architecture**: The art and science of designing and erecting buildings. Buildings and other large structures: the low, brick and adobe architecture of the Southwest. A style and method of design and construction: Byzantine architecture. Orderly arrangement of parts; structure: the architecture of the federal bureaucracy; the broad architecture of a massive novel; computer architecture.

**Arithmetic logic unit (ALU)**: Internal part of computer (found in CPU) that performs the arithmetic computations.

**ASCII**: American Standard Code of Information Interchange.

**Assembly language**: A hardware dependent symbolic language, usually characterized by a one-to-one correspondence of its statements with machine language instructions.

**Auxiliary storage**: Data storage other than main memory, such as that on a disk storage unit.

**Backup**: A duplicate copy of a file or program. Backups of material are made on disk or cassette in case something happens to the original.

**Backup position listing**: A list of personnel who can fill a given position, as well as alternate personnel who can fill the same position.

**BASIC**: Beginner's All-Purpose Symbolic Instruction Code. A popular computer language invented at Dartmouth for educational purposes. An easy-to-learn, easy-to-use language.

**Batch processing**: A mode of processing in which any program submitted to the computer is either run to completion or aborted. No interactive communication between program and user is possible.

**Baud**: Unit of measurement of transmission speed, equivalent to bits per second in serial transmission. Used by microcomputer.

**Binary number system**: Number system made up of the digits 0 and 1— "the language of the computer."

**Bit**: Binary digit (0 or 1).

**Browser**: A computer program which allows the user to search for data across the networks of computers which make up the Internet.

**Bubble memory (data)**: Thin film of synthetic garnet. The bubbles are microns in size and move in a plane of the film when a magnetic gradient is present. Viewed under a microscope with a linear polarized light, the bubbles appear to be fluid circular areas that step from space to space following fixed loops and tracks.

**Bug**: An error in a program or an equipment fault.

**Business Continuity Planning (BCP)**: An all encompassing, "umbrella" term covering both disaster recovery planning and business resumption planning.

**Business interruption**: Any event, whether anticipated (e.g., public service strike) or unanticipated (e.g., blackout) which disrupts the normal course of business operation at a corporate location.

**Byte**: Eight bits make up a byte (a letter, symbol, or number).

**CAD**: Computer-aided design.

**CAD/CAM**: Acronym for Computer-Assisted Design/Computer-Assisted Manufacturing, terms used by designers, engineers, and managers.

**CAI**: Computer-aided instruction.

**CAL**: Computer-aided learning.

**CAM**: Computer-aided manufacture.

**Care map**: A sequential or branching plan of the anticipated key treatments and diagnostic tests for a specific condition or medical diagnosis. IT may be used as a template for comparing the actual experience of a patient with that anticipated for the majority of patients with the same condition.

**CASE**: Computer Assisted Systems Engineering

**CD-ROM**: Compact Disk Read Only Memory. A compact disk is round, flat and silver in colour and can contain massive amounts of information (600 megabytes or more of data, text, graphics, video, or sound).

**Central processing unit (CPU)**: Internal part of the computer that contains the circuits which control and perform the execution of instructions. It is made up of Memory, Arithmetic/logic unit, and Control unit.

**Certified Disaster Recovery Planner (CDRP)**: CDRPs are certified by the Disaster Recovery Institute, a not-for-profit corporation, which promotes the credibility and professionalism in the DR industry.

**Chip**: An integrated circuit made by etching myriads of transistors and other electronic components onto a wafer of silicon a fraction of an inch on a side.

**CIPS**: Canadian Information Processing Society.

**Client/server**: An architecture that has computers in a network assume different roles and tasks based on their particular strengths. Thus, a computer might be identified as a file server or a database server.

**CNA**: Canadian Nurses Association.

**COACH**: Canadian Organization for Advancement of Computers in Health.

**COBOL**: Common Business-Oriented Language.

**Cold-site**: An alternate facility that is void of any resources or equipment except air conditioning and raised flooring. Equipment and resources must be installed in such a facility to duplicate the critical business functions of an organization. Cold-sites have many variations depending on their communication facilities, UPS systems, or mobility (Relocatable-Shell).

**COM**: Computer Output to Microfilm.

**Compiler**: A translation program which coverts high-level instructions into a set of binary instructions (object code) for direct processor execution. Any high-level program requires a compiler or an interpreter.

**Computer**: An electronic device capable of taking in, putting out, storing internally, and processing data under the control of changeable processing instructions within the device.

**Computer literacy**: A term used to indicate knowledge of what a computer can do, how it works, how it is used to solve problems, and the limitations of a computer.

**Contingency plan**: *See* Disaster Recovery Plan.

**Control key**: Key that executes commands, in conjunction with other keys pressed simultaneously.

**Control unit**: Internal part of computer (found in CPU) that monitors the sequence of operations for all parts of the computer.

**CP/M**: Control Program/Microprocessors.

**CPU**: Central processing unit.

**CR**: Change Request.

**Critical needs**: The minimal procedures and equipment required to continue operations should a department, main facility, computer center or a combination of these be destroyed or become inaccessible.

**CRT**: The Cathode-Ray Tube in a television set or video display monitor.

**CRUD**: Created, Read, Updated or Deleted.

**CSF**: Critical Success Factor.

**Cursor**: A patch of light or other visual indicator on a screen that shows you where you are in the text.

**DA**: Data Administrator.

**Data**: Recorded facts performing arithmetic and logical process on data.

**Data base**: An organized collection of data or information.

**DB**: Database.

**DBA**: Database Administrator.

**DBMS**: Database Management System.

**DCE**: Distributed Computing Environment.

**Decision support system**: A computer program devised to help a health care professional select the most likely clinical diagnosis or treatment.

**DFD**: Data Flow Diagrams.

**DI**: Diagnostic Imaging.

**Digital**: A computer that uses numbers to solve problems by performing arithmetic and logical processes on data.

**Disaster**: Any event creates an inability on an organization's part to provide critical business functions for some predetermined period of time.

**Disaster prevention**: Measures employed to prevent, detect, or contain incidents which, if unchecked, could result in disaster.

**Disaster prevention checklist**: A questionnaire used to assess preventative measures in areas of operations such as overall security, software, data files, data entry reports, microcomputers, and personnel.

**Disaster recovery**: The ability to respond to an interruption in services by implementing a disaster recovery plan to restore an organization's critical business functions.

**Disaster Recovery Coordinator**: The Disaster Recovery Coordinator may be responsible for overall recovery of an organization or unit(s).

**Disaster Recovery Plan**: The document that defines the resources, actions, tasks, and data required to manage the business recovery process in the event of a business interruption. The plan is designed to assist in restoring the business process within the stated disaster recovery goals.

**Disaster Recovery Planning**: The technological aspect of business continuity planning. The advance planning and preparations which are necessary to minimize loss and ensure continuity of the critical business functions of an organization in the event of a disaster.

**Disaster Recovery Software**: An application program developed to assist an organization in writing a comprehensive disaster recovery plan.

**Disk**: An external storage medium that is a flat, circular magnetic surface used to store data. The data is represented by the presence or absence of magnetized spots.

**Disk drive**: The device used to access or store information via a disk.

**Distributed processing**: Use of computers at various locations, typically interconnected via communication links for the purpose of data access and/or transfer.

**Documentation**: Refers to the orderly presentation, organization, and communication of recorded specialized knowledge, in order to maintain a complete record of reasons for changes in variables. Documentation is necessary, not so much to give maximum utility, as to give an unquestionable historical reference record.

**DOS**: Disk-operating system.

**DRGs**: Diagnosis Related Groups. A method of costing care and treatment by grouping together cases by diagnosis or treatment method.

**DSS**: Decision Support System.

**EDI**: Electronic Data Interchange.

**EDP**: Electronic Data Processing.

**EIS**: Executive Information System.

**E-mail**: Electronic mail. The messages created, sent, and read between networks of computer users without having to be printed on paper.

**EPROM**: Erasable Programmable Read-Only Memory. A type of ROM that can be changed by means of electrical erasing.

**Expert system**: A computer program that stores knowledge in a special data base by expressing it in the form of logical rules. The program can then logically reason, given that set of rules.

**FDDI**: Fibre Distributed Data Interface.

**File backup**: The practice of dumping (copying) a file stored on disk or tape to another disk or tape. This is done for protection case the active file gets damaged.

**FIPS**: Federal Information Processing Standard.

**Firmware**: Computer instructions that are located in Read-Only Memory (ROM). These instructions can be accessed but not altered.

**Floppy disk**: A flexible plastic disk enclosed in a protective envelope used to store information.

**Formal Decision Table**: A logical presentation of all decision paths available in the development of a computer system.

**FORTRAN**: Formula Translator.

**Friendly**: How easy a program or computer is to work with. A "user friendly" program is one that takes little time to learn, or that offers on screen prompts, or that protects the user from making disastrous mistakes.

**FTAM**: File Transfer, Access and Management.

**FTP**: File Transfer Protocol.

**FTS**: File Transfer Systems.

**GUI**: Graphical User Interface.

**Hard copy**: Computer output printed on paper.

**HDLC**: High-level Data Link Control.

**Head**: Part of magnetic storage unit (Disk drive) which reads and writes information on the magnetic media.

**High-level languages**: Programming languages that are as close to writing English statements as possible.

**HIS**: Hospital Information Systems (Chapter 5)—a term used to describe overall hospital use of computers. Examples would be nurse staffing, medical records, patient admittance and discharge, patient bed control, and so on.

**HMRI**: Hospital Medical Records Institute.

**Hot-site**: An alternate facility that has the equipment and resources to recover the business functions affected by the occurrence of a disaster. Hot-sites may vary in type of facilities offered (such as data processing, communication, or any other critical business function needing duplication). Location and size of the hot-site will be proportional to the equipment and resources needed.

**IC**: Integrated circuit.

**ICD-9-CM**: International Classification of Diseases—9th rev—Clinical Modification.

**IEW**: Information Engineering Workbench—Proprietary product.

**I/O (input/output)**: An Input device such as a keyboard feeds information into the computer. An Output device such as a printer or monitor takes information from the computer and turns it into usable form. Modems, cassettes, and disks work in both directions, so they are I/O devices. Input and output are also used as verbs: You input data from the keyboard.

**Input**: The data to be processed by the computer.

**Input device**: Device used to enter data to be processed by a computer (e.g., keyboard, light pen, touch screen).

**Interactive video disk**: A computer program uses a compact disk storing large amounts of data to provide video sequences on screen for the user to select the next sequence, or based on the answer given to a question.

**Interface**: A device or program that permits one part of a computer system to work with another, as when making a connection between a cassette tape recorder and the computer.

**Internal memory**: The internal storage of the computer. Made up of ROM and RAM.

**Internal hot-sites**: A fully equipped alternate processing site owned and operated by the organization.

**Internet**: A world-wide computer network, available via a modem and the telephone line that connects universities, government departments, and individuals. Users can send and receive e-mail, join in electronic conferences, and copy files.

**IMIA**: International Medical Informatics Association. It organizes a congress every three years and has a number of special interest groups composed of representatives drawn from member countries. The British Computer Society (BCS) is the member organization for the UK. The BCS Nursing Specialist Group nominates one member to the IMIA Nursing Specialist Group (SIGN).

**Interpreter language**: Language that converts the higher-level languages and assembler language to a language the computer (machine can understand).

**IPSE**: Integrated Product Support Environment.

**IRM**: Information Resource Management.

**ISDN**: Integrated Services Digital Network.

**ISO**: International Standards Organization.

**ISP**: Information Systems Professional.

**IT**: Information Technology.

**ITCH**: Information Technology for Community Health (Annual Conference).

**JADD**: Joint Application Design and Development.

**JCL**: Job control language.

**JIT**: Just-in-Time.

**K**: Symbol used to express 1000. Ir a computer context it is 1024. Example: 16K = 16,000 bytes; in reality it is 16,384 bytes.

**LAN**: abbreviation for **L**ocal **A**rea **N**etwork. Computing equipment, in close proximity to each other, connected to a server which houses software that can be accessed by the users. This method does not utilize a public carrier.

**Load**: To enter a program into the computer from cartridge, cassette, or disk.

**Loop**: A group of instructions that may be executed more than once.

**Low-level languages**: Programming languages that are less sophisticated than our normal English language.

**LPM**: Lines per minute.

**Machine language**: Language the computer actually understands. Nothing more than everything converted into the binary system. i.e., 0's and 1's, the presence or absence of electricity.

**Magnetic tape**: Flexible plastic tape, on one side of which is a uniform coating of dispersed magnetic material, in which signals are registered for subsequent reproduction. Used for registering television images, sound, or computer data.

**Mailbox**: An e-mail account or address, to which messages can be sent and stored, on a computer network such as Internet.

**Mainframe Computer**: A high-end processor, with related peripheral devices, capable of supporting large volumes of batch processing, high performance on-line transaction processing systems, and extensive data storage and retrieval.

**Mark sense card**: An input device that allows the operator to use a special pencil and computer readable card to input data.

**Medical informatics**: The discipline of applying computer science to medical processes.

**Megabyte**: 1 million bytes or 8 million bits.

**Memory**: Internal part of computer (found in the CPU) where programs and data are stored.

**Metathesaurus**: The combinations of several systematically arranged lists of words, their synonyms, and antonyms. A word finder to help in the identification of a language such as that used by nurses.

**Microcomputer**: A small inexpensive desk-top computer which uses floppy disks or small hard disk drives.

**Microprocessor**: Another name for the CPU chip.

**Minicomputer**: A larger and more powerful computer than a micro-computer, which uses large capacity hard disks, works at a greater speed and has several hundred K of memory.

**MIPS**: Millions of instructions per second.

**MIS**: Medical (or Management) Information System (Chapter 5). A term used interchangeably with HIS; however, it specifically applies to a computerized system related to patient care as opposed to a system used by the finance department for billing financial statements, and so on.

**Modem**: Modulator/Demodulator. A device used to change computer codes into pulses or signals that can travel over telephone lines.

**Monitor**: Video device; quality of display is better than that of a television set.

**MOS**: Metal-oxide semiconductor.

**Mouse**: An input device that can be moved around over a flat surface causing the cursor to move on the screen.

**MVS**: Multiple virtual storage.

**NANDA**: North American Nursing Diagnosis Association. Its conference proceedings are published and list the currently agreed diagnoses and their definitions. NANDA encourages research to identify and clarify diagnoses.

**Network architecture**: The basic layout of a computer and its attached systems, such as terminals and the paths between them.

**Neural network model**: A model on a computer system to mimic the way the human brain processes information using large numbers of neurons all working on one problem at the same time (parallel processing). Based on repeated patterns, connections are made across the computer's network of "neurons" to produce the same result each time.

**NFS**: Network File System.

**NIC**: Nursing Interventions Classification.

**NIS (Nursing Information System)**: A term used to describe overall nursing use of computers. Examples would include source data capture, patient care plans and use of expert systems.

**NIST**: National Institute of Standards and Technology.

**Node**: The name used to designate a part of a network. This may be used to describe one of the links in the network, or a type of link in the network (e.g., host node or intercept node)

**Nursing diagnosis**: A clinical judgment about individual, family, or community responses to actual or potential health problems or life processes. A nursing diagnosis provides the basis for the selection of nursing interventions.

**Nursing informatics**: The discipline of applying computer science to nursing processes.

**Nursing Minimum Data Set (NMDS)**: The agreed minimum number of items of data, such as patient and nursing care elements, to be collected for managerial and government purposes. In the United States, the term may be used for the data elements identified by Werley et al. in 1985.

**OA**: Office Automation.

**OCR**: Optical Character Recognition.

**OEM**: Original equipment manufacturer.

**Off-site storage**: The process of storing records at a location removed from the normal place of use.

**Omaha System**: Developed by the Visiting Nurses Association of Omaha for use in community health nursing, there are three components: a problem classification scheme, a problem-rating scale for outcomes, and an intervention scheme.

**On-line**: Being electronically connected, for example a computer linked to a printer so that it is ready to print, or one computer linked to another computer such as over the Internet.

**On-line terminal**: The operation of terminals, disks, and other equipment under direct and absolute control of the central processor to eliminate the need for human intervention at any stage between initial input and computer output.

**Operating Software**: A type of system software supervising and directing all of the other software components plus the computer hardware.

**OS**: Operating system.

**OSI**: Open Systems Interchange. A particular technical standard that allows computers of different origins to be linked together.

**OSE**: Open Systems Environment.

**OSF**: Open Standards Foundation.

**OSI**: Open Systems Interconnection.

**Output**: Information transferred from internal storage to output device.

**Output device**: Devices or machines that deliver information from the computer to the operator (e.g., CRT, tape, disk, keypunched card).

**Paper tape**: Refers to strips of paper capable of storing or recording information. Storage may be in the form of punched holes, partially punched holes, carbonization or chemical change of impregnated material, or by imprinting.

**Parallel interface**: A port that sends or receives the eight bits in each byte all at one time. Many printers likely to be used in homes use a parallel interface to connect to the computer.

**Parsing**: The computer science term for checking the correctness of each line and the action of putting the line into proper form for next phase of program execution.

**Patient classification system**: There are a variety of systems, some manual, that assign either a patient's nursing problems or the nursing activities required, to a defined level of dependency on nurses for care. Some systems use nursing care plans to calculate the number of minutes of nurse time needed in 24 hours.

**PC**: Personal Computer.

**PC-DOS**: IBM's name for the Disk Operating System used in the IBM Personal Computer.

**(PDQ) Cancer system**: Protocol Data Query. A data retrieval system for cancer material.

**Peripherals**: Accessory parts of a computer system not considered essential to its operation. Printers and modems are peripherals.

**Personal Health Number (PHN)**: A unique identifier given to individuals eligible for health services.

**Physical Prevention**: Special requirements for building construction as well as fire prevention for equipment components.

**PIR**: Post Implementation Review.

**POSIX**: Portable Operating System Interface for Computer Environments.

**Printer**: Transforms computer output into hard copy.

**Program**: Shortened form of "computer program." A set of stored instructions in a computer which directs the actions within the computer. See Application program.

**Programmable key**: Another term for user-defined key.

**Programming languages**: Much like French, English, and German—the grammar and punctuation accepted by the computer's input device that enables a user to communicate with the computer.

**PROM**: Programmable Read-Only Memory. A type of ROM that can be changed, but only with a high degree of expertise.

**Proprietary software**: A computer program belongs to its developer. Programs (generally) cannot be copied and freely given away, just as you cannot copy a book and give copies away.

**RAM**: Random-Access Memory or Read-Write Memory. This part of internal memory is known as temporary memory.

**RDBMS**: Relational Database Management System.

**Read**: To extract data from a computer's memory or from a tape or disk.

**Real-time**: An action or system capable of action at a speed commensurate with the time of occurrence of an actual process.

**Reset**: To reset the computer and its peripherals to a starting state before beginning a task. Done automatically by the disk operating system.

**RFD**: Request for Development.

**RFI**: Request for Information.

**RFP**: Request for Proposal.

**RISE**: Relationally Integrated Systems Engineering.

**Risk Analysis**: The process of identifying the risks to an organization, assess the critical functions necessary for an organization to continue operations, define controls to reduce exposure, and evaluate the cost of such controls. The risk analysis often involves an evaluation of the probabilities of a particular event. Associated terms: risk assessment, impact assessment, corporate loss analysis, risk identification, exposure analysis, exposure assessment.

**Risk management**: The discipline that ensures that an organization does not assume an unacceptable level of risk.

**Robotics**: General term for industrial robots used to increase production. An example is the use of computer-controlled robots in automobile assembly lines.

**ROM**: Read-only memory.

**RPG**: Report Program Generator.

**SAA**: Strategic Application Architecture.

**SCAMC**: Symposium on Computer Applications in Medical Care.

**Scroll**: To move a video display up or down, line by line, or side to side, character by character.

**SDE**: Systems Development Environment.

**SDLC**: Systems Development Life Cycle.

**Server**: A master computer into which other computers hook, so it controls a network of computers.

**Soft-function key**: See User-defined key.

**Software**: The general term for sets of computer instructions (programs) which manage the general facilities of the computer and control the operation of application programs.

**SNOMED**: Systematized Nomenclature of Medicine

**Source code instructions**: In many microprogrammed processors, source code instructions are interpreted in the instruction register as pointers to the microprocessor programs that emulate the particular instruction set being executed. In the conventional approach, on the other hand, each instruction is decoded and executed with specific control logic wired into the machine.

**SSA**: Strategic Systems Architecture.

**Stakeholder**: Any individual or organization with vested interest in the health system.

**Standards**: Documented agreements containing technical specifications or the precise criteria to be used consistently as rules, guidelines, or definitions of characteristics to ensure that materials, products, processes, and services are fit for their purposes.

**Storage**: Usually refers to long term storage, such as storage on tape or disk.

**Support**: Help available from computer and software merchants. Also used as a verb to describe what products are compatible with each other.

**System**: A group of actions or procedures which together are logically connected by their operation and products and which accomplish a connected set of organizational objectives.

**TCP/IP**: Transmission Control Protocol/Internet Protocol.

**Telematics**: The combination of telecommunications and computing. Data communications between systems and devices.

**Technical Threats**: A disaster causing event that may occur regardless of any human elements.

**Terminal**: Device used to transmit and receive data over communications lines to and from the computer.

**Top-down structure**: A logical method of presenting the structure of a computer application. The initial system is the head of the structure and is subdivided into each of its component parts ultimately ending in a detailed level that allows you to go directly to programming.

**TQM**: Total Quality Management.

**Turnkey**: A term used to describe a hardware-software combination that comes in a "package." There are no changes or options; the package must be run as it is. An example is a microcomputer with a generalized software package for nurse scheduling. A "turnkey" is the opposite of a "tailored" system developed specifically for a nursing department.

**Unique Lifetime Identifier (ULI)**: A unique identifier given to persons who receive or provide health services in Alberta.

**User-defined key**: A key whose function can be changed by which a command or sequence of commands can be executed with a single keystroke. Same as Programmable key and Soft-function key. Unlike a special-function key, a user-defined key may have a predefined purpose.

**VDU**: Visual display unit.

**VDT**: Video display terminal.

**Video terminal**: Computer terminal which shows data on a cathode ray tube (CRT), like a television tube, in letters, numbers, and so on.

**Warm-site**: An alternate processing site which is only partially equipped (as compared to a hot-site, which is fully equipped).

**Winchester disk**: A powerful form of backup storage for a computer. It is a rigid magnetic disk in a sealed container scanned by a head which does not quite touch the disk, therefore not wearing it out.

**Winchester drive**: A form of hard disk permanently sealed into a case.

**WLMS**: Work Load Measurement System.

**WMS**: Workload Measurement System.

**Write**: To enter information into memory or onto a tape or disk.

**WWW**: World Wide Web. A database made of linked hypertext documents originated by CERN, it exploded onto the computing scene during 1994. You call it up from a starter screen. An early browser was a program called Mosaic. WWW can provide graphics and sound but downloading these take time.

# Index

# Health Informatics Series
## *(formerly Computers in Health Care)*

Knowledge Coupling
*New Premises and New Tools for Medical Care and Education*
L.L. Weed